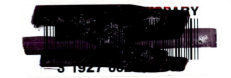

D0217788

Environmental Nutrition

Understanding

the Link between

Environment,

Food Quality,

and Disease

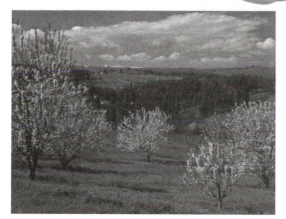

Buck Levin, Ph.D., R.D.

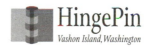

HingePin
Vashon Island, Washington

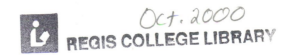

For my mother and father

Environmental Nutrition: Understanding the Link between Environment, Food Quality, and Disease
Buck Levin Ph. D., R. D.

HingePin Integrative Learning Materials
8021 SW 204th Street
Vashon Island, Washington 98070-6257
phone: (206) 463-1733
fax: (206) 463-1739
e-mail:contactus@hingepin.com
website: http://www.hingepin.com

Cover and interior photograph of orchard: "Blossoming cherry orchards on rolling hills of the Rowena plateau" © Terry Donnelly
Cover design, interior design and composition: Lynne Faulk

ISBN: 0-9671283-0-7
Library of Congress Catalog Card Number: 99-62180

Printed and bound in the United States of America.
03 02 01 00 99   5 4 3 2 1

Contents in Brief

Contents in Full

CHAPTER 2
The Impact of Non-Environmental Standards on Nutritional Practice *41*

CHAPTER 5

Impact of Food Toxins on the Body *177*

CHAPTER 5: **Part IV** *continued*

CHAPTER 6
The Challenge of Food Toxicity *245*

PREFACE

As a professor, practitioner, and student of nutrition, I have always felt an overwhelming sense of contradiction. On the one hand, physical nourishment has always seemed attractive to me, with much the same appeal as honest work and sound sleep. On the other hand, I've always wondered if physical nourishment was really that attractive, why do people get so stressed in their relationship to it? "I don't have time," "I can't afford," "I know it's bad," and "I know I shouldn't" are the most common statements I hear about people's relationships with food, and the most common strategy I see is one that wedges food into an overcrowded lifestyle by doing the drive-through at fast food restaurants and take-out from the corner store.

Contradiction has also characterized my experience of nutrition as a field of science. On one side of the stalemate has been absolute scientific proof that nourishment (including optimal intake of nutrients like vitamins, minerals, and proteins) is essential for health. On the other side of the impasse is the non-existence of nutrition courses at the majority of medical schools in the U.S. When asked, many medical school professors contend that the real science of nutrition is actually contained within the fields of biochemistry, physiology, and other basic sciences. It's a contention I've been unable to fully dismiss, since my own teaching and this text depend much more on research findings published in journals of general medicine or medical specialties (like gastroenterology, immunology or environmental medicine) than on findings published in journals inside the field of nutrition. In addition, if nutritional science is really that solid and dependable, why is the field so widely known for its endless and unresolved debates over issues like high-carbohydrate versus low-carbohydrate diets and butter versus margarine?

The final type of contradiction I've experienced has been clinical. If nutrition truly belongs in the category of honest work and sound sleep and exists as a well-established science, why do nutritional interventions play a role in so few common health problems? In the conventional practice of nutrition, many common health problems are still regarded as having no effective dietary treatment. These problems include Alzheimer's disease, asthma, atopic dermatitis, benign prostatic hyperplasia, cataracts, chronic fatigue syndrome, Crohn's disease, depression, eczema, fibromyalgia, glaucoma, hyperthyroidism, hypothyroidism, insomnia, irritable bowel syndrome, migraine and cluster headache, multiple sclerosis, Parkinson's disease, premenstrual syndrome, psoriasis, rheumatoid arthritis, serous otitis media, systemic lupus erythematosus, and ulcerative colitis. Finally, if conventional nutrition interventions are so scientifically sound, why don't more people get better?

This book is part of my search for a way around the contradiction, and writing it has convinced me that all the good routes run straight through the ecosystem. The further we extend nutrition out into the environment, the closer we're going to get to molecular events inside our cells. And the more we think about nourishment as a process directed at the planet as well as the body, the healthier we're all going to be.

How to Use this Book

While the six chapters in this text are largely self-contained, they are designed to be read sequentially and do not make complete sense when read out of order. Chapters 1 and 6 are intended to serve as a conceptual framework for the book, and specifically avoid the biochemistry and molecular biology featured in Chapters 3 and 5. While the entire text has been written at an introductory college level, every effort has been made to explain scientific concepts "from the ground up" in such a way that readers who lack prior exposure to these sciences can still follow the descriptions.

As an author, I have made no effort to remove my philosophical and ethical values from the text, although I have tried to limit exclusively personal statements to the boxed sections entitled "Back to Basic Concepts." The other category of boxed sections, called "Historical Perspectives," are the most free-standing of the text entries and need not be read to understand the basic themes introduced in the book.

About the chemical drawings in this text

All of the chemical structures appearing within this text have been drawn with ACD/ChemSketch, Version 3.60 (1998, Advanced Chemistry Development, Inc., 133 Richmond Street West, Suite 605, Toronto, Ontario, M5H 2L3, Canada). The structures have been modeled in two (versus three) dimensions to emphasize the role of specific elements and metabolic principles rather than the underlying molecular geometry that makes them possible.

Many of the structures appearing within the text are small and medium-sized hydrocarbons. These structures are primarily composed of hydrogen and carbon atoms. In the case of extremely simply molecules like propene (C_3H_6), all carbon and hydrogen atoms have been shown. In the case of more complex molecules like BHT ($C_{15}H_{24}O$), all carbon and hydrogen atoms have been hidden except those atoms involved in functional groups (like methyl groups) that play a unique role in the conceptual understanding of the molecule. In molecules depicted with hidden carbon and hydrogen atoms, all straight line intersections represent bonds leading to a carbon atom, and all hydrogen attachments necessary to fulfill carbon's full complement of four bonds have been assumed. In addition, all benzene rings depicted in the text have been drawn as traditional Kekulé structures, despite the fact that present-day physical measurements lend stronger support to other depictions showing the presence of delocalized π electron clouds.

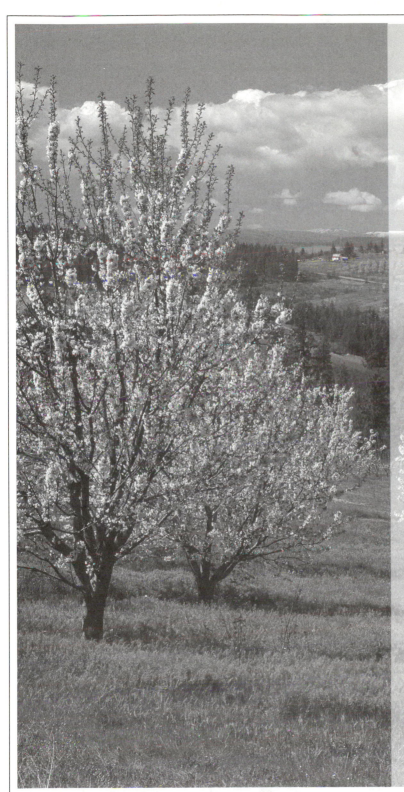

CHAPTER 1

Re-Establishing Environmental Standards in Nutrition

CONTENTS

Chapter 1: **Re-Establishing Environmental Standards in Nutrition**

Re-Establishing Environmental Standards in Nutrition

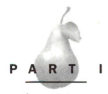

PART I

The Environment as an Intrinsic Standard in Nutrition

The Experience of Food

Although the title "Environmental Nutrition" appears for the first time in this text, the connection between nutrition and environment is familiar to anyone who eats. Nutrients come from food, and food comes from the environment. It's a common sense, two-part equation that hardly seems worthy of discussion.

While taken for granted at an intellectual level, this nutrient-food/food-environment equation is not something U.S. citizens experience first-hand in their everyday lives. The following section of this chapter looks in detail at the food experience of U.S. adults from a population-based perspective, as well as from the standpoint of individual and personal experience.

The Experience of Food in the United States

Heightened Awareness Through Media Exposure

During the past decade, U.S. consumers have been described as becoming increasingly aware of nutrition and diet. For example, according to a 1997 American Dietetic Association Survey, 92% of all respondents believed that fruits and vegetables had "very healthful effects"; 69% said they altered food purchases based on labels; 67% were aware of the Food Guide Pyramid; and 51% liked to hear about new dietary research.[1] These numbers represented all-time highs in consumer awareness of dietary issues.

Consumer awareness of dietary issues also appeared to be closely associated with food-related advertising and media exposure. Total dollars spent on food-related advertising reached an all-time high in 1997, with over $3 billion spent directly on food and food products. Over three quarters of that total was devoted to high-profile television ads, including network, spot, syndicated, and cable promotions.[2] An additional $3 billion in advertising was spent on restaurant and fast foods, $1.3 billion on beverages, $1.1 billion on confectionery and snacks, and $1.1 billion on alcoholic beverages.[3] Cumulatively, these food-related expenditures amounted to $10 billion, ranking food-related advertising as the third largest category of advertising in the U.S. (behind automobile and department/discount stores).[4]

In 1997, television was cited as the major source for nutrition information by 57% of all U.S. adults.[5] This reliance on television for food-related information represented all all-time high in the history of the survey, and a jump of 15% from 1995.

Self-Reported Lack of Knowledge

In contrast with increased levels of awareness among consumers was their self-reported lack of factual knowledge. For example, when surveyed in 1997 about their knowledge of food, approximately half of U.S. adults indicated that they were not knowledgeable.[6] Similarly, almost one third of the subjects indicated that they did not have the time or energy to try and understand the contents of their food.[7] In a similar nationwide survey also conducted in 1997, one fourth of all U.S. adults described confusion about nutrition as a major barrier that prevented them from eating well.[8]

These findings also matched closely with the results of a nationwide study conducted by the National Pork Producers Council in 1991, which showed three fourths of all subjects unable to pass a knowledge-based cooking test.[9]

Low Levels of Agricultural and Household Involvement

Lack of food knowledge among U.S. adults in the 1990s was paralleled by low levels of agricultural involvement in the U.S. population, and by low levels of household involvement with food-related activities and chores. In 1994, only 2% of the economically active population in the U.S. was involved in agriculture.[10] When total agricultural activity was averaged across the entire population, less than 17 hours per year were devoted to agriculture on a per capita basis.[11]

At the level of individual households and food-related activities like cooking and meal preparation, decreased food involvement was also reflected in statistical trends. In 1993, for the first time in U.S. history, dollars spent by U.S. adults on food outside the home matched dollars spent on food prepared inside the home.[12] This event was consistent with a 1992 meal preparation study conducted by the National Livestock and Meat Board in Chicago, Illinois. The study looked at the average number of meals prepared at home during a seven-day period. Out of 21 possible meals, 9–10 meals was the average number cooked by the 800 respondents. In summarizing the results of the study, authors listed a lack of knowledge about seasonings, sauces, and meat cuts as a basic finding. In addition, they concluded that the average U.S. adult had little knowledge of meats or meat cookery, little desire to become involved in cooking, and an unsophisticated cooking vocabulary.[13]

Lack of involvement with food-related activity at the household level was also reflected in national statistics involving land use and home gardening. At the beginning of the 1990s, approximately 890 million acres of land (including arable land, grassland, and pasture) were available for agriculture-related use in the U.S.[14] Only 1.3 million of these acres (approximately one seventh of one percent) were used for backyard vegetable gardens.[15]

The Experience of Food in Other Cultures

The separation of food awareness from food involvement that characterized of the experience of food in the U.S. in the 1990s was not an equally common characteristic of food experiences in other cultures. For example, in 1994, among all non-industrialized countries with a GNP (gross national product) per capita of less than $1,000, over half of all individuals were directly involved in agriculture.[16] Even in larger and partly industrialized countries, participation in agriculture was widespread. In 1990, for example, in India, China, and numerous African countries including Uganda and Zimbabwe over two thirds of the labor force was engaged in agricultural practice.[17]

In the summer of 1998, the largest agricultural country in the world, China, began its first nationwide farm survey. The survey planned to gather information from 300 million households, representing the vast majority of China's 1.2 billion population. Researchers designed the survey to include questions about types and amounts of crops grown, available land, and use of fertilizers and pesticides. The ability of most Chinese citizens to answer detailed survey questions about crops, land, fertilizer, and pesticides contrasted sharply with the self-reported food knowledge of U.S. citizens. Historically, this contrast dates back at least as far as 1957, when China's 500 million population was divided into 740,000 cooperatives of approximately 150–175 households each, and responsibility for food production was organized at the cooperative level.

Frequent At-Home Consumption

Examination of food expenditures as a percentage of total personal consumption expenditures also provides a cross-cultural contrast in the profile of food experience. In 1993, U.S. citizens spent less than 8% of their total personal consumption dollars on food and beverages consumed at home, the lowest of any country worldwide.[18] In several countries, including Bangladesh, India, and the Philippines, over 50% of total personal consumption dollars were spent on food and beverages consumed at home. Countries in which this percentage exceeded 33% included Mexico, Venezuela, and Pakistan.[19] While these percentages reflected the relative affluence of U.S. citizens in comparison with citizens in other countries and the higher percentage of discretionary dollars available to U.S. adults, they were also consistent with patterns of food-related activity in which household involvement was the norm in many countries but an exception within the U.S.

Personalized Involvement Through Ritual Practice

Direct contact with agricultural activity, routine food preparation, and at-home food consumption have not been the only points of difference between food experience in the U.S. and other countries. Unlike the U.S., many countries have maintained population-wide channels for acknowledging and placing value on the individual's personal experience of food. These channels have typically come in the form of ritual and religious practices and in the recognition of specific foods as sacred or taboo. Environmental standards have often played a key role in the establishment of food prohibitions and allowances. Considerations of climate, geography, and seasonality have all been included in these environmental standards.

In parts of South America, for example, the outdoor cooking of tortillas has traditionally been avoided due to the perceived environmental mismatch between cold air and the warmth of the cooking (and the cook's own body).[20] In traditional Chinese medical traditions, wind has traditionally been associated with spring, and susceptibility to wind influences during this season of the year has required increased intake of foods to reduce wind symptoms, including black soybeans, black sesame seeds, pine nuts, coconut, and spices like ginger, anise, and fennel.[21, 22]

Dietary Laws. The most striking connections between environment and personalized experience of food have come in the form of religious dietary laws. In this context, no tradition has been more careful in its "environmentalization" of food experience than the Tibetan tradition. Consumption of animal foods within this Tibetan tradition has been guided by an elaborate set of dietary laws that classify each animal according to its environmental habitat.In effect, this classification system has created environmentally-based animal food groups. Tibetan classifications of animal foods include: 1) animals that live in dry places like mountains, 2) those that live in wet places like oceans or lakes, and 3) those that live in both habitats. Animals that live in holes (like marmots, porcupines, toads, snakes, and badgers) fall into yet another dietary category. Birds that eat by power of dexterity (e.g., vultures, kites, owls) are differentiated from large birds that walk and obtain food by digging in the ground with their claws, and also from small birds that hop and obtain food by digging out food with their beaks.[23] Observation of these dietary laws by Tibetan people has acted as a cultural channel for personalizing the role of environment in food experience.

The Themes of Diversity and Wholeness

The role of environment as an intrinsic standard in nutrition is supported not only by the experience of food, but also by recognition of environmental themes that extend beyond the food realm. These themes include diversity and wholeness. As themes that characterize the essential nature of the ecosystem at all levels of function, the themes of diversity and wholeness become manifest in all geographical settings, including the ones that provide food for humans. The following sections look more closely at the themes of diversity and wholeness, and their implications for agricultural production and human nourishment.

The Theme of Diversity

The term "diversity" has its roots in the Latin *di* (apart) and *versus* (turning) and literally translates as "a turning apart." The term "diverse" has the same etymological structure as the term "universe" (*uni* + *versus*, "turning as one"), and together the two terms capture an essential feature of the ecosystem. As a "diverse universe," the ecosystem is characterized by a "turning together while at the same time divided." The word "ecology" focuses on the "turning together" aspect of the universe by combining the Greek words *oikos* (house) and *logos* (having been gathered together into a coherent form and made manifest). But what is equally implicit in the word "ecology" is the purpose of this housing: to provide a coherent and accomodating spot for the diversity of living organisms.

In a more practical sense, the term "biodiversity" has several specific ecologically-based meanings. When used within the context of a habitat or community, the term implies a richness of species found within the habitat. "Biodiversity" is also used, however, within the context of a single species. When used in this way, the term typically refers to a genetic richness within that species. Biodiversity can also refer to the number of communities being housed in a single habitat.

Geographical Aspects of Diversity

Geography forms the backdrop against which biodiversity is measured. At all geographical levels, diversity is a natural feature of the living world. At the broadest level, the earth itself is regarded as the geographical backdrop for diversity. To date, approximately 1.8 million species of plant, animal, and microbial organisms have been determined to exist on the earth, although most researchers believe that the actual number is much higher and may eventually be identified as closer to 50–70 million.[24] These 1.8 million species include approximately 350,000 species of plants. Over the course of human evolution, tens of thousands have been used by humans for food.

Within smaller geographical areas, diversity still remains a natural feature of the lifeworld. In the United States, for example, 7,098 varieties of apples (*Malus pumila*) were produced for food consumption between the years 1804 and 1904.[25] During this same time period, over 775 varieties of corn (*Zea mays*) were known to have been planted. (Only 50 still exist, and out of these 50, less than 10 are routinely planted and harvested).[26] The total number of edible plant and animal species indigenous to North America originally numbered well into the thousands.

Seasonal Aspects of Diversity

Like geography, seasonality forms a backdrop for measurement of diversity by establishing cyclical patterns characteristic of the living world. Cereal grains, for example, have evolved over centuries into "winter" (acclimatized) and "spring" (non-acclimatized) species. In acclimatized species, seasonal changes occurring in the fall (like decreasing day length) trigger metabolic changes that protect cells from dehydration. These changes often include increased deposition of free amino acids and synthesis of polyhydroxy compounds (PHCs) like glycerol and sorbitol.[27]

A widely-recognized feature of seasonality among farmers and gardeners is the frost-free period. This seasonal phenomenon is defined as the length of time between the last lethal frost of spring and the first lethal frost of fall. While cyclical, the frost free period can vary dramatically from year to year within a single location. For example, over a forty-five year period in the town of Moscow, Idaho, frost-free period ranged from 83 to 192 days.[28]

Interactive Aspects of Diversity

Maintenance of ecological diversity requires constant interaction between organisms and their environment. Interaction takes place simultaneously on a variety of levels. All forms of organisms (including microbes, plants, and animals) interact with each other, and researchers have studied these interactions in each of six possible categories: plant–microbe, animal–microbe, microbe–microbe, plant–plant, animal–plant, and animal–animal. Organisms also interact directly with their environment. (Some of these interactions have been described previously within the context of seasonality.) Direct interactions typically involve sensitivity on the part of organisms to environmental cycles like photoperiod (light–dark cycle) or thermoperiod (temperature cycle), as well responses to geomagnetic, gravitational, and electromagnetic patterns. In the remainder of this section, we will review several types of interaction that are necessary for the maintenance of diversity.

Plant–Microbe Interactions. Maintenance of ecological diversity requires constant interaction between organisms. In order to obtain nitrogen for the synthesis of proteins, for example, many plants must find a way to "fix" molecular nitrogen (N_2) available in the atmosphere. "Fixation" is a term used to describe the conversion of molecular nitrogen to into any compound. (Compounds are substances containing two or more different elements). The conversion of N_2 into NH_3 (ammonia) or NO_3 (nitrate) are examples of nitrogen fixation.

Although nitrogen fixation can occur both photochemically and electro-chemically, many plants rely on biological fixation using nitrogenase enzyme systems. These enzyme systems are often found not in the plants themselves, but in soil bacteria living in close proximity to the plant roots.

Rhizobium is the genus (or family subdivision) name for a type of bacteria that provide nitrogenase enzyme systems and nitrogen fixing capacities for many plants found in the legume (*leguminosae*) family. These plants include peas, clover, alfalfa, jicama, lima beans, fava beans, kidney beans, mung beans, soybeans, chickpeas, and tamarind. Within the *Rhizobium* genus of bacteria are found a wide variety of species, and specific *Rhizobium* species found in soil are uniquely matched up with specific legumes. These *Rhizobium* species leave the soil, move into the root hairs of the plant, and reproduce. As the root hairs grow, the bacteria and plants work together symbiotically to fix nitrogen needed for plant growth.

Animal–Plant Interactions. Like interaction between plants and microbes, interaction between animals and plants is also a prerequisite for diversity. Many grazing animals, like deer belonging to the genus *Odocoileus*, are able to live in vastly different climates and habitats by becoming carefully attuned to seasonal patterns. *Odocoileus* species inhabit parts of central America as low as the 17th parallel, but also inhabit parts of northern Canada as high as the 60th parallel. At the higher northern latitudes, breeding is limited to a single two-month period each year. At lower southern latitudes, breeding is continuous. The deer are able to maintain their species and habitat diversity by timing their breeding periods according to environmental cues. These cues are partly provided by the changing content of forage grasses. Particularly important in the content of the grasses are amino acid patterns, which change on a seasonal basis, but also remain synchronized to yearly fluctuations.[29] Similar relationships between forage proteins and the overall life strategies of animals have been observed in dairy cows[30] and laying hens.[31]

Animal–Light Cycle Interactions. As discussed previously within the context of seasonality, most organisms are sensitive to changes in dark–light cycle (photoperiod) and develop life strategies that remain synchronized with it. In humans, for example, production of the hormone melatonin is closely patterned after dark–light cycles in at least two of the body's organs. The first of these organs is the eye, where fluctuation in retinal synthesis of melatonin (requiring activity of the enzyme hydroxy-indole-O-methyl-transferase, or HIOMT) closely follows photoperiod.[32] In the pineal gland, a similar phenomenon has been observed.[33] Researchers have further observed that the release of excitatory amino acids (including glutamic acid

and aspartic acid) from the suprachiasmatic nucleus (SCN) in the hypothalamus of the brain is involved in moment-by-moment adjustments
made by humans to dark–light patterns.[34]

Sensitivity to dark–light cycles is one example of an interaction that
happens continuously and contributes to the remarkable genetic diversity
of human beings. In the absence of this direct environmental synchroniza-
tion, humans would have been unable to diversify in their selection of
habitats. They would also have been unable to develop flexibility in timing
of puberty[35] or length of sleep cycles.[36]

Experiential Aspects of Diversity

Diversity is a concept that can be experienced as well as studied, and the
experience of diversity is nowhere more accessible than in relationship to
food. Even in the produce section of a local, ethnic grocery, with its loquat,
daikon, bamboo shoots, jicama, tamarind, jackfruit, pak choi, kai laan, choi
sum, mizuna, Chinese artichoke, burdock root, juke, star fruit, jujube, lotus
root, lychee, and bitter mellon, the diversity of food can be experienced.
Travelers often experience this same diversity when moving from country to
country, and finding that quinces do best in Turkey and Iran, loquats, in
southern China and Japan, topi-tambo in the Caribbean, and naranjilla in
the Andes. Adventurers unexpectedly stumbling upon a patch of Morama
beans in the Kalahari desert, or edible sea greens in the nearly lifeless, alkaline salt water of Lake Chad 2,000 miles north also experience this diversity.

Outside the produce sections of local supermarkets, where the aesthetics
of food have been genetically or chemically altered to achieve uniformity
and predictability, the aesthetic diversity of food is also a universal human
experience. On the tree and in the garden, the looks of food are non-
uniform and unpredictable. Even within a single variety of a single species,
the color, size, and texture of a food can vary dramatically along with growing conditions and genetic input. We experience the diversity of food in the
unique appearance of each plant or fruit that looks blochy, splotchy, lop-
sided, or simply "unusual." The non-uniform or non-symmetrical appearance of a food is not the result of a defect or deficiency. It is evidence that
the food was adapted to its spot and adjusted to natural forces like angles of
light and amounts of rain, as well as to the presence of other organisms.

The Theme of Wholeness

Working together with the concept of diversity as a foundational component in ecology and in the human experience of food is the concept of
wholeness. The term "wholeness" points back etymologically to the Greek

holon, which originally meant both "universe" (*uni + versus*, "turning as one") and "organism" (*organon*, "means of function"). In Aristotelian philosophy, wholeness was used as a concept to explain how things came into being. In this context, wholeness was contrasted with "association" (*synkrisis*) and "dissociation" (*diakrisis*). Aristotle argued that things in the universe could not have come into being simply though the association (or combination) of smaller units into larger ones or through dissociation (splitting apart) of larger unit into smaller ones. He argued that the only force which could change "this" into "that" was the force of wholeness (*holon*).[37] More recently, recognition of a unique, unifying force in all organisms has become a focus of healthcare practitioners who ascribe to the principles of "holistic medicine." According to the American Holistic Health Association, headquartered in Anaheim, California:

"Rather than focusing on illness or specific parts of the body, holistic health considers the whole person and how it interacts with its environment. It emphasizes the connection of body, mind, and spirit. Holistic Health is based on the law of nature that a whole is made up of interdependent parts. The earth is made up of systems, such as air, land, water, plants, and animals ….When one part is not working at its best, it will impact all the other parts of that person …this whole person, including all of the parts, is constantly interacting with everything in the surrounding environment."[38]

Example of a Danish Dairy Farm

The concept of wholeness described above was designed to provide healthcare practitioners with a frame of reference for clinical practice. But it is a description that can also be applied to a broad spectrum of nutritional activities, including agricultural production of food. An agricultural research study conducted in 1988 on a small Danish dairy farm exemplifies the way that wholeness can be applied as a thematic framework for understanding nutrient dynamics. In the study, ecologists in Denmark observed nitrogen patterns associated with annual activity on an 80-acre dairy farm located within a sandy soil region near the town of Jutland. The farm housed 44 dairy cows and 60 younger calves who depended on forage crops raised onsite. A study of the farm's nitrogen ecology showed the mineral nitrogen to be present throughout the farm's environment: in the atmosphere, where it existed primarily in the form of dinitrogen gas (N_2); in soil microorganisms, where it entered as N_2 and became transformed into ammonia (NH_3) or nitrate (NO_3^{-}); and in the livestock, where it was found in a wide variety of inorganic and organic forms. From all sources, including nitrogen-containing fertilizer added to the pasture land each year, the farm was estimated to receive a total annual nitrogen input of 10,019 kilograms.[39] Nitrogen content of clover planted on the acreage was estimated at 1246 kilograms, and nitrogen content of annual meat and milk production was estimated at 1515 kilograms.[40] On an annual basis, loss of nitrogen to leaching and runoff was estimated at more than 8,000 kilograms.[41] The amount of nitrogen contained within any single farm source (e.g., soil microbes, pasture clover, or cow's milk) was determined to depend on the interaction of these organisms and on their collective interaction with events like fertilizer application or time of planting.

The documentation of nitrogen sources on the dairy farm and the tracking of nitrogen movement throughout the farm has important implications for the understanding of food quality. Rather than measuring food quality by looking strictly *inside* the cow's milk and the beef, this ecological approach also looks *outside* the foods to understand their nutritional content (in this case, protein). From the perspective of agricultural ecology adopted in this study, all organisms in the farm environment can be viewed as participating in the production of milk. Similarly, a disturbance anywhere in farm can upset milk and beef production. For example, in the absence of sufficient soil microbes to transform atmospheric nitrogen, livestock growth and milk output will decrease as a result of decreased protein availability. (Organic farmers often inoculate soils with nitrogen-fixing bacteria, like strains of the bacterium *Bradyrhizobium japonicum*, for precisely this reason).

Livestock and dairy production can also be disrupted by lack of year-round plant root systems for absorption of the nitrogen-containing compounds that have been created by soil bacteria. The planting of ground cover, particularly during times of the year when rainfall exceeds the absorptive capacities of air and soil, can help offset the loss of unabsorbed nitrogen to rainwater runoff.

Lack of organic matter available for decomposition in pastures and cropland can also upset milk and beef production. Plant material (like crop stubble) left on top of soil contains a higher ratio of carbon to nitrogen than the ratio found in soil microbes. As plant material decomposes, this difference in carbon-to-nitrogen ratio allows soil microbes to better absorb nitrogen and prevent its loss through runoff. Without this organic matter, nitrogen retention is reduced.

Productivity on the dairy farm can also be disrupted by nitrogen-related activities occurring at great distances from the farm. Industrial combustion of oil or coal releases nitrogen oxides (NO_x) into the air, and within several days, these oxides can be converted into nitric acid (HNO_3). Incorporation of nitric acid into rainfall increases rainfall acidity. Upon contact with the ground, acidic rainwater increases soil acidity, and along with it, the acidity of microbial and plant habitats. A farm lying miles downwind from an industrial nitrogen-oxide producer can have its nitrogen cycles and other nutrient cycles disrupted by these events.

The concept of wholeness captures the unified nature of these ecological events by assigning to each participant in the nitrogen-cycling process an inescapable and non-interruptible set of connections with other participants. Like the human body described by the American Holistic Health Association as being in constant interaction with everything in the surrounding environment, the Danish dairy farm and its two food products (milk and beef) are equally interconnected to the world outside.

The theme of wholeness that provides a framework for understanding the human body and the Danish dairy farm is a theme that has been eloquently described by U.S. engineer, designer, architect, and 1983 Medal of Freedom award-winner Buckminster Fuller. While defining the term "function" in his 1975 work, *Synergetics*, Fuller wrote the following description of wholeness and its relationship to function: "Functions occur only as inherently cooperative and accommodatively varying subaspects of synergistically transforming wholes."[42] Like holistic practitioners examining body function or agricultural researchers examining dairy farm operations, Fuller saw the ability to function as an ability based on wholeness.

Experiential Aspects of Wholeness

Like diversity, wholeness is part of our everyday food experience. Outside of the supermarket, where food has often been fragmented into unrecognizable remnants of its original form, what we eat draws us into a sense of connection with the entire universe from which it came. As something "found" on the tree, in the ground, or on the vine, food has always pointed beyond itself to the kind of soil in which it grew or the time of year in which it ripened. Considerations of this type have often found their way into our food-naming process: winter melon, summer spinach, swamp potato, tree ear mushroom.

Food has always struck us as part of something larger, some greater context, some grander scheme, some overriding set of events which made it possible. The "grander scheme" to which food belongs is a scheme characterized by wholeness.

When it is natural and not disordered, the experience of wholeness is also present in our experience of eating. When we need food, we do not say that our brains or our intestines are hungry. We say that *we* are hungry, and our hunger is something that engages us as whole persons.

If our sense of wholeness becomes disrupted, it is easy for our eating to become disrupted as well. The strongest appetite can be instantaneously lost upon hearing about the death of a close friend, or upon witnessing a tragedy or grave injustice. When our sense of wholeness is threated in a more deep-seated or chronic way, the disruption can lead to the development of an eating disorder. The experiences of anorexia or bulimia are often experiences related to wholeness, both in the sense of something threatened and something that needs to be protected. The idea of threatened wholeness is consistent with the experience of many individuals who have been diagnosed with eating disorders. The feeling of estrangement from family and friends, the unraveling of shared experience, and the unraveling of private experience are possible consequences of threatened wholeness. The threat to wholeness may be sufficiently strong to make a person with an eating disorder feel like he or she is standing outside of his or her own experience and losing touch with himself or herself. At the same time, the experiences of anorexia or bulimia can help protect and preserve a sense of wholeness by allowing individuals to disengage from lives that simply do not feel their own.

PART II

The Non-Environmental Nature of Current Standards

In Part I of this chapter, we review the intrinsic role of environment in the origination, cultivation, nutritional composition, and experience of food. We refer to environment as an intrinsic standard against which nutrition could be evaluated and understood. In Part II, we look at current standards for evaluating nourishment and see how environment has been widely abandoned as a standard in nutritional practice.

Loss of Interaction

Loss of an interactive environmental standard has become a hallmark of nutrition across its spectrum of practice. Except in the area of nutrient-drug interactions, where many clinicians have made a concentrated effort to address the impact of prescription medications on nutrient status, interaction is not a standard that has been adhered to in agricultural practice, food supply dynamics, public health recommendations, or clinical decision-making.

Nutrient Reference Books

A static, non-interactive view of food and nutrients has become the standard in nutritional reference books, nutrient databases, and product labeling. When ascertaining the vitamin C content of broccoli, for example, dietitians commonly refer to Bowes and Church's *Food Values of Portions Commonly Used*. In that reference source, raw broccoli is listed as containing 41 milligrams of vitamin C per half cup serving.[43] From an ecological standpoint, the idea of broccoli containing a fixed and static amount of vitamin C (or any other nutrient) is both illogical and scientifically unfounded. For example, at least twenty one studies have shown organically grown foods (including cruciferous vegetables like broccoli) to contain significantly greater amounts of vitamin C than their non-organically grown counterparts.[44] Similarly, nutrient content of foods have been shown to vary along with seasonal change, climate, soil conditions, seed stock, planting, harvesting, and storage methods.[45]

Nutrient Databases

Nutritional databases have also adopted a static, non-interactive standard for data inclusion. United States Department of Agriculture (USDA) Handbook No. 8, originally developed in 1950, has remained the primary source of food composition data in the U.S.[46] In its original release, this handbook contained information on 15 nutrients in 751 food products. As standards for obtaining accurate and reliable nutrient data, USDA researchers established a variety of sampling procedures as appropriate in the gathering of nutrient data. These sampling standards included single sampling, in which average nutrient content was calculated from several individual samples of a single food; single composite sampling, in which mixed samples of a food obtained at different times and places were combined, analyzed, and reported as a single food; and multiple composite sampling, in which different brands or cultivars of a food were combined, weighed to approximate a single food product as it would appear in the marketplace, and subsequently analyzed.

These sampling procedures virtually guaranteed a nutrient database that would remain indifferent to the environmental dynamics that shaped the nutrient content of foods contained within it. Random combining of cultivars, selection of samples without respect to seasonal or geographical variation, and restriction on the total number of samples were research decisions that produced a database insensitive to environmental standards and potentially non-representative of the nutrient content of foods actually being eaten by the U.S. public. As one representative of the Quaker Oats Company in Chicago, Illinois remarked in an address to the 14th National Nutrient Database Conference in 1989 in Iowa City, Iowa, "it is nearly impossible to keep up to date on any nutrient database which would adequately represent the foods now available to the American public."[47]

Clinical Recommendations

The Example of Fatty Acid Ratios

The abandonment of an interactive environmental standard in nutrition has also been exemplified in the area of clinical practice. While many aspects of the clinical decision-making process could serve as examples of this lost standard, neglect of fatty acids ratios stands out for two reasons. First is the total human dependence on diet for establishment of optimal fatty acid ratios. From an environmental standpoint, the position of humans with respect to fatty acid ratios is striking, since humans lack the delta 15 and delta 12 desaturase enzymes required to synthesize 3 and 6 fatty acids *de novo*, i.e., "from scratch." Many plants, including mosses, ferns, grasses, and trees, possess these enzymes. (They are also commonly found in algae and phytoplankton.) In the absence of *de novo* synthesis capability, or the presence of conversion enzymes, humans are completely dependent upon diet for establishment of optimal balance in omega 3 and omega 6 fatty acid ratios. While this dietary dependency obviously places a premium on the interaction between humans and their food, it also points to the importance of interactions that underlie the final fatty acid composition of food.

Omega 3:6 Ratio and Plant Development. A second reason for focusing on fatty acid ratios as an example of lost standards in clinical practice is the unique nature of fatty acid ratios in plant growth and development. Studies on plant development and nutrient content that have shown dramatic changes in fatty acid ratios occur within a three-week period after flowering.

These changes occur while young, growing plants make continual metabolic adjustments to their new environment. In corn oil, an omega 6:omega 3 fatty acid ratio of 3.8 has been shown to rise to 11.4 during this time.[48] In soybeans, during a one-week period, the same ratio has been observed to increase from 1.2 to 3.8.[49] These agricultural findings have suggested that the age at which fat-containing foods are harvested or consumed can make a significant difference in fatty acid balance, both for the plants and the human who consume them.

Omega 3:6 Ratio and Human Metabolism. An interactive standard is also maintained inside the body following ingestion and absorption of dietary fatty acids. Even if dietary ratios have been well-balanced, a wide variety of metabolic interactions are necessary in order for this balance to be maintained. Because most omega 3 and omega 6 molecules are highly unsaturated, long-chain fatty acids, oxidative metabolism must be optimally supported in order to avoid peroxidation of omega 3 and 6 fats. This support requires the presence of a wide variety of antioxidant nutrients. (Nutritional support of oxidative metabolism is discussed in detail in Chapter 5.) Successful elongation and desaturation of omega 3 and 6 family members also requires proper function of enzymes like delta 5 and delta 6 desaturase. These enzymes cannot function in the absence of additional nutrients, including vitamins B-3, B-6, C, and the minerals zinc and magnesium. Finally, maintenance of omega 3:6 balance in the body requires non-excessive conversion of fatty acid molecules into eicosanoid messengers by cyclo-oxygenase and lipoxygenase enzymes. Overactivation of these enzymes is often the result of exposure to prescription medicines and environmental toxins.

Omega 3:6 Ratio and Human Disease. The importance of these interactive aspects has been further solidified by establishment of omega 3:6 ratio as a major risk factor in human disease.[50] Decreased ratios (typically produced by deficient intake of omega 3 fatty acids) have been shown to be a risk factor in the development of neurological problems of infancy,[51] childhood hyperactivity,[52] and numerous chronic conditions of adulthood including coronary heart disease[53] and chronic obstructive pulmonary disease.[54] Yet in spite of these findings, omega 3:6 ratio has remained almost totally ignored in public health recommendations by nutritional organizations and by most dietitians in clinical practice.

Neglect of Omega 3:6 Ratio in Dietary Guidelines. Omega 3:6 fatty acid ratios were not mentioned in the United States Department of Agriculture's 1992 release of the Food Guide Pyramid.[55] (A 1997 survey showed this widely-publicized guide to be the single most recognized nutritional guideline in the U.S., acknowledged by more than two thirds of all U.S. adults).[56] Similarly, a 1998 American Dietetic Association position paper on fat intake and fat replacement made only one mention of omega 3 or omega 6 fatty acids.[57] This single mention involved the suggestion that deficiency symptoms could be prevented if 1–2% of total caloric intake was derived from omega 6 fatty acids and if 1% was derived omega 3 fatty acids.[58] The recommendation was not translated, however, into any food recommendations. More importantly, it ignored the reality of fatty acid intake by U.S. adults, who had already been estimated to receive approximately 6% of total calories from omega 6 fatty acid intake.[59]

In its most recent 1999 Nutrition Fact Sheets entitled "ABCs of Fats, Oils and Cholesterol" and "Fats and Oils in the Diet: The Great Debate," the American Dietetic Association once again made no mention of omega 3 or omega 6 fatty acids.[60] At a conceptual level, this ongoing failure to address a major risk factor for human disease might best be remedied by re-instituting an interactive environmental standard in nutritional practice that focuses attention on relationship between organisms, their environment, and food.

The Example of Nutrient Synergisms and Antagonisms

Absence of an interactive environmental standard in nutrition has also been witnessed by the neglect of nutrient synergisms and antagonisms. In 1988, Bodwell and Erdman published a 400-page textbook entitled *Nutrient Interactions*.[61] The text listed several hundred nutrient interactions falling into fourteen basic categories. (These categories included vitamin–vitamin interactions, mineral–mineral interactions, vitamin–mineral, carbohydrate–lipid, protein–mineral, and other types of interactions). The text also provided well over 1,000 indexed journal references.

Flavonoids and Vitamin C. Since publication of the Bodwell and Erdman text, well over one thousand additional studies have been published in the nutrition literature that shed light on nutrient interactions and their significance for human health. Flavonoids like dihydroquercitin, for example, have been shown capable of reducing ascorbyl radical, thereby protecting vitamin C and serving to enhance its effectiveness.[62] This finding has important implications for dietary intake. Many foods naturally high in vitamin C (like oranges or bell peppers) are also naturally high in dihydroquercitin. However, the parts of these foods normally eaten by U.S. adults (i.e., the juice-filled sections of the orange and the crunchy green casing of the bell pepper) are parts that contain vitamin C but not the dihydroquercitin. The flavonoid component of these foods is predominantly found in the white pulpy portion. Consumption of these foods in their whole form would be required for simultaneous intake of vitamin C and dihydro-quercitin. These aspects of vitamin C status have gone unmentioned, however, in all public health recommendations by nutritional organizations. Even in the forthcoming Dietary Reference Intakes (DRIs) for antioxidant nutrients being prepared by the Panel on Dietary Antioxidants and Related Compounds from the National Academy of Sciences in Washington, D.C., flavonoid intake will not be discussed or evaluated. According to the Panel, "Although phenols and polyphenols may be important dietary constituents, inefficient data are available at this time to warrant their inclusion in this evaluation."[63]

From an environmental standpoint, interactions involving nutrients like flavonoids and vitamin C are standard features of the earth's biogeochemical cycles, organic matter, and its flux through ecological communities. In ecology and plant biochemistry, substances like flavonoids are involved in a variety of life functions including screening of light, photosensitization and energy transfer.[64] Against this environmental backdrop, their interaction with vitamin C does not stand out as a novel or unexplored area of research. Instead, it exists alongside of other similar interactions as a commonplace event that sustains the health of organisms by aligning their resources with surrounding conditions.

Loss of Seasonality

The lack of an environmental standard in nutrition has also been demonstrated by loss of seasonality from the marketplace and from inattention to seasonality in food guidelines and clinical decision-making. Approximately 25,000 different food items have been estimated to exist on the shelves of grocery stores nationwide, and national distribution of these food items involves the operation of some 30,700 stores.[65] When combined together with the cost of energy required for crop production, the energy cost of processing, packaging, and distributing foods accounts for 17% of total energy expenditure in the U.S.[66] In oil-equivalent terms, over 1500 liters of oil per person per year are required for processing, packaging and distribution of food.[67]

More than half of all fruits and vegetables produced in the U.S. are produced for use in processing rather than direct consumption.[68] For some crops, like tomatoes, the percentage exceeds 90%.[69] Processing not only means displacement of food from its original shape and form, but also displacement of food from its natural timetable. Through the use of gases, ripening of foods can be accelerated or delayed.

Together with the use of food additives and preservatives, freezing, canning, and high-technology packaging, food processing has eliminated the natural timetable for food from the marketplace. Any food can be purchased and consumed at any time of year, and any food can be processed in such a way as to extend or shorten its natural lifespan. This marketplace reality stands in sharp contrast with the environmental standard of seasonal cycles and the strict dependency of food upon annual patterns in temperature, solar radiation, and rainfall. Within the environmental context, cucumbers like to be planted later in the year than corn. Carrots don't mind being planted early, even three weeks before the beginning of the frost-free period. Asparagus might not yield a harvest for 1–3 years. The natural timetable of foods is a seasonal timetable, and it varies along with seasonal changes. Most cultures have developed food practices that are closely synchronized with the passage of seasons, and nutrient intake within these cultures reflects this seasonal variation.

Seasonality is not only a natural process but a process that is essential for sustainable production of food. For example, during the winter, conditions favor increased nitrification (the process of converting ammonia to nitrate that takes place in soil with the help of soil bacteria). In the absence of seasonal changes that occur during winter months, nitrification becomes insufficient to provide enough nitrate in the spring for young, germinating plants.

The importance of seasonality in food production may also be reflected in the results of agricultural research studies showing significantly greater nutrient content in organically grown foods. (These studies are reviewed in Chapter 6, page 277, under "Organically-Grown Food"). While non-organic growing practices can often override the restrictions imposed by seasonality on the planting and harvesting of food, organic farming is usually well-synchronized with passage of the seasons. Non-organic food practices rely on input of synthetic fertilizers to sustain crop production from year to year, but successful organic farming often depends on seasonal transitions in which plants die, decompose, and become re-incorporated into the soil. These seasonal transitions that allow for natural recycling of plant materials may contribute to the nutritional superiority of organically grown foods.

Loss of Geographical Uniqueness

Like the loss of seasonality, loss of geographical uniqueness has also been a consequence of non-environmental standards in nutrition. Where food comes from has lost its relevance in the national food marketplace. Many foods indigenous to North America, including tepary beans, scarlet runner beans, paiute, and chiltepines have become virtually non-existent in the U.S. food supply. At the same time, other indigenous foods that could easily be produced within the U.S. have become the product of corporate operations in other countries. Beginning in the late 1950s, many U.S. food manufacturers began to expand production and processing operations to include locations outside of the U.S. This expansion came partly in response to the passage of labor laws that increased labor costs within the continental U.S. By the early 1970s, Cargill (the largest grain exporter and producer worldwide) had operations in Peru, Spain, France, Canada, El Salvador, Guatemala, the Philippines, the Netherlands, Argentina, Pakistan, Brazil, Taiwan, and South Korea. Del Monte owned facilities in over 20 countries, including Italy, Great Britain, South Africa, the Philipines, Ecuador, Venezuela, Mexico, and Brazil.[70]

The above combination of events served to remove geographical uniqueness as a factor in the U.S. marketplace. With local production of food removed as a restriction on dietary consumption, the food supply was freed to respond to global economic factors rather than remaining tied to geographical (or seasonal) factors.

Dietetic practitioners responded to this severed connection between food and geography in much the same way as the food supply itself. Dietary recommendations during the past three decades have focused upon selection of a variety of foods rather than consumption of foods produced locally or originally native to a person's locale. To date, no public or professional recommendation by the American Dietetic Association, National Academy of Sciences, U.S. Department of Agriculture, or Department of Health and Human Services has addressed the link between food and geography as a relevant aspect of dietary practice.

The disconnection of food production and food intake from geography sharply contrasts with environmental standards in which food is tied to its spot. Bananas retain their native home in southern Asia, and potatoes owe their beginning to the eastern coast of South America.[71] Greece is famous for its olives, and Tahiti for its breadfruit. Like its connection to seasonality, food's link to geography is a link to the uneven distribution of natural resources, and to conditions that are place-specific. As Michael Begon and his co-authors have written in their textbook on ecology, "All species are absent from almost everywhere,"[72] and the reason for this absence is geographical uniqueness.

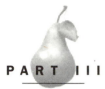

PART III
The Energy-Based Origin of Non-Environmental Standards

Nutrition as we now know it is a direct outgrowth of scientific research in the late 1800s and early 20th century. At that time, scientists were actively engaged in two fundamental endeavors, one involving chemistry and the other involving physics. Both of these endeavors were united in their focus on the concept of energy as a unifying factor in the investigation of phenomena from a scientific perspective.

The Concept of Energy in Western Science

Energy, referred to by some physicists as the most central idea in all of science,[73] is a concept familiar to many students of science within the context of Albert Einstein's well-known theory of relativity. This theory, proposed in 1905, produced the equation "$E = mc^2$" in which "E" stands for energy, "m" for mass, and "c" for the speed of light. Prior to the proposal of this theory, however, many scientists had performed experiments trying to determine the nature of energy and its relationship with matter and mass. These experiments often began with investigations involving the concept of "work." Work was defined as the application of force by one object to another object resulting in movement of the second object across some distance. "Energy" was defined as the quality of the first object that allowed it to apply force to the second.

Energy Theory in Physics

Between 1860 and 1910, physical scientists began to use the concept of energy to account for a wide variety of phenomena. For the first time in the history of science, phenomena like heat, light, electricity, magnetism, and radiation were all being investigated as forms of energy. James Clark Maxwell's deduction of electromagnetic waves in 1864, his kinetic theory of gases in the late 1870s, and Ludwig Boltzmann's mathematical testing of the kinetic theory of heat in the 1880s all exemplified the predominance of the energy concept during this period.

Elemental Theory in Chemistry

During this same period of time, chemical scientists working alongside of their counterparts in physics were in the process of identifying 16 new elements. The identification of fluorine in 1886, helium in 1895, neon in 1898, and radon in 1900 exemplify this expansion of elemental knowledge during the period 1860–1910. Simultaneous with the identification of these new elements were important refinements being made in the periodic table which had been developed to explain the relationship of these elements to each other.

Industrial Applications of Energy Theory

In his book, *Grammatical Man*,[74] author Jeremy Campbell has argued that these activities in chemistry and physics culminated in the invention of a machine for harnessing energy based on an understanding of the elements. That invention was the steam engine. Invention of the steam engine spawned an industrial revolution, changed population patterns, shifted environmental balances, and altered human work practices. Many of these changes brought about by the industrial revolution have continued to this day.

Energy-Thinking in Nutrition

Although Campbell's book, *Grammatical Man*, was not designed to address issues in the field of nutrition, many of the observations made in his book are applicable to that field, which emerged during this same time period. Nutrition was rarely mentioned as a field of science prior to the year 1898,[75] and the connection of diseases like beriberi and pellagra to dietary deficiency did not begin to be well-understood until the late 1890s. Calometric studies of foodstuffs became increasingly common in the 1880s, and by the turn of the century, human protein and mineral requirements were being studied by physiologic balance methods.[76]

Each of nutrition-related activities described above owed its occurrence to the concept of energy and to the identification of chemical elements. In the following section, we will look more closely at the role of energy and chemical elements in inaugurating the science of nutrition and in maintaining its current practice.

Caloric Energy

Like nutritionists at the turn of the century, most present-day dietitians still focus attention on the energy content of food. This energy content is measured in terms of calories through the process of bomb calorimetry. While the technology of bomb calorimetry has changed somewhat over the past century, the basic instrumentation has remained similar to the apparatus developed in 1903 by Atwater and Snell.[77] A small chamber containing food is floated on a known quantity of water with a known temperature of 14.5° centigrade in a sealed chamber at atmospheric pressure. Oxygen and an electrical spark are combined in the chamber, causing the food to combust and begin burning. As the temperature in the floating chamber rises, so does the temperature of the surrounding water. When the temperature in one gram of water has been increased by 1° centigrade (from 14.5° to 15.5°), combustion of the food is describe as having produced one calorie of energy.

Carbohydrates, fats, and to a lesser degree proteins, are still widely-regarded as the energy-containing parts of food. Each of these macronutrients is valued for its caloric contribution to the diet, and to a certain extent, each category of macronutrient has been looked upon as homogenous in light of its caloric contribution. Fats, for example, are often regarded as more problematic in the diet than carbohydrates because of their 9-calorie-per-gram contribution to caloric energy versus the 4-calorie-per-gram contribution of carbohydrates.

Food as Fuel

The idea that food contains caloric energy is closely paralleled by the idea that the human body is designed to combust it. Just as food can be viewed as a repository for caloric energy, the body can be viewed as an ingenious bomb calorimeter that heats food up through chemical means and then metabolically extracts calories from it. The concept of food as fuel owes its existence to this confluence of ideas.

Present-day nutritional researchers still conduct a large number of studies to determine exactly how food serves as fuel for human beings. For example, debates continue over the proper fuel mixture for human health. (These mixtures range from a 10:80:10 ratio of total dietary calories from protein:carbohydrate:fat to a 30:40:30 ratio of total caloric energy obtained from these macronutrients). This view of diet as a source of metabolic fuel has direct roots in the physics and chemistry of the late 1800s.

The Historical Value of Energy-Thinking in Nutrition

For scientists conducting research in western Europe in the late 19th century, the concept of energy was likely to have provided a unifying framework for integrating a wide array of experimental findings. Expansion of physics research into the realms of light, heat, electromagnetism and radiation, like expansion of chemistry research across a widening range of elements and elemental interactions, must have challenged the thinking pattern of scientists attempting to make sense of new discoveries and patterns. The ability of scientists to conceptualize light, heat, electromagnetism and radiation as forms of energy was likely to have provided them with a sense of intellectual congruity and wholeness.

The value of energy-thinking for nutritional researchers at the turn of the century was likely to have been equally significant. The concept of energy provided a comprehensive framework for understanding nourishment. It helped carve out a distinction between energy and non-energy nutrients; it established a systematic relationship between the macronutrients; and it provided a practical connection between diet and health.

The Problem with Energy-Thinking in Current Nutritional Practice

Unlike their scientific counterparts in the late 19th century, present-day nutritional researchers have been faced with an increasing variety of research findings that have been difficult to account for within the context of energy-thinking. Proteins, carbohydrates and fats have been easily classified as energy nutrients. Even vitamins and minerals have been readily incorporated into an energy-based paradigm, since they frequently play a role as enzymatic co-factors in the energy-based metabolism of food. But for an increasing number of nutrients, including carotenoids, flavonoids, short-chain fatty acids, oligosaccharides, and organic acids, energy-thinking seems to have become less and less capable of providing a comprehensive context for understanding the dynamics of nourishment.

Nowhere has this mismatch between energy-thinking and nutrition become more apparent than in the area of food toxicity. As described in detail in Chapter 4, over one hundred potential toxins in drinking water are currently being monitored by the U.S. Environmental Protection Agency. As of 1992, 73 pesticides authorized for agricultural use had been classified as potential carcinogens by the EPA.[78] Over 150 chemical residues in poultry and meat are now the subject of routine analysis by the Food

Safety and Inspection Service (FSIS) of the U.S. Department of Agriculture. In spite of these developments, however, the field of nutrition has been unable to cohesively address the issue of food toxins, or to incorporate toxic assessment into its everyday practice.

The Example of Dioxins

On July 8, 1997, for the first time in U.S. history, the U.S. Food and Drug Administration set a dioxin food standard. Dioxins are chlorine-containing, highly toxic, Class 1 carcinogens produced during the manufacture of herbicides, the bleaching of paper, and the burning of chlorine-containing organic materials. (A more lengthy and technical review of dioxins appears in Chapter 3, page 107, under "Dioxin.") The setting of this first-time, non-legally binding standard came in conjunction with the banning of commercial chicken shipments from hundreds of chicken producers, mainly in the state of Arkansas.

What had happened to create dioxin contamination of chicken products was simple. Near Sledge, Mississippi, at the end of a gravel road, there existed an open-pit bentonite clay mine. (Bentonite clay pits have long been favorite illegal dumping sites for toxins, since bentonite clay can chelate toxins and help prevent their detection by smell.) A local Mississippi manufacturing plant had illegally dumped toxic waste, including dioxins, into the bentonite clay pit. The bentonite clay (called "ball clay") had been sold to two chicken feed manufacturers in Arkansas for incorporation into chicken feed. The bentonite was being added to the feed to prevent clumping and improve flow through feeding troughs. Soon after ingesting the dioxin-tainted feed, chickens (and the eggs they produced) became contaminated with dioxin. Consumers ingesting the chicken and eggs were in turn affected with dioxin poisoning.

Present-day nutritional software programs cannot measure the dioxin content of food. (Prior to the summer of 1997, they could not have determined dioxin excess even if they had wanted to, since no standards had been set for safe levels of dioxins in food). The list of everyday food components that cannot be measured by current software systems is a ever-expanding list that is by no means limited to dioxin. Nutrition analysis programs cannot measure any of the 100 potential toxins found in drinking water, or the 150 chemical residues found in meat and poultry, or the 73 carcinogenic pesticides found in a variety of other foods. In addition, they are unable to measure any of the 300+ carotenoids or 4000+ flavonoids that are presently known to exist in food.

The inability of software programs to measure any of the nutritionally-related compounds described above is evidence of the increasing mismatch between energy-thinking and nutrition. Nutritional software programs haven't been set up to measure flavonoids, carotenoids, or toxins contain in food because nutritionists have been accustomed to thinking about diet in terms of energy. Flavonoids, carotenoids, and dioxins haven't lent themselves to energy-thinking.

Incorporation of phytonutrient and toxicity research into the field of nutrition requires an alternative conceptual framework that is capable of providing a more comprehensive context for understanding the dynamics of nourishment. In the final section of this chapter, we consider one alternative conceptual framework for evaluating research on phytonutrients and toxicity. This framework is based not on the concept of energy, but on the concept of information.

P A R T   I V

The Return of Environmental Standards Through Information-Based Thinking

Over the past 100 years, scientists have been continually re-interpreting biological events as events involving exchange of information. At the center of this information-based revolution in biology has been the field of genetics. Information has become the model for understanding DNA and the genetic code. The advent of genetic assessment, genetic counseling, genetic therapy, and cloning has added a controversial sociocultural dimension to the information paradigm. The concept of information has had a significant impact, however, on areas of science well outside of the genetic arena.

The Concept of Information in Western Science

In his book *Grammatical Man*, author Jeremy Campbell has likened the 20th century concept of information to the 19th century concept of energy. Just as energy-based thinking in the late 19th century culminated in the invention of the steam engine and spawned the industrial revolution, so has information-based thinking in the 20th century culminated in the invention of the computer and spawned the age of cyberspace.[79] The concept of information has led to the establishment of new fields of science, including cybernetics and informatics, and new sets of rules have been established for understanding information and its dynamics.

Information as an Interactive Concept

Information is typically defined as "knowledge communicated or received."[80] Implicit in this definition is an interaction between two parties. One of the parties is regarded as the sender of the information, and the other party is regarded as the receiver. Information systems always involve transmission of knowledge between parties. By its very definition, information is characterized as an interactive process that involves give and take between sender and receiver.

Equally important for nutrition and the body sciences as a whole is the nature of knowledge transferred from sender to receiver. This knowledge must always be understandable to both parties, and must be encoded in such a way as to make sense to both sender and receiver. If for example, components of edible plants are conceptualized as informational entities, then the botanical environment that "sent" them must share a biochemical common ground with the human body that "received them."

Information as a Unifying Concept

Equally important in information theory is the ability of any signal to be encoded and transferred between a sender and a receiver. Modern systems for information processing and transmission have turned more and more toward a digital framework for accomplishing this encoding process.

In digital information transfer, the key unit of information is referred to as a "bit," or binary digit. Binary digits are part of the binary number system. This system contains only two digits: 0 and 1. In digital information transfer, all information is translated into binary code.

Consider, for example, how the compass directions of north, east, south and west, could be encoded as digital information using only the digits "0" and "1." Provided that a sender and receiver knew that compass directions were the focus of the information transfer, a system could be set up in which a series of logical questions were answered with the digits 0 and 1. For example, a question could be asked, "Is the compass direction north or south?" A "0" code could mean "the compass direction is north," and a "1" code could mean "the compass direction is not north." Once a "1" digit were encoded, the receiver would know that the compass direction was not north. However, the receiver would not know which of the other compass directions were being referred to.

This shortcoming of the encoding process could be overcome by using two digits instead of one digit to describe the compass directions. For example, "00" could be used to designate "north," "01" for south, "10" for east, and "11" for west. Through this system, four discrete possibilities could be identified to the receiver with the use of only two digits, 0 and 1.

Digital information transfer uses this exact same logic to encode any type of message being sent from a sender to a receiver. The message could be a word, or a picture, or a sound. The more complicated the differentiation being made to the receiver, the more binary digits required to encode the message. For example, a five-digit code would be required to differentiate all the letters of the English alphabet, since a total of 26 possible letters would require 25 (or 2 x 2 x 2 x 2 x 2 = 32) binary digits. Encoding of music on a compact digital disc typically requires this same number of binary digits, and involves the transfer of 1,411,200 bits per second between the compact disc and the disc player that reads it.

At the same time as digital information transfer appears to divide knowledge up into discrete bits, it can also serve as a unifying principle insofar as it brings together all diverse types of experience into a single practical framework. Hearing, seeing, and speaking are not the only life events that can be viewed as congruous within the context of information theory. As explored in detail in Chapter 5, genetic transmission, intercellular communication, and cell cycles can also be brought together into a conceptually integrated framework through the application of information-related concepts.

Qualitative Aspects of Information

Unlike the concept of energy, which brings along with it a primarily quantitative orientation toward events, the concept of information involves qualitative as well as quantitative aspects. The quantitative aspect of information was illustrated in the previous paragraphs through the example of 1,411,200 binary digits being sent out every second between a compact disc and a compact disc player. The qualitative aspect of this information lies in these exact same 1,411,200 binary digits, but in the case of quality, the emphasis is not on the vast number of 0s and 1s, but on the unique pattern of 0s and 1s that represents a unique wavelength carrying a unique musical message. In digital information transfer, encodings are highly specific. A 32-bit encoding, for example, specifies one unique set of circumstances among 232 or 131,072 possible circumstances. A 64-bit encoding would specify one unique situation among 264 or 562,949,953,400,000 circumstances.

The interactive, unifying, and qualitative aspects of information make it a strong candidate for returning a set of environmental standards to the field of nutrition. They also make information-thinking a possible alternative framework for understanding the dynamics of nourishment in a way that goes beyond the concept of energy and energy dynamics.

The Application of Information-Thinking to Nutrition

The interactive, unifying, and qualitative aspects of information make it a particularly valuable concept for nutritional practice. This value comes in the non-discriminating character of information. In the same way that any sight, sound, or word can be digitally encoded, any food component can be examined for encoded message content. While 4000+ flavonoids presently known to exist in food have not lent themselves to an energy-based analysis, they have already received substantial research attention as molecules involved in cellular communication. (The communication-based role of one flavonoid family, called isoflavones, is reviewed later in this chapter).

Equally accessible to nutrition from an information-based perspective are the toxins found in drinking water and chemical residues found in animal products. Where an analysis of food as fuel has left little room for consideration of these food toxins, their impact on cellular communication and information-based processes in the body has already been well-established in medical research.

In summary, information-thinking has the potential to establish an understanding of food that no longer excludes flavonoids, carotenoids, and toxins because of their non-fuel role in nourishment.

Information-Thinking About Non-Toxic Aspects of Food

In the preceding section, we review the tendency of nutrition to view macronutrients as the energy-containing parts of food. We describe how carbohydrates, fats, and to a lesser degree proteins are valued for their caloric contribution to the diet, and how each of these three types of macronutrients could be looked upon as homogenous in light of their caloric contribution to the diet. Each of these observations is based on energy-thinking about diet.

If we replace energy-thinking with information-thinking, the role of these macronutrients looks different. If macronutrients are treated like units of information, they must also be regarded as transmitting messages from a sender to a receiver. Equally important, each message sent must be regarded as unique. To better understand the transition from energy-thinking to information-thinking, we will look closer at one type of macronutrient (carbohydrate) from an information-based perspective.

Carbohydrate

Energy-thinking about carbohydrate has taught us to look at this macro-nutrient as the body's main source of anaerobic energy, the primary substrate for glycolysis, and the overwhelming choice for caloric energy in diets worldwide. Thanks to the field of glycobiology, however, we have already witnessed a change in perspective about carbohydrate that can be classified as a shift from energy-based to information-based thinking. Carbohydrate has increasingly been recognized as a key player in cellular communication. Research has shown that cells cannot talk to each other, or at least not coherently, without the right glycoproteins attached to their surface.[81] (The "glyco" part of "glycoprotein" is the carbohydrate portion of the molecule, and it makes a unique contribution to the molecule's function.) Recognition of carbohydrates and their role in communication has also paved the way in immunology for recognition of Type I hypersensitivity reactions in which glycoproteins bind to Fc receptors on mast cells and trigger degranulation. (This topic is reviewed in more detail in Chapter 5, page 206, under "Mast Cell Degranulation").

One subset of glycoproteins, called lectins, are found in virtually all foods. These low molecular weight compounds have also been found capable of triggering mast cell degranulation, and may be the basis for urticaria (hive-like) reactions associated with intake of foods like strawberries that have high glycoprotein content.[82] Considered as a whole, all of the above observations establish a role for carbohydrate that goes far beyond its activity as a dietary fuel. In addition to providing a substrate for glycolysis, or a primary source of anaerobic energy, carbohydrate is also designed to promote intercellular communication.

Phytoestrogens

Phytoestrogens provide a second well-researched example of information-thinking in nutrition. Many foods, including soybeans, contain diphenolic compounds called isoflavones. Blood levels of isoflavones (including genistein and daidzein) have been found to be 100 to 1,000 times higher in Asian versus U.S. populations.[83] When isoflavones from soybeans are modified by intestinal bacteria and taken up into the blood, they can bind (weakly) onto the body's estrogen receptors.[84] The body recognizes this binding of its estrogen receptors as a signal to produce less of its own estrogen. Because of their ability to bind estrogen receptors and trigger feedback mechanisms that alter endogenous (originating inside the body) estrogen production, isoflavones like genistein and daidzein are often referred to as phytoestrogens. (The prefix "phyto" points back to the Greek word *phyton*, meaning "plant").

Estrogen receptor status is recognized as an important factor in the development of breast cancer,[85] and a factor of potential importance in autoimmune disease.[86] Among women diagnosed with breast cancer, Caucasian women have been determined to have a much higher percentage of five-year survival rates than African-American women, and at the same time, to have significantly lower levels of estrogens, including estrone, estradiol, free estradiol, and androstenedione.[87]

These observations have suggested a definite role for isoflavone-containing foods in breast cancer prevention. But they have also underscored the value of information-thinking in nutrition. From this cancer-prevention perspective, phytoestrogens in soy foods cannot be described as providing fuel. They can only be described as participants in an information-based process in which a component of food sends a signal to our cells that instructs the cells to decrease their production of estrogen.

Information-Thinking About Toxic Aspects of Food

As introduced earlier in this chapter, toxins have become routine components of the U.S. food supply. (Chapter 4 provides a detailed review of food toxins within seven basic food groups). Like flavonoids and carotenoids, toxins have not lent themselves to nutritional analysis from a food-as-fuel perspective. From the standpoint of information, however, toxins have been well-researched for the harmful effects upon cell communication and transmembrane signaling. In this section we will look at the information-disrupting effect of one specific member of the toxic heavy metals (mercury), and also at the disruptive effects of a larger group of food contaminants, namely, pesticides.

Mercury

Mercury-containing substances (called organomercuric compounds), are widely distributed in the U.S. food supply. Factors that contribute to mercury in food include the direct use of mercury in agriculture (approximately 400 metric tons per year); the coating of seed stocks with mercury to prevent growth of molds and fungi; the atmospheric release of mercury from coal burning, petrochemical production, and mercury vapor lights; the discarding of mercury-containing batteries, electrical equipment, and anti-mildew paints and caulks into landfills; and the industrial discharge of mercury into freshwater and seawater. (Even when this discharge involves inorganic mercury, microorganisms in the water convert this elemental mercury into organic compounds that are readily absorbed into the body.)

Intake of tuna contaminated with mercury provides a first example of cellular signaling and its disruption. A 1991 FDA analysis of 220 cans of tuna has shown an average of 170ppb (parts per billion) mercury in tuna, with levels as high as 750ppb.[88] From an information standpoint, when this tuna is eaten a multitude of signals are sent to the body. These signals include messages carried by proteins and vitamin B-6, both of which are plentiful in tuna. Also included is a mercury message. After 24 hours of exposure to methylmercuric chloride, apoptosis (genetically programmed cell death) occurs in 67% of human T cells when examined in the lab at specific serum concentrations. The presence of mercury by itself does not appear sufficient to throw T cells into programmed death. Other metabolic conditions must be present. But when they are, the mercury compounds signal the T cells to induce apoptotic genes.[89]

Low concentrations of mercuric chloride and methylmercury also send signals to brain astrocytes. (Astrocytes are brain cells that establish communication between the blood vessels and the nerves.) The presence of mercury tells astrocytes to alter their transmembrane ion gradients.[90] (Alteration of activity across the cells membranes of astrocytes has been associated with neurotoxicity and the development of neurological conditions like dementia).[91]

Pesticides

Pesticides provide a second example of toxic signaling to the body. A 1996 study by the Environmental Working Group examined supplies of drinking water in 748 U.S. towns. 96% of all samples contained the pesticide atrazine, and in 24 of the towns, risk of cancer related to atrazine exposure was 15 times higher than limits established under the Food Quality Protection Act of 1996.[92] At least 20 different pesticide residues, including organochlorine and organophosphate residues, have repeatedly been found in drinking waters throughout the U.S.[93]

When tap water is consumed, a variety of messages are sent to the body. Stimulation of the oropharynx by water tells the hypothalamus to stop secreting arginine vasopressin.[94] Hydration of the postgastric mucosa sends this same message.[95] When the water being consumed is water from municipal tap water in the U.S., pesticide messages are also sent. Pentachlorophenol and lindane tell the liver to synthesize more P450 CYP3A enzymes.[96] (This upregulation can increase the risk of oxidative stress, as discussed in detail in Chapter 5). Dieldrin tells nerve cells in the dorsal root ganglia to potentiate, and then switch off, GABAA receptor-chloride channels.[97] (This ultimate inhibition of GABA neurotransmitter activity, also discussed in Chapter 5, can increase the risk of oxidative stress through excessive elevation of glutamate:GABA ratios). Dioxins and pesticides also tell liver and brain cells to switch on protein kinase C enzymes.[98] (Overactivation of these enzymes, also addressed in Chapter 5, has been associated with increase risk of cancer).

Summary: A Paradigm Shift

The transition from energy-thinking to information-thinking represents a paradigm shift in the sciences. As in any paradigm shift, it is the piling up of anomalous observations (observations that don't seem to fit with the current framework for understanding) that initiates the process of change. It is precisely this piling up of anomalous observations that continues to occur in the field of nutrition, where the number of research studies on non-recognized nutrients like flavonoids has begun to exceed the number of studies on recognized nutrients like zinc or protein. The prevalence of toxins in the U.S. food supply has also become a factor in the initiation of change. Intake of common foods traditionally regarded as "healthy" by healthcare professionals has increasingly shown up as illness-producing in nutritional research, and toxic contamination has repeatedly been identified as the cause. These unexpected events have suggested the need for a new conceptual framework that can address food toxins and flavonoids as well as zinc and protein. Information-thinking about food is the emerging framework that harbors this potential.

---

1. American Dietetic Association. (1997). The American Dietetic Association (ADA) 1997 Nutrition Trends Survey. American Dietetic Association, Chicago, Illinois.

2. Advertising Age. (1998). Ad age marketplace. Total measured U.S. ad spending by category and media in 1997. Advertising Age, September 28. (Website location: http://www.adage.com/dataplace/archives).

3. *Ibid.*

4. *Ibid.*

5. American Dietetic Association. (1997). The American Dietetic Association 1997 Nutrition Trends Survey: key findings. American Dietetic Association, Chicago Illinois. (Website location: http://www.eatright.org/press090397d.html).

6. The Hartman Group. (1997). The Hartman report. Food and the environment: a consumer's perspective. Phase II. The Hartman Group, Bellevue, Washington, p.53.

7. *Ibid*, p.52.

8. American Dietetic Association, *op. cit. (see reference 1).*

9. Hall T. (1992). Johnny and Susie can't cook? Food experts see a growing trend. Journal American, January 22.

10. Pimentel D. (1994). Food, land, population and the U.S. economy. Carrying Capacity Network, Washington ,D.C., p.6.

11. *Ibid*.

12. Saporito B. (1994). Home cooking is off the boil. Fortune 129(6):15.

13. Beiulinsky M. (1992). Cooking in America: a waning art. Food and Nutr News 64(3):19–20.

14. *Ibid*, p. 15.

15. Conn C and Silverman I. (Eds). (1991). What counts: the complete Harper's index. Henry Holt and Company, New York, p. 140.

16. Pimentel D, *op. cit. (see reference 6)*, p. 7.

17. *Ibid*, p.30–31.

18. U.S. Bureau of the Census. (1998). Statistical abstract of the United States: 1998. 118th Edition. Washington, D.C., p.839.

19. *Ibid.*, p.839.

20. Farb P and Armelagos G. (1980). Consuming passions: the anthropology of eating. Wash-ington Square Press, New York, p. 118.

21. Kaptchuk TJ. (1983). The web that has no weaver. Understanding Chinese medicine. Congdon & Weed, New York, p.120.

22. Pitchford P. (1993). Healing with whole foods. Oriental traditions and modern nutrition. North Atlantic Books, Berkeley, California, p.288–289.

23. Donden Y. (1986). Hopkins J (Ed). Rabgay L (Transl). Health through balance: an introduction to Tibetan medicine. Snow Lion Publications, Ithaca, NY.

24. Begon M, Harper JL, and Townsend CR. (1996). Ecology. Third edition. Blackwell Science, Oxford, p. 914.

25. Fowler C and Mooney P. (1990). Shattering. Food, politics, and the loss of genetic diversity. The University of Arizona Press, Tucson, p. 63.

26. Fowler C and Mooney P. (1990). Shattering: food politics, and the loss of genetic diversity. The University of Arizona Press, Tucson, pp.54–89.

27. Franks F, Mathias SF, and Hatley RHM. (1990). Water, temperature and life. Phil Transact Royal Soc Series B 326: 517–533.

28. Begon M, Harper JL, and Townsend CR, *op. cit. (see reference 24)*, p.55.

29. Bronson FH. (1985). Mammalian reproduction: an ecological perspective. Biol Reprod 32:1–26.

30. Hansen WP, Otterby DE, Linn JG et al. (1991). Influence of forage type, ratio of forage to concentrate, and methionine hydroxy analog on performance of dairy cows. J Dairy Sci 74(4):1361–1369.

31. Koelkebeck KW, Parsons CM, Leeper RW et al. (1991). Effect of protein and methionine levels in molt diets on postmolt performance of laying hens. Poult Sci 70(10):2063–2073.

32. Raloff J. (1996). Eyes possess their own biological clocks. Sci News 149:245.

33. Tamarkin L, Baird CJ, and Almeida OFX. (1985). Melatonin: a coordinating signal for mammalian reproduction? Science 227:714–720.

34. Ding JM, Chen D, Weber ET et al. (1994). Resetting the biological clock: mediation of nocturnal circadian shifts by glutamate and NO. Science 266:1713–1717.

35. Tamarkin L, Baird CJ, and Almeida OFX, *op. cit. (see reference 33).*

36. Roush W. (1995). Chronobiology. Can ìresettingî hormonal rhythms treat illness? Science 269:1220–1221.

37. Peters FE. (1967). Greek philosophical terms. A historical lexicon. New York University Press, New York, p.84.

38. Walter S. (1999, forthcoming). Encyclopedia of Body Mind Disciplines. Rosen Publishing Group, New York. Reprinted on the AHHA Internet website location: http://www.healthy.net/ahha.

39. Bennekon G and Schroll H. (1988). Nitrogen budget for a dairy farm. Ecol Bulletins 39:134–135.

40. *Ibid.*

41. *Ibid.*

42. Fuller RB. Synergetics: Explorations in the Geometry of Thinking. New York, N.Y.: Macmillan Publishing; 1975;58.

43. Pennington JAT. (1994). Bowes and Church's food values of portions commonly used. 16th Edition. J.B. Lippincott, Philadelphia, p. 296.

44. Worthington V. (1998). Effect of agricultural methods on nutritional quality: a comparison of organic with conventional crops. Alt Ther 4(1):58–69.

45. Smith JL. (1994). Atwater to present: what have we learned about our food supply? J Nutr 124(suppl):1780S–1782S.

46. Southgate DAT and Greenfield H. (1992). Principles for the preparation of nutritional data bases and food composition tables. Wrld Rev Nutr Diet 68:27–48.

47. Hurt HD. (1989). Nutrient databanks: the role of the food industry. In: Stumbo PJ. (Ed). Proceedings of the fourteenth national nutrient databank conference. 1989 June 19–21. Iowa City, Iowa. The CBORD Group Inc., pp.11–15.

48. Bengmark S. (1998). Ecoimmunonutrition: a challenge for the third millennium. Nutr: Internatl J Appl Basic Nutr Sci 14(7/8):566.

49. *Ibid.*

50. Simopoulos A. (1991). Omega-3 fatty acids in health and disease and in growth and development. Am J Clin Nutr 54:438–463.

51. Makrides M, Neumann M, Simmer K et al. (1995). Are long-chain polyunsaturated fatty acids essential in infancy? Lancet 345:1463–1468.

52. Stevens L. (1995). Essential fatty acid metabolism in boys with attention-deficit hyperactivity disorder. Am J Clin Nutr 62:761–768.

53. Simopoulos A, *op. cit. (see reference 50).*

54. Shahar E, Folsom AR, Melnick S et al. (1994). Dietary n-3 polyunsaturated fatty acids and smoking-related chronic obstructive pulmonary disease. New Engl J Med 331:228–233.

55. Human Nutrition Information Service. (1992). USDA's Food Guide Pyramid. United States Department of Agriculture. Home Garden Bulletin 249. U.S. Government Printing Office, Washington. D.C.

56. American Dietetic Association, *op. cit. (see reference 15).*

57. American Dietetic Association. (1998). Position of the American Dietetic Association: fat replacers. JADA 98(4):463–468.

58. *Ibid*, p.464.

59. National Center for Health Statistics. (1996). Energy and macronutrient intakes of persons ages 2 months and over in the United States: Third National Health and Nutrition Examination Survey, Phase 1, 1988–1991. Available through the Centers for Disease Control Internet website at: http://www.cdc.gov/nchs/products/pubs/pubd/ad/260–251/ad255.htm.

60. American Dietetic Association. (1999). Nutrition fact sheets. ABCs of fats, oils, and cholesterol. (nfs2) and Fats and Oils in the Diet: The Great Debate (nfs82). Available at the Internet website http://www.eatright.org.

61. Bodwell CE and Erdman JW. (Eds). (1988). Nutrient interactions. Marcel Dekker, New York.

62. Bors W, Michel C and Schikora S. (1995). Interaction of flavonoids with ascorbate and determination of their univalent redox potentials: a pulse radiolysis study. Free Rad Biol Med 19(1):45–52.

63. Standing Committee on the Scientific Evaluation of Dietary Reference Intakes and Its Panel on Dietary Antioxidants and Related Compounds. (1988). Dietary reference intakes: proposed definition and plan for review of dietary antioxidants and related compounds. A report by the 63 Standing Committee on the Scientific Evaluation of Dietary Reference Intakes and Its Panel on Dietary Antioxidants and Related Compounds. Food and Nutrition Board, Institute of Medicine. National Academy Press, Washington, D.C., p.8.

64. Middleton E Jr. And Kandaswami C. (1993). The impact of plant flavonoids on mammalian biology: implications for immunity, inflammation and cancer. Chapter 15. In: Harborne JB. (Ed). The flavonoids: advances in research since 1986. Chapman and Hall, London., pp.619–620.

65. Emerich M. (1995). 1994:22.7% growth! Natural Foods Merchandiser XVI(6)1:62–73.

66. Pimentel D, *op. cit. (see reference 6)*, p.20.

67. *Ibid.*

68. Powledge F. (1984). Fat of the land. Simon and Schuster, New York, p.40.

69. *Ibid.*

70. Connor JM, Rogers RT, Marion BW et al. (1985). The food manufacturing industries. Lexington Books, DC Heath and Company, Lexington, Massachussetts.

71. Moore DM. (Ed). Green planet: the story of plant life on earth. Cambridge University press, Cambridge.

72. Begon M, Harper JL, and Townsend CR. (1996). *Op. cit.*,p. 3.

73. Hewitt PG. (1977). Conceptual physics. Third edition. Chapter 4: Energy. Little, Brown and Company, Boston, p.51.

74. Campbell, J. (1982). Grammatical man. Touchstone Books, Simon & Schuster, New York.

75. Todhunter EN. (1984). Historical landmarks in nutrition. Chapter 58. In: Olson RE. (Editorial Committee Chairman). Present knowledge in nutrition. Fifth edition. The Nutrition Foundation, Washington, D.C., p.871.

76. *Ibid*, p.876.

77. Atwater WO and Snell JF. (1903). Description of a bomb calorimeter and method of its use. J Am Chem Soc 25:659–699.

78. United States Environmental Protection Agency. (1992). Environmental Protection Agency list of food use pesticides evaluated for carcinogenicity. Chem Regul Reporter, EPA, Washington, D.C., Aug 28.

79. Campbell J, *op. cit. (see reference 75)*.

80. Urdang L. (Ed) (1968). The Random House dictionary of the English language. College Edition. Random House, New York, p. 684.

81. Sharon N and Lis H. (1993). Carbohydrates in cell recognition. Scient Amer 268(1): 82–90.

82. Roitt I, Brostoff J, and Male D. (1985). Immunology. C.V. Mosby, St. Louis, 19.8–19.9.

83. Adlercreutz H, Honjo H, Higashi A et al. (1991). Urinary excretion of lignans and isoflavonoid phytoestrogens in Japanese men and women consuming a traditional Japanese diet. Am J Clin Nutr 54:1093–1100.

84. Miksicek RJ. (1995). Oestrogenic flavonoids: structural requirements for biological activity. Proc Soc Exp Biol Med 208:44–50.

85. Harlan LC, Coates RJ, Block G et al. (1993). Estrogen receptor status and dietary intakes in breast cancer patients. Epidemiol 4:25–31.

86. Cutolo M, Sulli A, Seriolo B et al. (1995). Estrogens, the immune response and auto-immunity. Clin Exper Rheumat 13:217–226.

87. Woods MN, Barnett JB, Spiegelman D, et al. (1996). Hormone levels during dietary changes in premenopausal African-American women. J Natl Canc Inst 88:1369–1374.

88. Yess NJ. (1993). U.S. Food and Drug Administration survey of methyl mercury in canned tuna. J AOAC Int 76(1):36–38.

89. Shenker BJ, Datar S, Mansfield K et al. (1997). Induction of apoptosis in human T-cells by organomercuric compounds: a flow cytometric analysis. Toxicol Appl Pharmacol 143(2):397–406.

90. Aschner M, Rising L, and Mullaney KJ. (1996). Differential sensitivity of neonatal rat astrocyte cultures to mercuric chloride (MC) and methylmercury (MeHg): studies on K+ and amino acid transport and metallothionein (MT) induction. Neurotoxicol 17:107–116.

91. Aschner M. (1996). Methylmercury in astrocytes—what possible significance? Neurotoxicol 17:93–106.

92. Environmental Working Group. (1996). Executive summary. Tough to swallow. Washington, D.C.

93. Rea WJ. (1996). Pesticides. J Nutr Environ Med 6:55–124.

94. Figaro MK and Mack GW. (1997). Regulation of fluid intake in dehydrated humans: role of oropharyngeal stimulation. Am J Physiol 272(6 Pt. 2):R1740–1746.

95. Davis JD and Sayler JL. (1997). Confining ingested fluid to the stomach increases water and decreases saline intake in the rat. Physiol Behav 61(1):127–130.

96. Dubois M, Plaisance H, Thome JP et al. (1996). Hierarchical cluster analysis of environmental pollutants through P450 induction in cultured hepatic cells. Ecotoxicol Environ Saf 34(3):205–215.

97. Narahashi T, Carter DB, Frey J et al. (1995). Sodium channels and GABAA receptor-channel complex as targets of environmental toxicants. Toxicol Lett 82–83:239–245.

98. Bagchi D, Bagchi M, Tang L et al. (1997). Comparative in vitro and in vivo protein kinase C activation by selected pesticides and transition metal salts. Toxicol Lett 91(1):31–37.

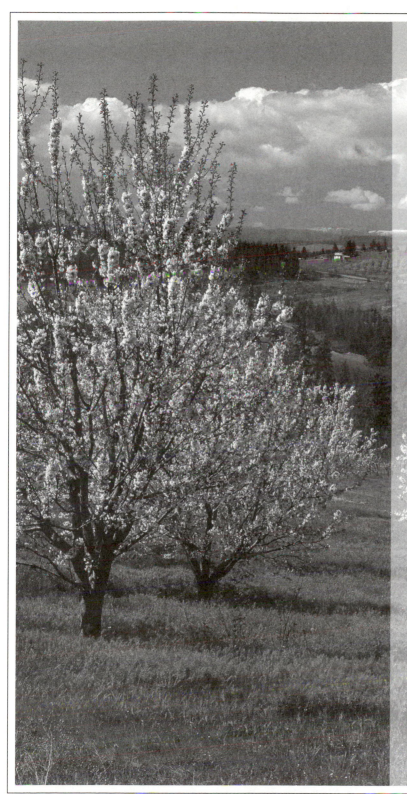

2 CHAPTER

The Impact of Non-Environmental Standards on Nutritional Practice

PART I
Measuring the Impact on Nutritional Policies and Procedures

PART II
Measuring the Impact in a Sample Diet

CONTENTS

Chapter 2: **The Impact of Non-Environmental Standards on Nutrition Practice**

The Impact of Non-Environmental Standards on Nutritional Practice

PART I

Measuring the Impact on Nutritional Policies and Procedures

The non-environmental nature of current standards in nutrition has had a measurable impact on every aspect of the field. This chapter examines the nature of that impact in two general areas of nutritional practice. The first area involves development of nutritional policies and procedures, and includes a review of Dietary Reference Intakes (DRIs). The second area involves assessment of dietary intake through computer analysis of a 24-hour diet diary. In both areas, the impact of non-environmental standards on nutritional practice will be evaluated for clinical relevance and potential effects on everyday nourishment.

Narrowed Nutrient Selection

Textbooks of nutrition typically define the term "nutrient" as any substance obtained from food and used in the body to promote essential life processes including growth, maintenance, or repair.[1] If the criteria established by this definition were used to evaluate the current status of nutrients in the field of nutrition, the actual number of nutrients would be staggering. The number of unique biochemical substances found in the body and in food extends well into the tens of thousands. Within the human genome, for example, are found approximately 100,000 genes. Approximately 80–90% of these genes have been estimated to be "non-coding." (Non-coding refers to the lack of a specific protein being synthesized in the cell as a result of gene expression). All cells in the body possess a full set of all 100,00 genes. As a result, since 20% of those genes have the potential to be expressed into unique proteins, each of the body's 100 trillion cells has the theoretical potential to produce approximately 20,000 unique proteins. Additionally, because each one of these proteins has the potential to act as an enzyme and facilitate the conversion of one substance (the "substrate") into another (the "product"), each cell has the potential not only to create 20,000 different proteins, but to take 20,000 unique, additional substances (substrates) and convert them into 20,000 new substances (products).

A single food like garlic (*Allium sativum*) can be equally complex in terms of its chemistry. Several hundred potentially nutritive components have already been identified in garlic's chemical composition. These components have included cysteine sulfoxides, alk(en)yl-cysteins, glutamylpeptides, thiosulfinates, ajoenes, dulfides, vinylithiins, amino acids, proteins, fatty acids, lipids, steroids, steroidal glycosides, saccharides, vitamins, minerals, organic acids, glycoproteins, and lectins.[2] Many of the most active constituents of plants cannot be placed within the simple categories of proteins, carbohydrates, fats, vitamins and minerals. These components include alkaloids, carotenoids, coumarins, flavonoids, glycosides, iridoids, mucilages, polyphenolic acids, quinones, resins, saponins, and terpenes.

When foods are considered as a group, their chemical diversity is even more far-reaching. For example, over 4,000 chemically unique flavonoids (the color-giving pigments of most plants) have already been identified in the laboratory.[3] Similarly, over 600 different carotenoids (another category of plant pigment) have been previously identified.[4] In their two-volume textbook entitled *Food Phytochemicals for Cancer Prevention*, editors Huang and Osawa addressed more than 1,000 unique compounds in food with documented health-related activity.[5]

DRIs

Against this backdrop of thousands of nutritive substances contained in food has been a focus on fewer than 35 nutrients by the National Academy of Sciences in its establishment of nutrient guidelines for the general public. In

1989, the Food and Nutrition Board (FNB) of the National Research Council (NRC) of the National Academy of Sciences (NAS) released its tenth and final version of the Recommended Dietary Allowances (RDAs).[6] These nutrient guidelines for the general public, adopted by most public health organizations in the U.S. including the American Dietetic Association, provided information on 7 minerals (calcium, iodine, iron, magnesium, phosphorus, selenium, and zinc) and 11 vitamins (B-1, B-2, B-3, B-6, B-12, folate, A, C, D, E, K). A supplemental list of nutrient guidelines, referred to as the Estimated Safe and Adequate Daily Dietary Intake (ESADDI) guidelines, provided additional information about 2 vitamins (biotin and pantothenate) and 5 minerals (chromium, copper, fluoride, manganese, and molybdenum).[7]

In 1995, the NAS undertook reorganization of the RDA guidelines.[8] Jurisdiction over guideline development was transferred from the National Research Council to the Institute of Medicine (IOM), and a committee on Dietary Reference Intakes (DRIs) was set up to begin consideration of new standards. In August 1997 the DRI committee released its first set of new guidelines for 5 nutrients (calcium, phosphorus, magnesium, fluoride, and vitamin D). In the spring of 1998, an additional 9 nutrient guidelines were released for the family of B-complex vitamins including B-1, B-2, B-3, B-6, B-12, pantothenate, folate, biotin, and choline. The IOM has planned release of additional guidelines for approximately 10 additional DRI nutrients, including vitamins C and E; the minerals chlorine, iron, potassium; selenium, sodium, and zinc; fiber; and phytoestrogens. Cumulatively, these additional guidelines will create a total of 24 DRI nutrients.

Included and Excluded Nutrients

Historically, the NAS has followed two basic strategies in its nutrient selection process. The first strategy has been elimination from the selection process of all nutrients that lack clearly-established age-specific and gender-specific requirements.[9] The second strategy has involved the refusal to issue guidelines for known nutrients if the available nutrient data has been judged to be "provocative and promising…yet not solid enough to serve as the basis for setting recommendations."[10] When combined, these two standards have been largely responsible for the narrowing of selection to approximately two dozen nutrients from a known nutrient pool of several thousand health-related food molecules and compounds. The NAS has itself acknowledged the omission of essential nutrients from its recommendation list.[11]

The Examples of Molybdenum and Boron. Treatment of the minerals molybdenum (a DRI nutrient) and boron (a nutrient excluded from the

DRIs) illustrates the narrowing of the nutrient selection process as followed by the NAS. While the exact roles of boron in human health has remained uncertain, the number of indexed journal studies on boron (n=608) during the past thirty years has closely paralleled the number of indexed journal studies on molybdenum (n=625).[12] In addition, these journal studies have verified metabolic functions for both nutrients. Boron has repeatedly been shown to be a natural constituent of body tissue and to alleviate effects of vitamin D deficiency,[13] particularly when other minerals like copper or magnesium are minimally present.[14] Boron has also repeatedly been shown to inhibit the activity of oxidoreductase enzymes that require pyridine or flavin nucleotide cofactors,[15] and to be a biochemical acceptor of hydroxyl ions by acting as a Lewis acid.[16] These metabolic functions of boron can be viewed as parallel to metabolic functions of molybdenum, which has been determined to act as a cofactor in dehydrogenase and oxidase reactions. The only difference in our research-based understanding of these minerals appears to involve identification of a cofactor form for molybdenum (molybopterin), with no such cofactor form yet identified for boron.[17]

Despite the research-based similarity between boron and molybdenum, NAS treatment of the two minerals has been dramatically different. Molybdenum was adopted in 1989 as a recommended essential nutrient with a 75–250 microgram Estimated Safe and Adequate Daily Dietary Allowance (ESADDI).[18] Ten years later, boron has yet to receive any official NAS recognition. Exclusion of minerals like boron from DRI status can reduce the efficacy and scope of dietary recommendations by ignoring known beneficial effects of metabolically active nutrients.

The Clinical Relevance of Narrowed Selection

Since 1995, the volume of research on officially-recognized nutrients has begun to drop below the number of studies on non-recognized nutritive substances. For example, studies on the tripeptide glutathione (n=12,408) have exceeded studies on iron (n=11,155), zinc (n=8,992), or vitamin C (n=3,084) in number.[19] Studies on non-essential amino acids like serine (n=16,881) have surpassed the number of studies on essential amino acids like cysteine (n=12,846), and investigations of non-essential fatty acids like butyric acid (n=1,072) have exceeded the number of studies on essential fatty acids like linolenic acid (n=374).[20] Since 1995, the same number of studies have been conducted on the officially unrecognized nutrient glutamine (n=4,553) as on vitamins B-6, B-12, and folate combined (n=4,622).[21] Inattention to this groundswell of research on unrecognized nutritive components of food has also had clinical consequences, since

Bleached, Refined Flour and Forgotten Wholeness

The narrowed range of nutrients that has become characteristic of public health recommendations and clinical nutrition practice has also become a standard feature of the food production process. No area of food production better illustrates this nutrient narrowing than the production of wheat products.

Products made from bleached, refined wheat flour constituted approximately 18% of total caloric intake for U.S. adults in the late 1980s.[22] These products were all made from the genus *Triticum*, a member of the grass (*Graminae*) family that also contains corn, oats, rice, barley, rye, lemon grass, and bamboo. Two species (*Triticum aestivum* and *Triticum turgidum*) accounted for production of virtually all wheat products. As of 1980, almost 95% of all wheat products were not only made from two species of wheat, but also from flour bleached and processed at an extraction rate of 70–75%.[23]

Whole grain wheat has been shown to be a significant source of at least 17 nutrients, including the vitamins B-1, B-2, B-3, B-6, E, pantothenate, and folate; the minerals calcium, copper, iron, manganese, phosphorus, selenium, and zinc; the essential fatty acid linoleic acid; and various types of fiber.[24] Well over half of these nutrients have been shown to be lost in the course of 75% flour extraction.[25]

Enrichment of flour, mandated by the U.S. government in 1941, involves re-addition of only four nutrients (vitamins B-1, B-2, B-3 and iron) to processed flour.[26] At the time of the enrichment decision, during a symposium in Toronto, Canada, held by the American Institute of Nutrition, one opponent to enrichment was reported to remark, "it seems a little ridiculous to take a natural foodstuff in which the vitamins and minerals have been placed by nature, submit this food stuff to a refining process which removes them, and then add them back to the refined product at an increased cost....If this is the object, why not follow the cheaper, more sensible, and nutritionally more desirable procedure of simply using the unrefined, or at most, slightly refined natural food."[27]

The image of bleached, refined wheat flour that accounts for 18% of U.S. caloric intake is the image of forgotten wholeness. While satisfying consumer demand, shelf life requirements, and government standards, bleached, refined wheat flour has emerged as a product that contains less than half of its original nutrient content and less than one third of its original nutrient variety. Highlighted in this image are all the features of narrowed nourishment and loss of wholeness. Also highlighted is the unsuccessful outcome of an exploitative approach (extraction) that attempts to re-constitute wholeness without addressing the injustice of its own action. ■

many officially unrecognized substances have been shown to have beneficial health effects. For example, flavonoids have been shown to be clinically useful in prevention of coronary heart disease[28] and skin cancer,[29] and in the treatment of acute viral hepatitis,[30] toxic alcoholic liver disease,[31] and venous insufficiency.[32] In vitro studies of flavonoids have also shown these compounds to have inhibitory effects on replication of human immunodeficiency virus.[33] Similarly, supplementation of the officially unrecognized nutrient glutamine has been shown to be clinically effective in treatment of intensive care patients,[34] postoperative patients,[35] bone marrow transplant patients,[36] premature infants,[37] and cancer patients undergoing chemotherapy.[38]

By narrowing nutrient selection, nutritional organizations have made it impossible for clinical findings like those cited above to be considered in the promotion of health. From a conceptual standpoint, restoration of environmental standards in nutrition would automatically help restore these lost opportunities, since such standards would bring an automatic focus on the diversity of nutrients, and the uniqueness of each nutrient in supporting health.

Loss of Functional Orientation

Narrowed nutrient selection has not been the only problematic impact of inattention to environmental standards in the field of nutrition. Neglect of environmental standards and their emphasis on interaction has also resulted in the loss of a functional orientation in nutritional practice.

The term "function" is derived from the Greek word ergon which literally translates as "the kind of action or activity proper to a person or thing; the purpose for which something is designed or exists."[39] In early Greek philosophy, *en-ergia*, the source for our English word "energy," originally meant functioning or "being in purposeful activity." A functional orientation to nutrition, or any other field of study, means an orientation that focuses on purpose in actions and events. It also means an orientation that treats events as designed and intended, rather than haphazard or arbitrary.

The Neglect of Food-Nutrient Dynamics

Loss of a functional orientation in nutrition has been illustrated by the neglect of food-nutrient dynamics in agriculture, as well as in compilation of food databases used to analyze the nutrient content of diets, recipes, and commercial products. The following sections look more closely at the loss of a functional orientation in the growing of broccoli, corn, soy and garlic, and as well as in the development of the most widely used food database in the U.S., United States Department of Agriculture (USDA) Handbook No. 8.

Agricultural Aspects

From a functional perspective, the nutrient content of any food is expected to be unique. While two plants of the same species, variety, and strain may inherit the same genetic composition, the expression of genes is expected to differ according to environmental circumstances. A wide variety of factors are assumed to be responsible for this uniqueness. These factors include source of seed stock, time of planting, soil conditions, atmospheric conditions, frequency of watering, intensity of watering, fluctuation in temperature, and interaction with other organisms (including soil bacteria or nearby plants and animals). A plant grown in low-selenium soil, for example, is not expected to contain as much selenium as the same species of plant grown in high-selenium soil. In addition, the amount of selenium contained within a plant is expected to depend upon the purpose that would be served by maintaining a higher or lower amount of the mineral inside the cells.

The Example of Broccoli and Vitamin C. According to the most widely-used reference book supplying data on nutritional contents of food (Bowes and Church's Food Values of Portions Commonly Used), one half cup of chopped raw broccoli contains 41 milligrams of vitamin C.[40] This same value is reported in Nutritionist III,[41] a version of the computer software most widely-used by dietitians to analyze patient diets. When using either of these two resources to determine the vitamin C content of a broccoli-containing diet, dietitians and other healthcare professionals approach these 41 milligrams of vitamin C as a fixed amount. Any half-cup of broccoli is assumed and expected to contain 41 milligrams of vitamin C.

From a functional perspective, this assumption and expectation are unwarranted. A functional orientation expects the vitamin C content of broccoli to be a constantly changing amount. These changes are assumed to be an intrinsic part of broccoli's design. Like any nutrient within any plant, the vitamin C in broccoli is assumed to serve a variety of purposes and to serve them by undergoing constant change.

Research on fluctuations in the vitamin C content of plants supports this functional point of view. Synthesis of vitamin C is a basic metabolic activity of most plants. Plants make vitamin C from sugar, using enzymes that still exist in a wide variety of animals, but are no longer expressed by human genes. Vitamin C is found in particularly high concentrations in the leaves and chloroplasts of plants.[42] (Chloroplasts are parts of plant cells containing chlorophyll, the green pigment required for photosynthesis. When a plant needs energy and new substances in its cells, it uses photosynthesis to take the energy of sunlight and convert it into usable compounds, especially sugar.) The high concentration of vitamin C in plant chloroplasts suggests that plants not only make vitamin C from sugar, but that vitamin C may be involved in the process of photosynthesis itself.

A plant's vitamin C content is related to its state of activity. When a seed germinates (i.e., begins to sprout), it triples its vitamin C content.[43] Presumably, this increase is related to the increased stress (both physical and chemical) placed on a sprout as it grows upward through the soil. A key component of the sprout's stress is oxidative stress, i.e., the challenge of increased metabolic activity involving oxygen. Plants, like people, have more capacity to withstand oxidative stress when they have an ample supply of vitamin C. In fact, when herbicides (like methyl viologen) are sprayed on plants, the plants increase their genetic expression of antioxidant-related enzymes (like glutathione reductase) and their synthesis of vitamin C.[44] Similarly, infection around the root nodules of soybeans, peas, and clover has been shown to trigger increased production of the vitamin C-related enzyme ascorbate peroxidase,[45] presumably to help lessen the oxidative stress caused by infection. At the other end of the spectrum, when plants cells die, large percentages of antioxidant compounds become oxidized and unavailable for stress resistance. Vitamin C, for example, decreases fourfold during leaf necrosis in tobacco plants.[46]

Changes in a plant's vitamin C content have also been shown to vary with soil composition. In comparison with crops grown by conventional agricultural methods, organically grown crops have been shown to have as much as 28% more vitamin C.[47] This finding is consistent with the results of more than 30 published studies showing the overall nutrient content of organically grown foods to be higher than the nutrient content of their non-organically grown counterparts.[48]

The Example of Fatty Acids and Time of Harvest. Research on the fatty acid content of plants has shown the same purposeful fluctuations observed for vitamin C. As previously discussed in Chapter 1 (page 18, under "Omega 3:6 Ratio and Human Metabolism"), fatty acid composition of certain plants undergoes substantial change particularly within the first three-week period after flowering. This change occurs as young, growing plants make metabolic adjustments to their new environment. In corn, an omega 6:omega 3 fatty acid ratio of 3.8 has been shown to rise to 11.4 during this time.[49] In soybeans, during a one-week period, the same ratio has been observed to increase from 1.2 to 3.8.[50] These altered fatty acid

Monocropping and the U.S. Corn Blight of 1970–1971

Monocropping

"Monocropping" is a non-technical term that refers to the cultivation of a single plant species in isolation from other species or types of crops. (The term "monoculture" is also used to describe plants which are cultivated in this way.) Monocropping also serves as the agricultural standard within the U.S. In 1987, for example, approximately 300 million total acres of land were planted and harvested.[51] About 20% of this land (59 million acres) was planted with corn. Each acre produced an average of 119 bushels, for a 7 billion bushel total.[52]

In contrast with this enormous amount of corn, however, was the extremely limited number of corn varieties. One hundred years ago, over 775 varieties of corn (*Zea mays*) were known to grow within the United States. Only fifty still exist, and out of these fifty, only a handful were planted and harvested on the 59 million acres.[53]

For many staple crops the situation has been identical to that of corn. Virtually all potatoes produced in the U.S. belong to a single genus-species, *Solanum tuberosum*. Twelve varieties within this one species account for 85% of the U.S. harvest. Even within these twelve varieties there is a lack of true diversity, since Russett Burbank is by far the most widely planted of the 12 varieties.[54]

The monocropping of corn and potatoes represents an unnatural narrowing of biodiversity, since hundreds of plant varieties would normally be present on U.S. acreage. Without a full spectrum of plant species to maintain nutrient and energy flow throughout the habitat, risk of ecological disruption is greatly increased. The U.S. corn blight of 1970–1971 illustrates the ecologically disruptive consequences of lost diversity.

The U.S. Corn Blight of 1970–1971

As documented by Jack Doyle in his book *Altered Harvest*, the U.S. corn blight epidemic of 1970–1971 involved the replication of a fungus, *Helminthosporium maydis*, on 10% of all corn crops in the U.S.[55] The extensive damage done by this fungus was partly a function of the fungus itself, which could reproduce within 60 minutes after landing on a plant and could withstand cold temperatures as low as -20° Fahrenheit. But this damage was also a function of monocropped acreage in which corn plants were universally susceptible to the fungus because of their identical genetic profile.

The corn blight epidemic had immediate agricultural and economic consequences for the U.S. food supply. Immediate ramifications included a lack of seed stock, and drastically reduced cultivation of corn in 1971.

Agricultural Response to the Corn Blight

After recognizing the connection between monocropping and increased susceptibility to microbial damage, many companies involved in agricultural research in the 1970s moved immediately in two directions to try and ♦

ratios also characterize the oils extracted from these plants, thereby linking dietary differences in fatty acid consumption not only to the type of food ingested (e.g., soy oil or corn oil) but also to the timing of the plant harvest (e.g., weeks after flowering). (The critical importance of fatty acid ratios for human health is discussed in Chapter 1, page 18, under "Omega 3:6 Ratio and Human Disease.")

The Example of Garlic and Allicin. A final example of food-nutrient dynamics involves garlic (*Allium sativum*) and fluctuations in its content of sulfur-containing compounds. Garlic, a member of the lily (*Lilaceae*) family, is propagated exclusively through vegetative means because of its sterility and has been shown to be highly sensitive in its nutrient composition to soil status. When grown in soil that has been fertilized with

---

HISTORICAL PERSPECTIVES: Monocropping and the U.S. Corn Blight of 1970–1971

CONTINUED

prevent future blights. One of these directions involved genetic engineering to try and create microbe-resistant varieties of corn. The other direction involved creation of pesticides to kill corn-threatening microbes directly. Particularly important in this regard was the development in the 1970s of the organochlorine pesticides. Twenty years later, soils from our U.S. corn belt continue to contain residues of DDT, DDD, DDE, cis-chlordane, trans-chlordane, heptachlor, heptachlor epoxide, dieldrin, alpha-hexachlorocyclohexane, and trans-nonachlor.[56] (These ten compounds are all organochlorine pesticides and are reviewed in greater detail in Chapter 3, pg 84, under "Pesticides and Other Substances.")

Today, these two types of industrial response have been combined to include direct genetic breeding of pesticide-like compounds into cultivated crops. Pesticidal agents, like the endotoxin gene from *Bacillus thuringiensis*, are now bred directly into

crops.[57] Many plants are also transgenically altered to become pesticide resistant.[58]

The transgenics-plus-pesticides reaction to monoculture-based problems has had far-reaching impact. In the plant world, this impact has involved transfer of genetically engineered characteristics from target to non-target species. Because field crops are typically surrounded by indigenous plants that are botanically related, engineered characteristics like pesticide resistance can get transferred from cultivated crops to native plants.[59] In addition to this risk of cross-species transfer is the potential for pathogenicity in the target plants themselves. For example, plant scientists attempted to combine genetic material from a fungus (*Rhizopogon sp.*) with genetic material from a bacterium (*Azobacter vinelandii*) in order to create a genetically unique nitrogen-fixing bacterium that could help promote the growth of pine trees (*Pinus radiata*). When the newly engineered bacterium was applied to pine tree seedlings, ▶

sulfur-containing compounds, garlic has been shown to release 48% more allicin.[64] Allicin is the main odor-producing compound in garlic. It is also a compound demonstrated to have significant health-protective properties. Along with its sulfur-containing derivatives, allicin has been shown to lower serum and liver levels of lipids, scavenge free radicals, decrease platelet aggregation, inhibit bacterial, viral, and fungal activity, and to exhibit antitumor and antimutagen effects.[65]

Collectively, these observations on broccoli, corn, soy and garlic support a functional approach to food that assumes fluctuation in nutrient content in accordance with environmental conditions and purposes served in the lives of the plants. These observations also raise into question the use of fixed nutrient values in food databases.

HISTORICAL PERSPECTIVES: Monocropping and the U.S. Corn Blight of 1970–1971

CONTINUED

however, several of the seedlings died. Fearing potential pathogenicity of the genetically engineered microbe, plant researchers destroyed all of the remaining seedlings and genetically engineered microorganisms.[60]

In the human world, extensive use of organochlorine pesticides on monocropped corn has been directly linked to the increased risk of chronic disease. For example, men working in the corn wet-milling industry, particularly around production processes required to convert corn starch into corn syrup, have been shown to have increased incidence of chronic nephritis, bladder cancer, death from diabetes, death from pancreatic cancer, and death from leukemia.[61] While other factors have been acknowledged to contribute to the health problems of these workers (including workplace factors like exposure to toxic solvents and toxic airborne particulates), a clear role has also been established for the contribution of corn pesticides to these health problems.[62]

Forgotten Wholeness

From a philosophical perspective, monocropping is a practice founded on forgotten wholeness. What is forgotten in the process of planting a single species or variety of plant in isolation from all other species or varieties is the belonging of all species to a lifeworld that is indivisibly whole. For example, most crop plants cannot survive in the absence of pollinators. Most pollinators cannot survive in the absence of plant diversity. If plant diversity is lost, pollinators are lost, and a new process (e.g., importation of bees) must be introduced to provide for pollination.

Like monocropping, use of pesticides to kill a crop-destroying fungus is also a practice philosophically founded on forgotten wholeness. In research on cucumbers, for example, it has been shown that genetic engineering to confer resistance to chrysomelid cucumber beetles simultaneously increases susceptibility to damage by red spider mites.[63] ■

Food Database Aspects

Dietitians rely heavily on computerized dietary analysis to evaluate nutrient intake. In a 1997 survey of dietitians belonging to three clinically-focused dietary practice groups (Dietitians in General Clinical Practice, Dietitians in Nutrition Support, and Clinical Nutrition Management), over 98% of respondents reported use of computerized dietary assessment.[66] This reliance on computerized assessment was in full consonance with the expressed goal of the American Dietetic Association to promote computerized assessment as a tool in nutritional analysis.[67]

Although the 1992 International Network of Food Data Systems (INFOODS) directory lists over 150 food composition tables available for research use,[68] a single database has served as the basis for virtually all dietary analysis by dietitians and other healthcare professionals in the U.S. This database, referred to as the Nutrient Database for Standard Reference, is a computerized version of the U.S. Department of Agriculture (USDA) Handbook No. 8, originally developed in 1950 and maintained by the USDA since that year. Handbook No. 8, also entitled "Composition of Foods: Raw, Processed, Prepared," contained information on 105 nutrients (or nutrient-related variables, like calories) in 5,976 foods in its twelfth, computerized, standard release version of 1998.[69]

As previously described in Chapter 1 (page 16, under "Nutrient Databases"), development of Handbook No. 8 involved solicitation of nutrient information from a variety of sources including research laboratories at colleges and universities, private laboratories, and the USDA itself.[70] However, approximately 85% of all values in the database were obtained from food manufacturers or from previously published studies.[71] A variety of sampling procedures were used to gather data, including: 1) single sampling, in which average nutrient content was calculated from several individual samples of a single food; 2) single composite sampling, in which mixed samples of a food obtained at different times and places were combined, analyzed, and reported as a single food; and 3) multiple composite sampling, in which different brands or cultivars of a food were combined, weighed to approximate a single food product as it would appear in the marketplace, and subsequently analyzed.

From a functional perspective, it is easy to understand how single sampling could result in misrepresentation of a food's nutrient content. Samples of the same food planted at different times of year, or under different soil, water, or atmospheric conditions would be likely to have altered nutrient content in comparison to the sample analyzed. However, this variation in nutrient content would go unaccounted for in the database.

While single composite sampling would be more sensitive to variation in nutrient content according to time of planting or environmental conditions, this variation would be lost when the mixed samples were combined and reported as a single food. This method of sampling would also make inevitable a certain degree of nutrient misrepresentation, since the averaged database values would not actually apply to most individual foods. Random combination of cultivars as described in the third sampling method would further complicate this misrepresentation by failing to differentiate between the nutrient contents of genetically different plants.

The validity of USDA Handbook No. 8 information has been questioned by numerous researchers. For example, a 1993 study by the General Accounting Office (GAO) of the United States concluded that in some cases, "data have been accepted with little or no supporting documentation on the testing and quality assurance procedures used to develop the data."[72] In some instances, the GAO found that published values differed from other research findings by as much as 750%.[73]

From a functional perspective, even if quality assurance procedures had been better implemented by the USDA in construction of its food composition tables, environmental variation would have assured fluctuation in nutrient values and would have raised questions about the fixed values established in Handbook No. 8. Return of environmental standards to nutrition would require a re-thinking of database construction well beyond the issues of quality assurance and standards of documentation.

The Neglect of Variability in Human Requirements

Loss of a functional orientation in nutrition has also been illustrated by the neglect of variability in human nutrient requirements. This variability includes differences between one person and another (inter-individual variabilty), as well as differences occurring within the life of any one person (intra-individual variability).

Inter-Individual Variability

During the period 1943–1989 in its release of Recommended Dietary Allowances (RDAs) for the U.S public, the National Academy of Sciences (NAS) repeatedly cautioned against clinical use of the RDAs to determine nutrient deficiency in specific individuals. As described in the ninth edition of the RDAs in 1980, "RDAs are recommendations for the average daily amounts of nutrients that population groups should consume over time. RDA should not be confused with requirements for a specific individual. Differences in the nutrient requirements of individuals are ordinarily unknown."[74] For the first, time, however, in the tenth edition of the RDAs released in 1989, the NAS sanctioned limited clinical use of the RDAs in determining individual deficiency by stating: "Although RDAs are most appropriately applied to groups, a comparison of individual intakes, averaged over a sufficient length of time, to the RDAs allows an estimate to be made about the probable risk of deficiency for that individual."[75]

From a functional perspective, individual differences in nutrient requirements are expected and fundamental to maintenance of health and recovery from illness. When faced with toxic exposure, for example, humans require increased nutrient protection particularly in the areas of oxidative metabolism and liver function. Like plants sprayed with herbicidal toxins, humans facing toxic insult (for example, following exposure to cigarette smoke) require increased amounts of vitamin C, at levels tripling normal requirements.[76]

Supporters of the RDAs have frequently pointed out that recovery from illness has never been a situation that the guidelines were intended to address. This point was underscored in the tenth edition of the RDA guidelines, which described the RDAs as intake levels "considered adequate to meet the needs of most healthy people in the United States under usual environmental stresses."[77] However, even in circumstances where illness or unusual stress has not been found to be present, nutrient requirements have repeatedly been shown to vary substantially from individual to individual.

Researchers in Leuven, Belgium, for example, examined bloodwork and cellular activity in 449 subjects to determine the relationship between aging and vitamin status for vitamins B-6, B-12, and folate. Healthy subjects varied by as much as 400% in their serum B-12 and B-6 concentrations, by as much as 300% in their serum folate.[78] Also notable in their research was the finding that even though the percentage of healthy subjects showing deficient blood concentrations of nutrients was low (ranging from 5–9%), the percentage showing deficient nutrient-related metabolism inside their cells was high (occurring in 63% of healthy subjects).[79] This intracellular evidence was regarded as underscoring the importance of individual differences in healthy subjects who would have otherwise been lumped together as "normal."

The findings of Joosten and colleagues with respect to B-complex vitamins have been matched by research results involving vitamin E and vitamin C. A 1993 vitamin E research review published by VERIS, the Vitamin E Research and Information Service, reported a minimal five-fold difference in vitamin E requirements for healthy adults.[80] The report estimated this inter-individual variability to be substantially higher when polyunsaturated fat intake varied greatly between individuals.[81] Similarly, Mark Levine and colleagues, working out of the National Institutes of Health in Bethesda, Maryland, have determined that plasma ascorbate levels in healthy adults vary by approximately 30%, but may hide differences in cellular requirements that are much greater.[82] Collectively, these studies point to inter-individual variability as a defining characteristic in nutrient requirements among individuals.

Intra-Individual Variability

Variation in nutrient requirements occurs not only between healthy individuals, but also within healthy individuals. Numerous factors contribute to this intra-individual variability, including genetic and lifestyle factors. Also contributing to intra-individual variability are factors that extend outward into the distant environment, rather than being contained within the immediate life world of the individual. These factors include a wide variety of well-documented biorhythms that link nutrient status in an individual to changing patterns of events in the solar system. Circadian rhythms involve variability over a 24-hour period, and are primarily linked to daylight cycles (called photoperiods) involving the earth's rotation around its axis. Circumannual rhythms involve variability occurring over a 12-month period and are primarily linked to the earth's orbit around the sun. Both types of rhythms are common contributors to intra-individual variability in nutrient status. For example, plasma tyrosine has been shown to follow a clear circadian pattern,[83] while plasma vitamin D patterns have been shown to be circumannual, dropping to the 9–16 nanogram/milliliter level in winter and reaching 25–50 nanograms/milliliter in summer.[84]

Numerous studies on intra-individual variability in nutrient status have shown changes unrelated to circadian or circumannual rhythms, however. In healthy women, serum ferritin (an iron storage protein) has been found to vary intra-individually as much as 18%, and intracellular superoxide dismutase (an oxidative enzyme requiring copper and zinc for its function) as much as 17%.[85] Similarly, intra-individual variability in serum homocysteine status has been determined to reach a level of 60% in healthy adults who were supplemented with 1 milligram of folic acid for 8 days.[86] In this study, focused on methods for determining subclinical levels of folate deficiency, researchers concluded that the effect of intra-individual variability was so great that determination of folate deficiency could not be made within their experimental framework. Similarly high levels of intra-individual variability in healthy subjects have also been reported for vitamins B-1 and B-2.[87]

The phenomenon of intra-individual variability has also been shown to include instances of metabolic challenge to an individual. During these instances, increased nutrient pools are required to allow execution of metabolic response. For example, the process of inflammatory response triggers an acute need for increased presence of vitamin C in neutrophilic cells. Neutrophils, the most abundant type of white blood cells, play a critical role in inflammation. In the presence of microbial infection and other dangers to the body, neutrophils become activated. Depending upon their activation state, neutrophils can raise their internal vitamin C concentrations to ten times the normal level.[88] Individuals with mild but chronic inflammation can have their nutrient status impacted through this mechanism.

The above-cited findings on intra-individual and inter-individual variability in nutrient status emphasize the importance of a functional orientation to nutrition and health. Without consideration of circadian or circumannual, variation in nutrient need, and without accounting for individual uniqueness in metabolism, actual requirements at any one point in time can be significantly misrepresented. The consequences of this misrepresentation are examined in the following section.

The Clinical Relevance of a Non-Functional Orientation

Neglect of human variability in nutrient requirements, together with neglect of food-nutrient dynamics in agriculture and food databases, has restricted the effectiveness of clinical protocols in nutrition. This restriction has come in three basic forms. First has been the total absence of dietary protocols for many conditions in which basic nutrient needs appear to have been met but have actually gone unmet due to underestimation of inter-individual variability. For example, daily intake of vitamin E at the 15 IU (International Unit) level has been estimated to meet or exceed the requirements of 95% of healthy U.S. adults. For this reason, adults attaining this amount in their daily diet have been regarded as having little risk of vitamin E-related health problems. Similarly, when health problems have been studied epidemiologically to determine whether vitamin deficiencies were associated with their onset, conditions associated with vitamin E intake above the 15 IU level have typically been categorized as conditions unrelated to vitamin E status. Both of these conclusions would be incorrect, however, for individuals with vitamin E needs significantly greater than 15 IU. Particularly in the area of skin conditions (including skin cancers), prior conclusions about the sufficiency of vitamin E intake may need to be revisited.

A second type of restriction imposed by neglect of variability has involved a failure to recognize the potential magnitude of nutrient needs in individuals with health problems.. This second type of restriction is discussed below under the heading "Inattention to the Potential Benefit of High-Dose Supplementation."

Neglect of variability has also imposed a third type of restriction upon clinical practice. This third type of restriction has involved inattention to the use of conditionally essential nutrients. Because the category "conditionally essential" is particularly important in establishing a functional orientation for nutritional practice, it is explored in detail on the following page, under "Inattention to the Potential Benefit of Conditionally Essential Nutrients".

Inattention to the Potential Benefit of High-Dose Supplementation

When the relationship of diet to disease is viewed from a non-functional perspective, many diseases appear to lack a research-verifiable dietary intervention. Nutrition textbooks offering protocols for disease treatment have simply omitted from discussion numerous conditions affecting large numbers of individuals. For example, Zeeman's *Clinical Nutrition and Dietetics* is a widely-used textbook on dietary intervention for disease and contains treatment recommendations for over 75 named conditions.[89] In this text, 59 pages are devoted to treatment of diabetes mellitus, and 47 pages to intervention in the case of renal failure. But many chronic conditions affecting large numbers of individuals in the U.S. are either mentioned in the text without establishment of specific protocols, or omitted altogether. Autoimmune conditions like rheumatoid arthritis (RA), systemic lupus erythmatosus (SLE), and multiple sclerosis (MS) are mentioned by Zeeman but described as having no dietary intervention other than use of small frequent meals or tube feeding if required.[90] Psychiatric conditions, including depression and schizophrenia, are also mentioned but described as having no dietary intervention.[91] Other disorders affecting large numbers of individuals including otitis media (ear infection) in children, fibromyalgia in adults, and premenstrual syndrome (PMS) in women receive no mention in the text.[92]

When the magnitude of potential nutrient need in specific individuals is considered, all of the above conditions can be re-examined and re-evaluated for possible connections to nutrient deficiency. In keeping with a functional perspective on nutrient status, some individuals might be expected to require intake of nutrients at levels dramatically higher than the Dietary Reference Intakes (DRIs). This expectation has been met in a number of research studies showing effectiveness of nutrient doses at 10–3,000 times the DRI level. For example, in the case of psychiatric conditions like depression, supplementation of folate at 15 milligrams per day, or approximately 37 times the current DRI level, has been shown to enhance recovery in a double blind study.[93] With schizophrenic patients, vitamin B-3 supplementation at the level of 3–8 grams per day, or approximately 200–533 times the current DRI level, was demonstrated to improve numerous aspects of the condition in a placebo-controlled study.[94]

In the case of autoimmune conditions like systemic lupus erythematosus, rheumatoid arthritis, and multiple sclerosis, high-dose supplementation has also been shown to be beneficial. Lupus patients have been shown to benefit from supplementation of pantothenic acid (vitamin B-5) in the form of calcium pantothenate at levels of 10–15 grams per day, or approximately 2,000–3,000 times the current DRI.[95] Beneficial effects following daily supplementation of this same nutrient at the 2-gram level have also been demonstrated for rheumatoid arthritis patients.[96] Twenty-gram daily doses of linoleic acid, or approximately 10 times the standard dietary recommendation of 1% total calories, have been shown to have therapeutic benefit for acute remitting multiple sclerosis patients.[97]

Inattention to the Potential Benefit of Conditionally Essential Nutrients

The distinction between essential and non-essential nutrients has long been a mainstay of nutritional practice. According to this distinction, certain nutrients, classified as essential, cannot be synthesized in the body *de novo* (i.e., "from scratch") and must therefore be obtained from the diet. Other nutrients, classified as nonessential, can be synthesized in the body *de novo* and are therefore not necessary to have included in the diet. All categories of macronutrients and micronutrients have traditionally been divided according to this essential-nonessential principle. In the case of fatty acids, for example, only two have been classified as essential, even though approximately 100 are routinely present in the body. In the case of amino acids, only ten have been classified as essential. Ten more have been shown to be commonly present in human proteins, to be joined there by several dozen other amino acids that are metabolic modifications of these initial twenty. In the case of carbohydrates, none have been classified as essential.

The same essential-nonessential distinction has been applied to minerals and vitamins. RDAs have been established for only 7 minerals found in the body, despite the fact that 26 are widely distributed in the body and have been studied for their role in supporting health. The case of vitamins has been unique, since vitamins have been defined as "organic compounds essential for specific metabolic reactions that cannot be synthesized by human tissue cells."[98] In keeping with this definition, all vitamins have been considered essential. Only 11 substances were classified as RDA vitamins, however, in the tenth edition of the RDAs,[99] and in the most recent DRI guidelines, only 3 (pantothenic acid, biotin, and choline) have been added to the list.[100] These 14 substances currently recognized as vitamins constitute less than half of the total number of substances that have historically been given vitamin names and numbers.[101]

The distinction between essential and nonessential nutrients is inconsistent with a functional perspective based on human variability and metabolic uniqueness. From this perspective, the human body is viewed as varying in its capacities, including its capacity to synthesize, transport, metabolize and store nutrients, as well as its capacity to respond to challenges and stress. A body working at peak vitality with optimal nutrient stores and optimal ability to transport and metabolize nutrients would be expected to meet most challenges and stresses. A body working below peak vitality with sub-optimal stores and sub-optimal metabolic balance would not. Within this context, the degree of an individual's reliance upon diet for nutrients would be viewed as a function of that individual's degree of vitality, metabolic balance, and nutrient supply, rather than a function of the nutrient itself. Dietary provision of a nutrient might be essential under one set of circumstances, but nonessential under other conditions. The body's theoretical ability to synthesize a nutrient would not be a factor in determining the nutrient's essential or nonessential nature, since a body theoretically able to synthesize a nutrient might still be unable to do so under particular circumstances. From a functional perspective, all nutrients would therefore be categorized as "conditionally essential."

The classification of nutrients as conditionally essential is consistent with current research findings in clinical nutrition, where supplementation of nonessential nutrients has repeatedly been shown to improve health. Examples of effective nonessential nutrient supplementation include use of boron in osteoarthritis;[102] treatment of fibromyalgia with malic acid;[103] treatment of congestive heart failure with taurine[104] and coenzyme Q;[105] use of lipoic acid following cerebral ischemia;[106] treatment of rheumatoid arthritis with glucosamine sulfate;[107] use of n-acetyl-cysteine and glutathione in lung cancer;[108] treatment of non-insulin-dependent diabetes with vanadium;[109] treatment of multiple trauma with glutamine;[110] and treatment of myocardial infarction with carnitine.[111]

PART II

Measuring the Impact in a Sample Diet

Part I of this chapter examines the impact of missing standards on nutritional policies and procedures, with special emphasis on DRIs and food database composition. This second part of this chapter looks at the impact of missing standards on actual dietary intake as demonstrated by analysis of a 24-hour diet diary.

*Table 2-1. **The sample diet***

Breakfast

1.5 cups	Homemade granola
1.0 cups	2% cow's milk
0.5 cups	Fresh strawberries

Mid-morning snack

1.0 cup	Grapes
2.0 cups	Water

Lunch

Tuna sandwich

2.0 slices	Rye bread
4.0 oz.	Water-packed tuna
2.0 slices	Leaf lettuce
1.0 cup	Beef barley soup
8.0 oz.	Ginger ale

Mid-afternoon snack

1.0 cups	Grapes
2.0 cups	Water

Dinner

1.0	Poppy seed roll
1.0	Pat of butter

stir-fry:

1.0 tbs	Olive oil
2.0 tsp	Soy sauce
0.5 cups	Carrots
0.5 cups	Turnip greens
3.0	Chili peppers
1.5 cups	Egg noodles

Evening

1.0 cups	Water

The sample diet chosen for analysis is presented opposite in *Table 2-1*. Included in the diet were three meals and two snacks. With the exception of one canned soda, no prepackaged food was included. In terms of specific foods, the diet contained: three servings of fresh fruit, stir-fried vegetables with leafy greens, three types of grains and grain products at each meal, five cups of plain water, one reduced-fat dairy product, and olive oil. Only one high-fat item (a pat of butter) was included within the diet.

Macronutrient Analysis

The entire day's food described in *Table 2-1*, was analyzed with the computer software program, *Nutritionist III*.[112] Reported in *Table 2-2* are results of the analysis for macronutrients contained in the diet. As indicated in this table, all macronutrient guidelines were met or exceeded in the diet, including guidelines for calories, protein and fiber. While percentage of calories obtained from carbohydrate (52%) was basically consistent with national health guidelines, percentage calories obtained from fat (33%) was slightly higher than most recommendations, although lower than actual intake by the average U.S. adult.

Amino Acids

When compared to World Health Organization (WHO) standards for daily amino acid intake, the sample diet far exceeded WHO standards for all essential amino acids (*Table 2-3*, on the following page). Particularly plentiful was the aromatic amino acid phenylalanine, the uncharged polar amino acid threonine, and the branched chain amino acid leucine.

*Table 2-2. **Macronutrients in the sample diet***

Macronutrient	Amount	% RDA[a]
Protein	86 grams	172%
Carbohydrate	297 grams	108%
Fat	84 grams	115%
Fiber	42 grams	191%
Calories	2226	101%
% Protein	15%	
% Carbohydrate	52%	
% Fat	33%	

[a] Based on the 10th Edition of the Recommended Dietary Allowances, Food and Nutrition Board, National Research Council, National Academy of Sciences, National Academy Press, 1989. Guidelines established for females 25–50 years of age were used in computer calculations.

Table 2-3. Amino acids in the sample diet.

Amino acid	amount	%WHO[a]
Tryptophan	1196 mg	478%
Threonine	4226 mg	939%
Isoleucine	4865 mg	748%
Leucine	7683 mg	809%
Lysine	5846 mg	731%
Methionine	2207 mg	519%
Cysteine	1541 mg	363%
Phenylalanine	4706 mg	991%
Tyrosine	3040 mg	640%
Valine	5715 mg	879%
Histidine	2539 mg	462%

[a] Based on the World Health Organization (WHO) Energy and Protein Requirements. Report of a Joint FAO/WHO/UNU Expert Consultation. Technical Report Series 724. Geneva, Switzerland, World Health Organization, 1985. Guidelines established for adults were used in all computer calculations. A body weight of 70 kilograms was used to convert per kilogram requirements into total body requirements.

Micronutrient Analysis

Vitamins

With two exceptions (vitamins D and E), analysis of RDA vitamins in the sample diet showed intake surpassing the established requirements *(Table 2-4)*. Four out of ten vitamins (A, K, B-1, and folate) were present at 199% or more of the RDA.

Minerals

Analysis of the sample diet for RDA minerals also showed outstanding results *(Table 2-5)*. All 10 minerals analyzed were present at 80% of the RDA or greater, and only one mineral (manganese) fell below the 90% level.

Toxic Analysis

Simultaneous with its ability to exceed virtually all macronutrient and micronutrient guidelines was the ability of the sample diet to contain a potentially vast array of food toxins. In the above statement, the word "potentially" is of critical importance, for two reasons. First, no computerized software capable of estimating toxic content existed at the time of the analysis. All estimations of toxic content were therefore derived from published food science research rather than a single composite database. Second, the research used to derive toxic content was international rather than national in scope. The results may therefore have been misrepresentative of toxic residues found in foods available to U.S. consumers. These methodological limitations should be kept in mind when reviewing toxicity results.

Table 2-4. *Vitamins in the sample diet*

Vitamin	Amount	% RDA[a]
A	2221 mcg RE	278%
D	2.58 mcg	52%
E	5.3 mg	66%
K	502 mcg	773%
B-1	2.2 mg	200%
B-2	1.7 mg	130%
B-3	20.9 mg	135%
B-6	2.1 mg	132%
B-12	3.5 mcg	178%
Folate	359 mcg	199%

[a] Based on the 10th Edition of the Recommended Dietary Allowances, Food and Nutrition Board, National Research Council, National Academy of Sciences, National Academy Press, 1989. Guidelines established for females 25–50 years of age were used in computer calculations.

Table 2-5. *Minerals in the sample diet*

Mineral	Amount	% RDA[a]
Calcium	729 mg	91%
Phosphorus	1692 mg	212%
Magnesium	452 mg	161%
Iron	16.5 mg	110%
Zinc	10.8 mg	90%
Copper	2.3 mg	90%
Manganese	2.9 mg	82%
Selenium	354 mcg	643%
Sodium	2404 mg	100%
Potassium	2905 mg	145%

[a] Based on the 10th Edition of the Recommended Dietary Allowances, Food and Nutrition Board, National Research Council, National Academy of Sciences, National Academy Press, 1989. Guidelines established for females 25–50 years of age were used in computer calculations.

Breakfast

Potential toxins contained in the sample breakfast included three pesticides and two heavy metals *(Table 2-6)*. In addition, each component of the breakfast contributed to its potential toxicity.

Lunch

Potential toxins in the sample lunch included two heavy metals, two packaging migrants, several pesticides, a food additive, and several antibiotics *(Table 2-7)*. The widest variety of potential toxins were contained in the beef barley soup, even though the water portion of the soup was not analyzed for potential toxicity.

Dinner

Like the sample lunch, the sample dinner contained a variety of potential toxins, including heavy metals, pesticides, packaging migrants, fumigants, and food additives *(Table 2-8)*.

*Table 2-6. **Potential toxins in the sample breakfast***

Amount	Food	Residue	Toxin
1.5 cups	Granola	11.56 mcg	Lead[113]
		9.18 mcg	Cadmium[114]
1.0 cup	2% cow's milk	190 ppb	DDE[115]
0.5 cups	Strawberries	150 ppb	Captan[116]
		40 ppb	Folpet[117]

*Table 2-7. **Potential toxins in the sample lunch***

Amount	Food	Residue	Toxin
2.0 slices	Rye bread	912 ng	Lead[118]
		513 ng	Cadmium[119]
4.0 oz.	Tuna (water-packed)	170 ppb	Mercury[120]
2.0 slices	Leaf lettuce	131 ng	Total PAH[121]
1.0 piece	Shrink-wrapping	191 mcg	ESBO[122]
1.0 cup	Beef barley soup		
	Beef	0.89 ppt	Dioxins[123]
		trace	Neomycin[124]
		trace	Tetracyclin[125]
		trace	Gentamicin[126]
		trace	Oxytetracycline[127]
		trace	Penicillin[128]
	Barley	10 ppt	Terbufos[129]
		143 ppm	THI[130]
8.0 oz.	Ginger ale	Micromol	Aluminum[131]

Snacks

Although both the grapes and the water consumed for mid-morning, mid-afternoon, and evening snacks contained potential toxins, the greatest variety of potential toxins was associated with the water *(Table 2-9)*. Eight pesticides, a fumigant, a heavy metal, and a silicate were among the potential toxins brought into the diet by inclusion of tap water.

Table 2-8. Potential toxins in the sample dinner

Amount	Food	Residue	Toxin
1 piece	Poppy seed roll		
	Poppy seed	10 mcg	Cadmium[132]
	Wheat flour	10 ppb	Terbufos[133]
		4.42 ppm	HCH[134]
1 pat	Butter	1.19 ppm	HCH[135]
1 Tbs	Olive oil	500 ng	PAH[136]
		1 ppm	HCH[137]
2 tsp	Soy sauce	143 ppm	THI[138]
0.5 cup	Carrot	100 mcg	Phorate[139]
0.5 cup	Turnip greens	6 ppm	Permethrin[140]
3.0	Chili peppers	480 ppb	HCH[141]
1.5 cups	Egg noodles	13.6 mg	Methyl bromide[142]

Table 2-9. Potential toxins in the sample snacks

Amount	Food	Residue	Toxin
1.0 cup	Grapes	80 ppb	Captan[143]
		500 ppb	Folpet[144]
		Above MRL	Dithiocarbamate[145]
		Above MRL	Dicarboximide[146]
		Above MRL	Methylcarbamate[147]
		Above MRL	EBDC[148]
		Above MRL	Dicofol[149]
2.0 cups	Water	1M fibers/L	Asbestos[150]
		8 ng	EDB[151]
		423 ng	Xylenes[152]
		2.5 mcg	Arsenic[153]
		2.0 mcg	Nitrates[154]
		3.7 ppb	Atrazine[155]
		2.1 ppb	Cyanazine[156]
		260 ppt	Simazine[157]
		190 ppt	Acetachlor[158]
		3.65 ppb	Alachlor[159]
		4.34 ppb	Metalochlor[160]
		90 ppt	Metribuzin[161]

Summary

A summary of the potential toxins contained in the sample diet is presented in *Table 2-10*. Listed by category, these potential toxins included antibiotics, colorings, metals, pesticides, petrochemicals, plastics, and silicates. A total of 37 potential toxins were associated with the total day's intake.

The ability of the sample diet to exceed virtually all macronutrient and micronutrient guidelines, while at the same time containing potential toxins in virtually all of its foods, can be viewed as reflecting the impact of non-environmental standards on nutritional practice. In the following chapter, we look more closely at each of these individual toxins and exposure to them from everyday consumption of the U.S. food supply.

Table 2-10. **Summary of potential toxic exposure**

Antibiotics
  Neomycin
  Tetracyclin
  Gentamycin
  Oxytetracyclin
  Penicillin

Colorings
  Tetrahydroxybutylimidazole (THI)

Metals
  Aluminum (Al)
  Arsenic (As)
  Cadmium (Cd)
  Lead (Pb)
  Mercury (Hg)

Petrochemicals
  Polycyclic aromatic hydrocarbons (PAHs)
  Xylenes

Plastics
  Epoxidised soya bean oil (ESBO)

Silicates
  Asbestos

Pesticides
  Acetachlor
  Alachlor
  Atrazine
  Captan
  Cyanazine
  Dichlorodiphenyldichloroethylene (DDE)
  Dicarboximide
  Dicofol
  Dithiocarbamate
  Dioxins
  Ethylene dibromide (EDB)
  Ethylenebisdithiocarbamates (EBDCs)
  Folpet
  Hexachlorohexane (HCH)
  Metalochlor
  Methylcarbamate
  Metribuzin
  Permethrin
  Phorate
  Simazine
  Terbufos

1. Whitney EN, Cataldo CB and Rolfes SR. (1991). Understanding normal and clinical nutrition. Third edition. West Publishing Company, St. Paul, p.2.

2. Sendl A. (1995). Allum sativum and allium ursinum: part 1. Chemistry, analysis, history, botany. Phytomed 4:323–339.

3. Middleton E Jr and Kandaswami C. (1993). The impact of plant flavonoids on mammalian biology: implications for immunity, inflammation, and cancer. Chapter 15. In: Harborne JB. (Ed) The flavonoids: advances in research since 1986. Chapman and Hall, London, p.619.

4. Krinsky NI. (1993). Actions of carotenoids in biological systems. Ann Rev Nutr 13:561–587.

5. Huang M-T, Osawa T, Ho C-T et al. (Eds). (1994). Food phytochemicals for cancer prevention I and II. American Chemical Society, Washington, D.C.

6. Food and Nutrition Board, National Research Council, National Academy of Sciences. (1989). Recommended dietary allowances. Tenth edition. National Academy Press, Washington, D.C.

7. *Ibid.*

8. National Academy of Sciences. (1997). Origin and framework of the development of dietary reference intakes. Nutr Rev 55(9):332–334.

9. National Academy of Sciences. (1980). Recommended dietary allowances. Ninth edition. National Academy of Sciences, Washington, D.C., p.6.

10. Institute of Medicine (1998). Adults need to increase intake of folate; some women should take more. Press Release, April 7, 1998, Institute of Medicine, National Research Council, Washington, D.C.

11. Institute of Medicine (1998). Adults need to increase intake of folate; some women should take more. Press Release, April 7, 1998, Institute of Medicine, National Research Council, Washington, D.C., p.1.

12. Numbers derived from searches of the United States National Library of Medicine's MEDLINE(database using the Internet Grateful Med Version 2.6 (1998), Internet Grateful Med Development Team, National Library of Medicine, 8600 Rockville Pike, Bethesda, Maryland 20894. (Website location: http://www.igm.nlm.nih.gov).

13. Hunt CD. (1994). The biochemical effects of physiologic amounts of boron in animal nutrition models. Environ Health Perspect 102 Suppl 7:35–43.

14. Nielson FH, Shuler TR, and Gallagher SK. (1990). Effects of boron depletion and repletion on blood indicators of calcium status in humans fed a magnesium-low diet. J Trace Elem Exp Med 3:45–54.

15. Nielson FH. (1994). Ultratrace minerals. In: Shils ME, Olson JA and Shike M. (Eds). Modern nutrition in health and disease. Lea and Fabiger, Philadelphia, pp.269–286.

16. Loomis WD and Durst RW. (1992). Chemistry and biology of boron. BioFactors 3:229–239.

17. Kramer SP, Johnson JL, Ribeiro AA et al. (1987). The structure of the molybdenum cofactor. J Biol Chem 262:16357–16363.

18. National Research Council. (1989). Recommended dietary allowances. Tenth edition. National Academy Press, Washington, D.C., pp.243–246.

19. Numbers derived from searches of the United States National Library of Medicine's MEDLINE(database using the Internet Grateful Med Version 2.6 (1998), Internet Grateful Med Development Team, National Library of Medicine, 8600 Rockville Pike, Bethesda, Maryland 20894. (Website location: http://www.igm.nlm.nih.gov).

20. Numbers derived from searches of the United States National Library of Medicine's MEDLINE(database using the Internet Grateful Med Version 2.6 (1998), Internet Grateful Med Development Team, National Library of Medicine, 8600 Rockville Pike, Bethesda, Maryland 20894. (Website location: http://www.igm.nlm.nih.gov).

21. Numbers derived from searches of the United States National Library of Medicine's MEDLINE(database using the Internet Grateful Med Version 2.6 (1998), Internet Grateful Med Development Team, National Library of Medicine, 8600 Rockville Pike, Bethesda, Maryland 20894. (Website location: http://www.igm.nlm.nih.gov).

22. Food and Agriculture Organization (FAO). (1991). Food balance sheets 1984–1986 averages. Food and Agriculture Organization of the United Nations, Rome, Italy.

23. Davis RD. (1981). Wheat and nutrition— part 1. Nutr Today 16(4):16–21.

24. Pedersen B, Knudsen KEB, and Eggum BO. (1989). Nutritive value of cereal products with emphasis on the effects of milling. Wrld Rev Nutr Diet 60:1–91.

25. *Ibid.*

26. Lepkovsky S. (1944). The bread problem in war and peace. Physiol Rev 24:239–276.

27. *Ibid.*

28. Hertog MG, Feskens EJM, Hollman PCH et al. (1993). Dietary antioxidant flavonoids and risk of coronary heart disease: the Zutphen Elderly Study. Lancet 342:1007–1011.

29. Picard D. (1996). The biochemistry of green tea polyphenols and their potential application in human skin cancer. Alt Med Rev 1(1):31–42.

30. Piazza M, Guadagnino V, Piccioto L et al. (1983). Effect of (+)-cyanidanol-3 in acute HAV, HBV, and non-A, non-B vital hepatitis. Hepatol 3(1):45–49.

31. Abonyi M, Kisfaludy S, and Szalay F. (1984). Therapeutic effect of (+)-cyanidanol-3 in toxic alcoholic liver disease and chronic active hepatitis. Acta Physiologica Hungarica 64(3–4):455–460.

32. Meyer OC. (1994). Safety and security of Daflon 500mg in venous insufficiency and hemorrhoidal disease. Angiol 45(6)Pt2:579–584.

33. Takayama H, Bradley G, Lai PK et al. (1991). Inhibition of human immunodeficiency virus foward and reverse transcription by PC6, a natural product from cones of pine trees. AID Res Hum Retro 7:349–357.

34. Griffiths RD, Palmer TE, and Jones C. (1996). Parenteral glutamine supply in intensive care patients. Nutr 12(11/12) Suppl:S73–S75.

35. Byrne TA, Morrissey TB, Ziegler TR et al. (1992). Growth hormone, glutamine, and fiber enhance adaptation of remnant bowel following massive intestinal resection. Surg Forum 43:151–153.

36. MacBurney M, Young L, Ziegler TR et al. (1994). A cost-evaluation of glutamine-supplemented parenteral nutrition in adult bone marrow transplant patients. JADA 94:1263–1266.

37. Lacey JM, Crough JP, Benfel K et al. (1996). The effects of glutamine-supplemented parenteral nutrition in premature infants. JPEN 20:74.

38. Rouse K, Nwokedi E, Woodliff JE et al. (1995). Glutamine enhances selectivity of chemotherapy through changes in glutathione metabolism. Ann Surg 221:420–426.

39. Urdang L and Flexner SB. (1968). Random House dictionary of the English language. Random House, New York, p.535.

40. Pennington JAT. (1994). Bowes & Church's Food values of portions commonly used. Sixteenth edition. J.B. Lippincott, Philadelphia, p.296.

41. N-Squared Computing. (1991). Nutritionist III, Version 7.0. N-Squared Computing, Salem, Oregon.

42. Wheeler GL, Jones MA, and Smirnoff N. (1998). The biosynthetic pathway of vitamin C in higher plants. Nature 393(6683):365–369.

43. Sattar A, Badshah A, and Aurangzeb. (1995). Biosynthesis of ascorbic acid in germinating rapeseed cultivars. Plant Foods Hum Nutr 47(1):63–70.

44. Foyer CH, Souriau N, Perret S et al. (1995). Overexpression of glutathione reductase but not glutathione synthetase leads to increases in antioxidant capacity and resistance to photoinhibition in poplar trees. Plant Physiol 109(3):1047–1057.

45. Dalton DA, Joyner SL, Becana M et al. (1998). Antioxidant defenses in the peripheral cell layers of legume root nodules. Plant Physiol 116(1):37–43.

46. Willekens H, Chamnongpol S, Davey M et al. (1997). Catalase is a sink for H2O2 and is indispensable for stress defense in C3 plants. EMBO J 16(16):4806–4816.

47. Schuphan W. (1974). Nutritional value of crops as influenced by organic and inorganic fertilizer treatments. Qualitas Plantarum 23:333–358.

48. Worthington V. (1998). Effect of agricultural methods on nutritional quality: a comparison of organic with conventional crops. Alt Ther 4(1):58–69.

49. Bengmark S. (1998). Ecoimmunonutrition: a challenge for the third millennium. Nutr: Internatl J Appl Basic Nutr Sci 14(7/8):566.

50. *Ibid*.

51. United States Department of Agriculture. (1989). 1989 Fact Book of Agriculture. USDA Department of Public Affairs, Miscellaneous Publication Number 1063, p. 42.

52. *Ibid*, p.131.

53. Fowler C and Mooney P. (1990). Shattering: food politics, and the loss of genetic diversity. The University of Arizona Press, Tucson, pp.54–89.

54. Doyle J. (1985). Altered harvest. Viking Penguin, New York.

55. *Ibid*.

56. Aigner EJ, Leone AD and Falconer RL. (1998). Concentrations and enantiomeric ratios of organochlorine pesticides in soils from the U.S. corn belt. Envir Sci & Technol 332(9):1162–1168.

57. Vaeck M, Reynaerts A, Hofte H et al. (1987). Transgenic plants protected from insect attack. Nature 328:33–37.

58. May RM. (1993). Resisting resistance. Nature 361:593–594.

59. Levin SA. (1988). Safety standards for the environmental release of genetically engineered organisms. Tree 3(4); Tibtech 6(4):S49.

60. Doyle J, *op. cit. (see reference 50)*, pp.243–244.

61. Thomas TL, Krekel S and Heid M. (1985). Proportionate mortality among male corn wet-milling workers. Int J Epidemiol 14(3):432–437.

62. Rea WJ. (1996). Pesticides. J Nutr Environ Med 6:55–124.

63. DaCosta CP and Jones CM. (1971). Cucumber beetle resistance and mite susceptibility controlled by the bitter gene in Cucumis sativus. Sci 172:1145–1146.

64. Sendl A. (1995). Allium sativum and allium ursinum: part 1. Chemistry, analysis, history, botany. Phytomed 4:323–339.

65. Reuter HD. (1995). Allium sativum and allium ursinum: part 2. Pharmacology and medicinal application. Phytomed 2(1):73–91.

66. Biesmeier C and Chima CS. (1997). Computerized patient record: are we prepared for our future practice? JADA 97:1099–1104.

67. American Dietetic Association. (1996). Position of the American Dietetic Association: vitamin and mineral supplementation. JADA 96(1):73–77.

68. Simopoulos AP. (1992). International food data bases and information exchange. Wrld Rev Nutr Diet 68: preface.

69. United States Department of Agriculture. (1998). Nutrient database for standard reference. Nutrient Data Lab, Agricultural Research Service, Beltsville Human Nutrition Research Center, United States Department of Agriculture, Beltsville, Maryland.

70. Southgate DAT and Greenfield H. (1992). Principles for the preparation of nutritional data bases and food composition tables. Wrld Rev Nutr Diet 68:27–48.

71. Katch FI. (1995). U.S. government raises serious questions about reliability of U.S. Department of Agriculture's food composition database. Internatl J Sports Nutr 5:62–67.

72. U.S. Government Accounting Office. (1993). Food nutrition: better guidance needed to improve reliability of USDA's food composition data. Letter Report, 10/25/93, GAO/RCED-94-30, Washington, D.C.

73. *Ibid.*

74. National Academy of Sciences. (1980). Recommended dietary allowances. Ninth edition. National Academy Press, Washington, D.C.

75. National Academy of Sciences. (1989). Recommended dietary allowances. Tenth edition. National Academy Press, Washington, D.C.

76. Tribble DL, Giuliano LJ, and Fortmann SP. (1993). Reduced plasma ascorbic acid concentrations in non-smokers regularly exposed to environmental tobacco smoke. Am J Clin Nutr 58:886–890.

77. National Academy of Sciences, *op. cit. (see reference 75).*

78. Joosten A, van den Berg A, Riezler R et al. (1993). Metabolic evidence that deficiencies of vitamin B12 (cobalamin), folate, and vitamin B6 occur more commonly in elderly people. Am J Clin Nutr 58:468–476.

79. *Ibid.*

80. VERIS. (1993). Vitamin E research summary. An overview of vitamin E efficacy in humans. Vitamin E Research and Information Service, LaGrange, Illinois.

81. *Ibid.*

82. Levine M, Cantilena CC, and Dhariwal KR. (1993). In situ kinetics and ascorbic acid requirements. Wrld Rev Nutr Diet 72:114–127.

83. Fernstrom JD. (1979). The influence of circadian variations in amino acid concentrations on monoamine synthesis in the brain. In: Krieger DT. (Ed). Endocrine rhythms. Raven Press, New York.

84. McLaughlin M, Fiarney A, Lester E et al. (1974). Seasonal variations in serum 25-hydroxycholecalciferol in healthy people. Lancet 1:536–538.

85. Gallagher SK, Johnson LK, and Milne DB. (1989). Short-term and long-term variability of indices related to nutritional status. I. Ca, Cu, Fe, Mg, and Zn. Clin Chem 35(3):369–373.

86. Santhosh-Kumar CR, Deutsch JC, Ryder JW et al. (1997). Unpredictable intra-individual variations in serum homocysteine levels on folic acid supplementation. Eur J Clin Nutr 51(3):188–192.

87. Van Dokkum W, Schrijver J and Wesstra JA. (1990). Variability in man of the levels of some indices of nutritional status over a 60-d period on a constant diet. Eur J Clin Nutr 44(9):665–674.

88. Washko PW, Wang Y, and Levine M. (1993). Ascorbic acid recycling in human neutrophils. J Biol Chem 268(21):15531–15535.

89. Zeeman FJ. (1991). Clinical nutrition and dietetics. Second edition. Macmillan Publishing Company, New York.

90. *Ibid*, pp.737, 165, 732.

91. *Ibid*, p.736.

92. *Ibid.*

93. Godfrey PS, Toone BK, Carney MW et al. (1990). Patients with major depression and low red cell folate improved significantly over six mo. with methylfolate supplementation. Lancet 336:392–395.

94. Ananth JV, Vacaflor L, Kekhwa G et al. (1972). Nicotinic acid in the treatment of newly admitted schizophrenic patients: a placebo controlled study. Int J Clin Pharmacol 5:406–410.

95. Welsh AL. (1954). Lupus erhthematosus: treatment by combined use of massive amounts of pantothenic acid and vitamin E. Arch Dermatol Syphilol 70:181–198.

96. General Practitioner Research Group. (1980). Calcium pantothenate in arthritic conditions. A report from the General Practitioner Research Group. Practitioner 224:208–211.

97. Bates D, Fawcett PRW, Shaw DA et al. (1978). Polyunsaturated fatty acids in treatment of acute remitting multiple sclerosis. Br Med J ii:1390–1391.

98. Mahan KL and Escott-Stump S. (1996). Krause's food, nutrition, and diet therapy. 9th edition. W.B. Saunders, Philadelphia, p.78.

99. National Academy of Sciences, *op. cit. (see reference 75).*

100. Yates AA, Schlicker SA, and Suitor CW. (1998). Dietary Reference Intakes: the new basis for recommendations for calcium and related nutrients, B vitamins, and choline. J Am Diet Assoc 98:699–706.

101. Newstrom H. (1993). Nutrients catalog. McFarland & Company, Jefferson, North Carolina.

102. Travers RL, Rennie GC and Newnham RE. (1990). Boron and arthritis: the results of a double-blind pilot study. J Nutr Med I:127–132.

103. Abraham GE and Flechas JD. (1992). Management of fibromyalgia: rationale for the use of magnesium and malic acid. J Nutr Med 3:49–59.

104. Azuma J, Sawamura A, and Awata K. (1992). Usefulness of taurine in chronic congestive heart failure and its prospective application. Jpn Circ J 56:95–99.

105. Lampertico M and Comis S. (1993). Italian multicenter study on the efficacy of coenzyme Q10 as an adjuvant therapy in heary failure. Clin Investig 71:S129–S133.

106. Prehn JH, Karkoutly C, Nuglisch J et al. (1992). Dihydrolipoate reduces neuronal injury after cerebral ischemia. J Cereb Blood Flow Metab 12:78–87.

107. Tapadinhas MJ, Rivera IC and Bigmini AA. (1982). Oral glucosamine sulfate in the management of arthrosis: report on a multi-centre open investigation in Portugal. Pharmather 3(3):157–168.

108. Van Zandwijk N. (1995). N-acetylcysteine (NAC) and glutathione (GSH): antioxidant and chemopreventive properties, with special reference to lung cancer. J Cell Biochem Suppl 22:24–32.

109. Boden G, Chen X, Ruiz J et al. (1996). Effects of vanadyl sulfate on carbohydrate and lipid metabolism in patients with non-insulin-dependent diabetes mellitus. Metabol 45:1130–1135.

110. Houdijk APJ, Rijnsburger ER, Jansen J et al. (1998). Randomised trial of glutamine-enriched enteral nutrition on infectious morbidity in patients with multiple trauma. Lancet 352:772–776.

111. Singh RB, Niaz MA, Agarwal P et al. (1996). A randomised, double-blind, placebo-controlled trial of L-carnitine in suspected acute myocardial infarction. Postgrad Med J 72:45–50.

112. N-Squared Computing, *op. cit. (see reference 35)*.

113. Tahvonen R and Kumpulainen J. (1993). Lead and cadmium in some cereal products on the Finnish market 1990–91. Food Addit Contamin 10(2):245–255.

114. *Ibid.*

115. Trotter WJ and Dickerson R. (1993). Pesticide residues in composited milk collected through the U.S. Pasteurized Milk Network. J Assoc Off Anal Chem Int 76(6):1220–1225.

116. Gilvydis DM, Walters SM, Spivak ES et al. (1986). Residues of captan and folpet in strawberries and grapes. J Assoc Off Anal Chem 69(5):803–806.

117. *Ibid.*

118. Tahvonen R and Kumpulainen J. *op. cit. (see reference 113)*.

119. *Ibid.*

120. Yess NJ. (1993). U.S. Food and Drug Administration survey of methyl mercury in canned tuna. J Assoc Off Anal Chem 71(1):36–38.

121. Wickstrom K, Pyysalo H, Plaami-Heikkila S et al. (1986). Polycyclic aromatic hydrocarbons (PAC) in leaf lettuce. Z Lebensm Unters Forsch 183(3):182–185.

122. Castle L, Mayo A, and Gilbert J. (1990). Migration of epoxidised soya bean oil into foods from retail packaging materials and from plasticised PVC film used in the home. Food Addit Contam 7(1):29–36.

123. Ferrario J, Byrne C, McDaniel D et al. (1996). Determination of 2,3,7,8-chlorine-substituted dibenzo-p-dioxins and -furans at the part per trillion level in United States beef fat using high-resolution gas chromatography/high-resolution mass spectrometry. Anal Chem 68(4):647–652.

124. Gibbons SN, Kaneene JB, and Lloyd JW. (1996). Patterns of chemical residues detected in US beef carcasses between 1991 and 1993. J Amer Vet Med Assoc 209(3):589–593.

125. *Ibid.*

126. *Ibid.*

127. *Ibid.*

128. *Ibid.*

129. Westcott ND. (1988). Terbufos residues in wheat and barley. J Environ Sci Health 23(4):317–330.

130. Houben GF, Abma PM, van den Berg H et al. (1992). Effects of the colour additive caramel colour III on the immune system: a study with human volunteers. Food Chem Toxicol 30(9):749–757.

131. Duggan JM, Dickeson JE, Tynan PF et al. (1992). Aluminium beverage cans as a dietary source of aluminium. Med J Aust 156(9):604–605.

132. Hoffmann J and Blasenbrei P. (1986). Cadmium in poppy seeds and poppy seed-containing products. Z Lebensm Unters Forsch 182(2):121–122.

133. Westcott ND, *op. cit. (see reference 129).*

134. Kaphalia BS, Takroo R, Mehrota S et al. (1990). Organochlorine pesticide residues in different Indian cereals, pulses, spices, vegetables, fruits, milk, butter, Deshi ghee, and edible oils. J Assoc Off Anal Chem 73(4):509–512.

135. *Ibid.*

136. Menichini E, Bocca A, Merli F et al. (1991). Polycyclic aromatic hydrocarbons in olive oils on the Italian market. Food Addit Contam 8(3):363–369.

137. Kaphalia BS, Takroo R, Mehrota S et al, *op. cit. (see reference 134).*

138. Houben GF, Abma PM, van den Berg H et al, *op. cit. (see reference 130).*

139. Suett DL. (1986). Insecticide residues in commercially-grown quick-maturing carrots. Food Addit Contam 3(4):371–376.

140. George DA. (1985). Permethrin and its two metabolite residues in seven agricultural crops. J Assoc Off Ana Chem 68(6):160–163.

141. Kaphalia BS, Takroo R, Mehrota S et al, *op. cit. (see reference 134).*

142. Cova D, Molinari GP, and Rossini L. (1986). Residues after fumigation with methyl bromide: bromide ion and methyl bromide in middlings and final cereal foodstuffs. Food Addit Contam 3(3): 235–240.

143. Gilvydis DM, Walters SM, Spivak ES et al, *op. cit. (see reference 116).*

144. *Ibid.*

145. Frank R, Braun HE, and Ripley BD. (1990). Residues of insecticides, fumigants, and fungicides in fruit produced in Ontario, Canada, 1986–1988. Food Addit Contam 7(5):637–648.

146. *Ibid.*

147. *Ibid.*

148. *Ibid.*

149. *Ibid.*

150. Millette JR, Clark PJ, Stober J et al. (1983). Asbestos in water supplies of the United States. Environ Health Perspect 53:45–48.

151. Washington State Department of Agriculture. (1991). Washington State Agricultural Chemicals Pilot Study. Pesticides in Groundwater. Report No. 3. Washington State Department of Agriculture, Olympia, Washington.

152. Washington State Department of Agriculture. (1991). Washington State Agricultural Chemicals Pilot Study. Pesticides in Groundwater. Report No. 2. Washington State Department of Agriculture, Olympia, Washington.

153. *Ibid.*

154. *Ibid.*

155. Environmental Working Group (1997). Weedkillers by the Glass Study. Environmental Working Group, Washington, D.C. (Website location: http://www.ewg.org).

156. *Ibid.*

157. *Ibid.*

158. *Ibid.*

159. *Ibid.*

160. *Ibid.*

161. *Ibid.*

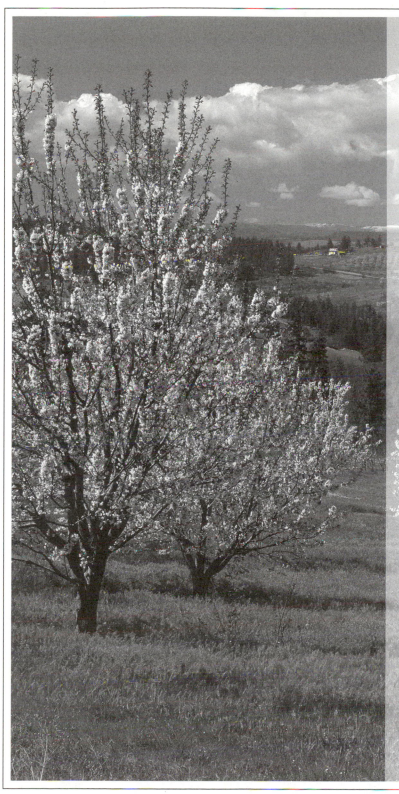

CHAPTER

Classification of Food Toxins

CONTENTS

Chapter 3: **Classification of Food Toxins**

Classification of Food Toxins

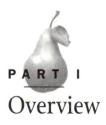

PART I
Overview

Definition of a Toxin

In textbooks of toxicology, toxins are defined as substances that cause harm to organisms.[1] The word "toxin" has its roots in the Greek word *toxikon*, literally "by smearing arrows." This connection dates back to a time when plant resins, like the curare resin obtained from *Strychnos toxifera*, were rubbed on tips of arrows to poison victims. (Curare has long since been identified as a nicotinic receptor blocking agent that prevents nerve signals from being effectively relayed to muscles. The result is paralysis, and at high doses, failure of other sensory systems.)

In the above definition of a toxin, there are only two basic factors. Those factors are *harm* and *organism*. The presence of two simple components might make the concept of a toxin also seem simple, but that is not the case. At a strong enough dose, anything can cause harm to an organism. Even water, when ingested for several hours at a rate greater than 16 milliliters per minute, can cause swelling of brain cells, convulsions and coma.

(This phenomenon is known as *water intoxication*). Because anything can be toxic at a high enough dose, we cannot evaluate the harmfulness of a substance without talking about its dose.

To further complicate matters, the guarantee of harm at a high enough dose has its corollary at the other end of the spectrum. At a low enough dose, virtually nothing is harmful. In a sufficiently small dose, the same substance that would otherwise be harmful to the body is eliminated or used for a beneficial purpose.

Exposure to Toxins: The Example of Arsenic

Arsenic is a tin-white, easily tarnished element found in arsenopyrite, cobaltite, orpiment, realgar, niccoline, and many other mineral formations throughout rocky landscapes in North America. Arsenic-containing compounds occur naturally in geology, but they also occur naturally within the human body. Inside of the body, these compounds appear to part of the body's methyl metabolism,[2] and our required daily intake of arsenic has been estimated at 12–15 micrograms.[3]

This dose of arsenic is infinitesimal, however, in comparison to the amount of arsenic that can be obtained through exposure to automobile exhaust; some colored chalks and plasters; and older toys, curtains, and carpets dyed with Paris green, a previously used color pigment. In manufacturing facilities, particularly facilities required for alloy making, bleach manufacturing, bronzing, canning, gasoline refining, smelting, and wood processing, exposure to arsenic can pose acute risk. The Occupational Safety and Health Act (OSHA) of 1970 currently allows for 500 micrograms of arsenic (30 times the estimated essential intake level) in every cubic meter of workplace air.[4]

These non-food sources of arsenic exposure still do not account for a high percentage of our total toxic risk. Over 70% of that risk comes from exposure to arsenic when we drink water, or when we eat meat, fish or poultry that contain residues from arsenical pesticides or arsenical antibiotics.[5] (Arsenicals are one category of antibiotic and are commonly used in treatment of parasitic infection, especially involving amoebae.) The U.S. Environmental Protection Agency (USEPA) currently restricts the arsenic content of drinking water to 50 micrograms per liter, but an estimated 350,000 persons in the U.S. may be routinely drinking tap water that exceeds this amount.[6]

The example of arsenic adds a new wrinkle to our definition of toxins as substances that harm organisms. Earlier we said that harm depends upon

Arsenic and Forgotten Wholeness

The example of arsenic illustrates a truth about toxins and their "safety." This truth is the truth of wholeness. The journey of arsenic through insects, parasites, drinking water, cows, fish, and chickens suggests that these beings are not separate entities lined up like books on a shelf. It suggests that they are, instead, actors in the same drama who share a common script. What any one does with his or her time onstage appears to directly transform the other. The resources available to fish are co-determined by the movement of water, and by the grazing practices of cows, and by the livestock feeding practices of farmers. When arsenic steps on stage, everything changes. It doesn't matter whether arsenic is stage left or stage right. The fish, the water, the cow, and the farmer must all co-operate and accommodate arsenic's presence. This accommodation must occur both spontaneously and co-operatively.

Along with the stage debut of arsenical pesticides comes an irony in the drama. Humans manufacture arsenical pesticides in order to kill insects that might damage the food supply. A damaged food supply might mean a food shortage. This shortage in turn could damage human health. Arsenic is added as an actor in the drama because it can bind to enzymes in insects and shut down their metabolic activity. But when the arsenic intended for insects cycles back into soil and groundwater and gets uptaken into an increasing number of foods, human exposure to arsenic broadens and becomes quantitatively increased. If this widening of arsenic exposure ends up shutting down the metabolic activity of human enzymes, the arsenic that was added was to protect human health instead returns to damage it.

At one level, scientific thinking has always acknowledged this possible irony. Use of arsenic as an insecticide and antibiotic has never been based on the scientific belief that it would act only as a protection and would pose no risk of harm. Scientists have always acknowledged that arsenic could harm humans as well as insects. To a certain extent, this acknowledgment has also stood as a recognition of wholeness. By acknowledging potential harm not only to insects but also to humans, scientists have recognized a connection between arsenic and all living things.

Yet while embracing a concept of wholeness, scientists have simultaneously adopted a position that has differentiated among organisms and predicted an equally differentiated response to arsenic. They have argued that different kinds of organisms will be harmed by different doses of arsenic, and they have predicted that insect-killing will occur at an astronomically lower dose of arsenic than human-killing (or even human-harming).

In this prediction scientists have been 100% correct. Insects are killed by doses of arsenic that do not bring harm to humans if human exposure to these doses is limited to one single, isolated moment. But ethically ▸

BACK TO BASIC CONCEPTS: Arsenic and Forgotten Wholeness

CONTINUED

and philosophically, this fact should never have been used as the basis for a decision about arsenicals, because it is a fact that separated more than it united. It is a fact that acknowledged a shared status between humans and insects, but then went on to treat humans and insects as fundamentally separate entities that could be dealt with like books on a shelf, first one and then the other. The separatist fact of a dose-different response led scientists to a logically separatist conclusion: kill parasites at a low enough dose of arsenic, and escape harmful consequences for humans. Humans 1, Parasites 0.

The philosophical problem with this scorecard was the problem of forgotten wholeness. After arsenic killed insects, it had to go *somewhere*. It surged up again (*surgere*, the Latin root for the word "resource") in the form of altered re-sources. The amount of arsenic that killed an insect wouldn't have harmed us if we had been standing next to the insect and had ingested the same amount at the same moment. But what about moments later on? What if we considered the ecological event that took place years downstream?

Taking into account the rest of the drama would have meant factoring in exposure to arsenic compounds cycling through air, water, food, and beverages. If these dramatic events had been factored in, the average adult exposure to arsenic would have become about 30 micrograms per day.[7] This amount would have been at least 2–3 times as higher than the estimated human

arsenic requirement. For persons consuming large amounts of fish, arsenic exposure might have been 70–100 times higher than the estimated requirement.[8]

Factoring in downstream events is precisely the role of environmental nutrition. Finding toxicity risk in tap water is not some vigilante crusade, political agenda, or fall into bad science. It stems from recognition of wholeness. Environmental nutrition finds toxicity risk in tap water because it sees arsenic, water, fish, cows, and farmers as participants in the same drama, co-operatively accommodating each other's presence. Environmental nutrition sees the problematic association of increased cancer[9] and vascular disease[10] following lifelong consumption of high-arsenic tap water as problems of forgotten wholeness. They are problems that encourage recognition of a bigger picture. They suggest that harm done by a food supply is not the kind of harm that can be treated like a single, one-time event in which "a little bit won't hurt you" and "everything's fine in moderation." Chronic problems associated with intake of high-arsenic tap water reflect a truth of wholeness that must be addressed across the entire spectrum of food-related activities. This spectrum includes agricultural practices, manufacturing practices, lifestyle, and eating habits. Finally, the arsenic story suggests a philosophical root for all toxicity: disregard for wholeness. Philosophically, it is this disregard that brings with it disruption, dysfunction, and disease. ■

dose. Now we are pointing out that dose is not simply the amount of a substance that someone is intentionally given (like a medical prescription), but the total amount to which a person is cumulatively exposed. A person might deliberately eat oysters to increase his or her arsenic intake, but if that person is working in a canning facility, living near a smelter, or drinking high-arsenic tap water, the oysters play a small role in total arsenic exposure.

Furthermore, once we open the door to total exposure, we raise the equally troubling question of time. If harm depends upon dose, and dose depends upon total exposure, over what period of time should exposure be measured? Is our goal to determine how much arsenic an individual is exposed to in one day? In one week? Over the course of a lifetime? For substances (including arsenic) that can be stored in the body over long periods of time, risk of toxicity can be virtually impossible to determine. Total exposure can change dramatically with a change in jobs or place of residence, and many individuals make several such changes in relatively short periods of time.

Prevalence of Food Toxins

The number of non-naturally occurring toxins present in the U.S. food supply is staggering and difficult to assess accurately. Some simple categories are helpful in understanding the magnitude of the problem, and the range of substances that make a contribution. One particularly long list of substances having potential for toxicity is the list of commercial additives available to food processors and manufacturers. This list of additives includes substances used as acidulants, antimicrobials, anticaking agents, buffers, chelating agents, clarifying agents, coloring agents, emulsifiers, enzymes, fillers, flavoring agents, flavor enhancers, gases, leavening agents, nutritive and nonnutritive sweeteners, propellants, preservatives, salts, sequestrants, stabilizers, thickeners, texturizers, and tracers. Over 2,000 of these substances are in common use worldwide,[11] and the total number of available substances may be three to four times higher.

Food Additives

Food additives do not always pose a practical risk of toxicity. In fact, the federal government established the GRAS (Generally Recognized As Safe) List of food additives in 1958 to exempt risk-free substances from toxicity testing. (This list was part of the 1958 Food Additives Amendment to the Food Drug and Cosmetic Act of 1938.) However, even within this original GRAS list and its 675 exempted substances can be found numerous

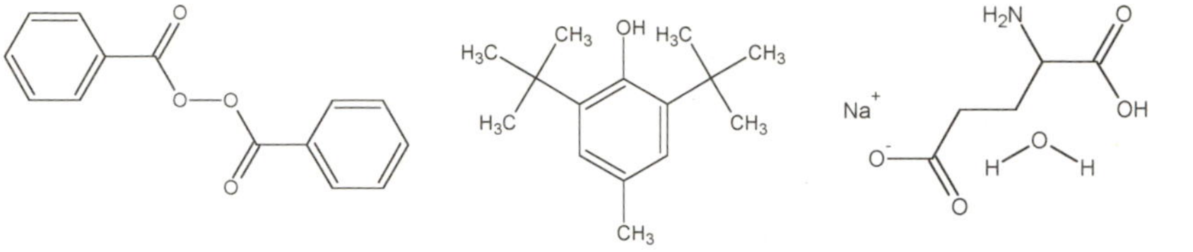

Benzoyl peroxide   Butylated hydroxytoluene   Monosodium glutamate

Figure 3-1
GRAS-listed additives

compounds that carry with them substantial risk of toxicity. These compounds include benzoyl peroxide,[12,13] butylated hydroxytoluene,[14] monosodium glutamate,[15] sodium benzoate,[16,17] and sodium bisulfite[18] (*Figure 3-1*). While the risk of toxicity associated with these substances has been clearly established, they remain on the GRAS list and continue to be commonplace additions to the food supply.

Pesticides and Other Substances

Pesticides constitute a second group of highly varied and potentially toxic compounds found in food. Approximately 400 different pesticides are currently registered for use on food,[19] and in 1988, 845 million pounds were used directly on food crops in the U.S.[20] Because of the virtually universal presence of pesticides in U.S. adult urine samples, the Centers for Disease Prevention and Control in Atlanta, Georgia have actually set up reference ranges for pesticide analytes in urine.[21]

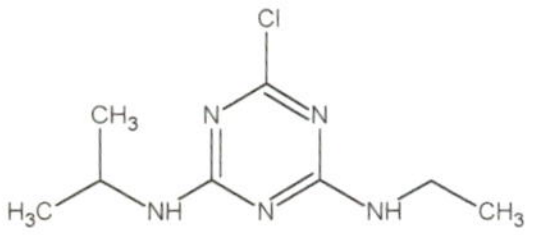

Figure 3-2
Atrazine

A 1996 study by Environmental Working Group (a not-for-profit content provider for public interest groups founded in 1993 in Washington, D.C). examined the presence of pesticides in the drinking water of 748 U.S. towns. Present in 96% of all water supplies was the pesticide atrazine (*Figure 3-2*), and in 24 towns, risk of cancer related to atrazine exposure was 15 times higher than limits established under the Food Quality Protection Act of 1996.[22] At least 20 different pesticide residues, including organochlorine and organophosphate residues, have repeatedly been found in municipal drinking waters throughout the U.S. Since 1974, under the Safe Water Drinking Act, the U.S. EPA has been charged with regulation of 83 different toxic substances known to be present in U.S. tap water.

Although less diverse in terms of the sheer numbers, other types of substances pose risk of toxicity and are normal constituents of the U.S. food supply. These types of substances include heavy metals and migrants from packaging (especially plastics). Considered in combination, this collection of food additives, pesticides, heavy metals, and packaging migrants poses an overwhelming task for clinical decision-making and even for intellectual analysis. With over 3,000 high-risk toxins routinely present in the U.S. food supply, some basic method for organizing both research and intervention becomes essential.

PART II

Classification of Toxins by Source of Exposure

In the field of toxicology (not specifically focused on food and diet) several different organizing principles are commonly used to place toxins into categories that can be helpful in research and public health. From a public health standpoint, the most common method for classifying toxins is classification by source of exposure. A brief description of exposure sources appears below.

Indoor Air

Indoor air includes air in both the home and workplace. Air quality can be compromised by a wide variety of different factors, including poor ventilation, presence of pollens and molds, presence of microorganisms, release of chemical fumes and gases, smoke, burning of indoor fuels, and faulty filtration. "Tight building syndrome," in which the design of a workspace prevents adequate exchange and circulation of air, and sick building syndrome," in which poor air circulation and exchange are combined with the presence of toxic materials, are two common clinical syndromes caused by poor indoor air quality. The term "sick building syndrome" dates back to 1982 in an EPA study commissioned by the U.S. Congress following increased complaints from U.S. workers about job-related symptoms including headache, irritation of the eyes, nose, and throat, irritability, depression, and forgetfulness.[23]

Specific substances found in polluted indoor air can themselves be classified according to source of release. For example, the burning of natural

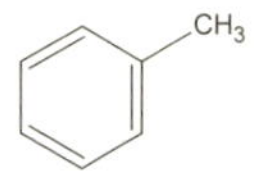

Toluene

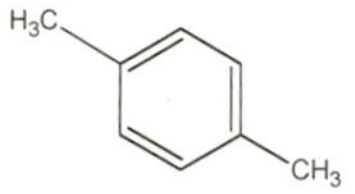

Xylene

Figure 3-3
Volatile organic compounds (VOCs)

gas generates high amounts of combustion gases including carbon monoxide (CO) and nitrogen dioxide (NO_2). If wood is burned, benzo(a)pyrenes are added to the list, along with numerous other hydrocarbons. From indoor burning of coal or oil, sulfur dioxide (SO_2) becomes a further pollutant.

Synthetic materials can also contaminate indoor air. Volatile organic compounds (or VOCs) are exceptionally common indoor air contaminants. VOCs are most commonly found in adhesives, soft plastics, caulks, sealants, paints, and varnishes. They include benzene derivatives like toluene and xylene (*Figure 3-3*) found in carpet, carpet adhesive, wallpaper adhesive, baseboard adhesive, vinyl flooring, glues, epoxies, latex paints, roofing, and polyurethane wood finish.

Cleaning products used indoors (or materials brought into contact with cleaning products) also act as contaminants. The storage of dry-cleaned clothes inside of a home can raise air concentrations of tetrachloroethylene (a VOC) to 300 micrograms per cubic meter within a 12-hour period.[24] Acetone, benzene, and benzyl alcohol are similar types of compounds frequently found in cleaning products and readily dispersed into air.

Outdoor Air

In comparison to pollutants of indoor air, outdoor air pollutants are more likely to be present in food and drinking water since natural events and cycles connect outdoor air to water, earth and plants. Atmospheric inversions (in which the natural upward movement of warmer air into the cooler and denser air above it becomes slowed or stopped) is one example of a natural event that can leave pollutants trapped at ground level and increase risk of toxicity to both persons and plants. Downwind transport (in which a plume of polluted air can be carried for miles by winds at ground level) is another example of a natural event that can heighten toxicity risk.

Extremely small particles (smaller than one micron in diameter) may stay suspended indefinitely in outdoor air, but gravity can carry larger particles directly downward and into the soil. The way that most airborne contaminants get deposited in soil, however, is by way of raindrops (or snowflakes), which assist in both the passage downward and inward among the soil's pores and crumb structure.

Researchers in Finland have determined that up to 94 micrograms of polycyclic aromatic hydrocarbons (or PAHs) may be present in a kilogram of leaf lettuce when the only source of these PAH particles is polluted air circulating above and around the growing plants.[25] Similarly, dioxin levels of up to 480 picograms per kilogram of beef have been traced by researchers in the U.S. Environmental Protection Agency (USEPA) to air vapor.[26] These researchers have postulated an "air-to-beef" food chain model in which 80% of all dioxin-like toxic particles found in beef can be traced to air vapor and can be shown to have transferred from air to soil to plants to grazing cattle.

Drinking Water

No component of human nourishment is more susceptible to toxic insult than drinking water. As described earlier in this chapter (page 84, under "Pesticides and Other Substances"), a 1996 study by the Environmental Working Group examined the prevalence of pesticides in the drinking water of 748 U.S. towns and determined virtually all of them to be contaminated with pesticide residues. Municipal drinking waters in the U.S. have also been determined to contain arsenic,[28] asbestos,[29] cadmium,[30] lead,[31] mercury,[32] nitrates, nitrites, and other N-nitroso compounds,[33] trichloroethylene,[34] and halogenated hydrocarbons including trihalomethane.[35] National standards for water quality were set for the first time in 1974 with Congressional passage of the Safe Water Drinking Act (SWDA). Under the act, MCLs, (maximal contaminant levels) were established for approximately 80 different contaminants, including volatile and non-volatile organics, inorganics, radioactive substances, and coliform bacteria. Enforcement of MCLs was assigned to the U.S. Environmental Protection Agency. A complete listing of these drinking water standards is presented in *Appendix A*.

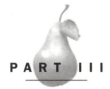

PART III

Classification of Toxins by Chemical Group: Organic Compounds

From a research and technical standpoint, the most common method of classifying toxins is by chemical group. Because this classification method will be used throughout the remainder of the text, the following pages provide a closer look at the chemical groups used to classify food toxins.

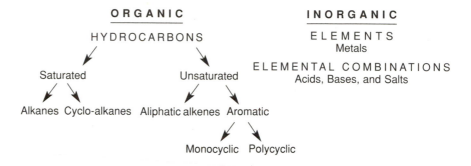

Figure 3-4
Chemical categorization of toxins

As indicated in *Figure 3-4*, toxicologists make a basic and first-level distinction between food supply toxins that are organic versus inorganic. In this context the word "organic" simply means containing the element carbon. "Inorganic" designates the opposite and refers to toxins that do not contain carbon.

Hydrocarbons

The simplest of all organic, carbon-containing compounds that we will examine in the food supply are hydrocarbons, that is, compounds composed solely of hydrogen and carbon atoms. When all of the atoms in a hydrocarbon are joined together by single covalent bonds, the hydrocarbon is referred to as saturated. A single covalent bond between atoms occurs when each of the atoms decides to share one electron with the other. In this case, the two atoms are said to be sharing a "single electron pair." The sharing of this electron pair draws the nuclei of the two atoms together by a net electrochemical force of attraction.

Saturated Hydrocarbons

Acyclic Alkanes

Alkanes constitute the simplest group of saturated hydrocarbons. These substances are composed exclusively of single-bonded carbon and hydrogen atoms, and do not tend to interact with other molecules. For this reason they are often referred to as parrafins or parrafinic hydrocarbons (from the Latin *parrum affinis*, or "little affinity"). The most likely event to take place with saturated hydrocarbons is burning, as occurs with candles made of parrafins.

Alkanes are generally divided into two structural categories. Acyclic alkanes are straight-chain, saturated hydrocarbons that do not form ring shapes. Cyclic alkanes, typically called cycloalkanes, are saturated hydrocarbons that exist as rings. *Figure 3-5* illustrates the chemical structure of methane, the simplest of all acyclic alkanes that contains a single carbon atom. *Table 3-1* lists names and formulas for the eight simplest alkanes. The name for an alkane always ends with the letters "-ane," and the first letters of the name indicate the number of carbon atoms in the alkane. The first letters of the name are used as prefixes not only for alkanes, but for many kinds of carbon-containing compounds.

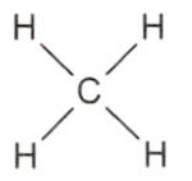

Figure 3-5
Methane

n-Hexane. In the petroleum industry, parrafinic hydrocarbons constitute one category of crude oils. Along with the categories of asphaltic and mixed crude oils, paraffinic oils can be distilled under high heat to produce a wide variety of petroleum solvents, including *n*-hexane. *n*-hexane (the 6-carbon alkane illustrated in *Figure 3-6*) is a colorless, volatile liquid whose most common food use is in the extraction of soy oil from soybeans.[36]

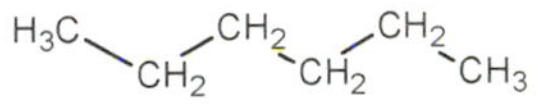

Figure 3-6
n-Hexane

For workers in the soy processing industry, as well as other industries involving use of *n*-hexane solvents, occupational exposure may reach 1800 milligrams/cubic meter of air.[37] *n*-hexane has been shown to induce neuropathy in humans when occupational exposures reach the 100ppm (parts per million) level, and measurement of urinary 2,5-hexanedione can be measured to monitor *n*-hexane exposure.[38] The toxicity of *n*-hexane is at least partly related to its induction of metallothionein-synthesizing enzymes in the liver. Research has demonstrated increased accumulation of metallothionein (MT) in the liver following exposure to *n*-hexane, and this increased MT concentration has been associated with increased inflammatory response.[39]

Table 3-1. ***Alkanes***

Name	Carbons	Hydrogens	Formula
Meth*ane*	1	4	C_1H_4
Eth*ane*	2	6	C_2H_6
Prop*ane*	3	8	C_3H_8
But*ane*	4	10	C_4H_{10}
Pent*ane*	5	12	C_5H_{12}
Hex*ane*	6	14	C_6H_{14}
Hept*ane*	7	16	C_7H_{16}
Oct*ane*	8	18	C_8H_{18}

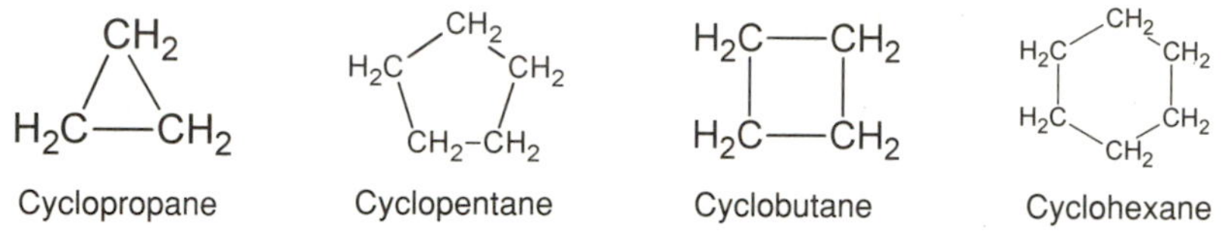

Figure 3-7
Cycloalkanes

Cycloalkanes

In contrast to the straight-chain structure shown for *n*-hexane in *Figure 3-6*, alkanes can also form rings. Ring-shaped alkanes are referred to as cycloalkanes. *Figure 3-7* shows the basic structure of the cycloalkanes containing 3-8 carbon atoms. Unless substituted (as discussed in the following paragraphs), the cycloalkanes have more industrial uses outside the food industry than inside it. Out of 3.38 million gallons of cyclohexane produced in 1992, for example, over 90% was used in the manufacturing of nylon. Similarly, cyclopropane is used primarily as a fuel in gas stoves and other heating equipment.

Halogenation of Alkanes

Table 3-2 shows the family of naturally-occurring elements referred to as the halogens. The atomic number of each halogen is shown in the far left-hand column. This number refers to the number of protons contained within the nucleus of the atom. An atom of fluorine, for example, contains 9 protons in its nucleus. The six columns on the far right of the table, labeled letters *k-p*, refer to the electron shells within the atoms. These shells are imagined as primary energy levels wrapped concentrically around the nucleus. Each level has a fixed number of electrons that it can accommodate, and the distance of a level from the nucleus determines how much

Table 3-2. **The halogens**

Number	Symbol	Name	*k*	*l*	*m*	*n*	*o*	*p*
9	F	Fluorine	2	7				
17	Cl	Chlorine	2	8	7			
35	Br	Bromine	2	8	18	7		
53	I	Iodine	2	8	18	18	7	
85	At	Astatine	2	8	18	32	18	7

energy it takes for electrons to reside there. The further a level is located from the nucleus, the more energy it takes for electrons to reside there. The *l* level, for example, can hold 8 electrons, and it takes more energy for electrons to reside there than inside level *k*, closer to the nucleus.

According to the atomic theory developed by Danish physicist Niels Bohr in the early 1900s, the energetics of an element and its relationship with other elements depend heavily on the number of electrons residing in the element's outermost energy level. All halogens, for example, have 7 electrons in their outermost energy level (even though for fluorine this outermost level is level *l*, while for bromine it's level *n*).

Energy levels help explain how halogens like fluorine can interact with hydrocarbons and become incorporated into their structure. The *l* level of fluorine can hold a maximum of 8 electrons. Under normal circumstances, however, this *l* level contains only 7. If fluorine can find another element willing to share one of its electrons, fluorine can bring the electron count in its *l* level up to 8, completely fill its outermost energy level, and favorably alter its energetics. One of the ways for fluorine to accomplish this feat is by replacing one of the hydrogen atoms in a hydrocarbon. Once the fluorine atom has taken over the hydrogen's spot, it can begin sharing an electron with the carbon atom to which the hydrogen was previously attached. Since fluorine is classified as a halogen, this process is referred to as halogenation. Even more specifically, it is referred to as fluorination, since the specific halogen involved is fluorine. Chlorination (substituting a chlorine for a hydrogen), bromination (substituting a bromine), and iodination (substituting an iodine) are also examples of halogenation reactions.

Halogenated compounds are pervasive in the U.S. food supply, and as a group, may pose the largest risk of food-related toxicity. Compounds that have been halogenated with the element chlorine are particularly problematic. Halogenation is possible not only for saturated hydrocarbons like alkanes, but for unsaturated hydrocarbons as well. (The term organochlorines is often used to refer collectively to all organic molecules containing chlorine). While most of the halogenated hydrocarbons that pose high risk of food-related toxicity are unsaturated and aromatic (reviewed later in this chapter, pages 100–108), there are several halogenated alkanes that also pose substantial risk.

Dichloromethane. Dichloromethane, also known as methylene chloride, methane dichloride, and methylene bichloride, is one such halogenated alkane. The substitution of two chlorine atoms for two hydrogen atoms on methane results in the production of a highly toxic compound that is

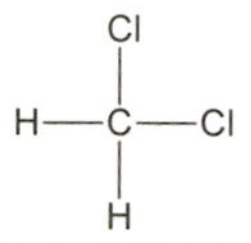

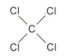

Figure 3-8
Dichloromethane

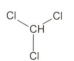

Figure 3-9
Carbon tetrachloride

readily absorbed from the intestine and can also cross the blood brain barrier. Current U.S. Food and Drug Administration (USFDA) standards permit up to 220ppm of dichloromethane in brewing hops, 30ppm in spice extracts, and 10ppm in decaffeinated coffee. (Prior to the use of dichloromethane as a coffee decaffeinating agent, the most common hydrocarbon extraction method involved trichloroethylene, in which three chlorine atoms were substituted for three hydrogen atoms on an unsaturated, two-carbon hydrocarbon, and tetrachloroethylene, which involved the substitution of four chlorines). *Figure 3-8* depicts the structure of dichloromethane.

Carbon Tetrachloride.   Carbon tetrachloride, also known as methane tetrachloride, requires the substitution of four chlorine atoms for all four hydrogen atoms in methane. *Figure 3-9* illustrates the structure of carbon tetrachloride. Although no longer permitted within the U.S. as a direct grain fumigant due to its well-documented toxicity, carbon tetrachloride is still widely used in the workplace and passes on into the food chain via airborne transport. (Fumigants are a category of hydrocarbons that exist as gases at room temperature. Their predominant agricultural use is the killing of insects found in the soil, or more commonly, in the air when foods have been stored within confined spaces such as silos, grain elevators, or warehouses).

EDB and EDC.   Ethylene dibromide (EDB) and ethylene dichloride (EDC) are two additional food fumigants that also fall into the category of halogenated alkanes. In the case of EDB, two bromine atoms are substituted for two hydrogens on a two-carbon ethane molecule. In the case of EDC, two chlorines are substituted (*Figure 3-10*). Although more likely to be used in the production of vinyl chloride (the precursor of many plastics) or in the manufacture of "anti-knock" gasoline, EDC and EDB not only remain in direct use as food fumigants but also make their way into the food supply through contamination of air and water.

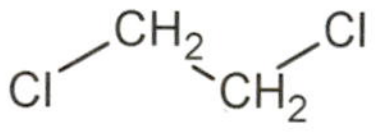

Chloroform.   A final halogenated alkane with important food-related toxicity is chloroform. Also called trichloromethane, methyl trichloride, or formyl trichloride, chloroform is a substituted alkane in which three chlorines have taken the place of three hydrogen atoms in the molecule (*Figure 3-11*). Because the vast majority of public drinking waters in the U.S. are chlorinated, widespread exposure to chloroform comes from consumption of simple tap water. The USEPA has estimated an average daily intake of 64–136 micrograms of chloroform per day based solely on intake of tap water. Because chloroform is produced industrially in large quantities (approximately 150,000 tons per year), atmospheric release and workplace-based exposure are also common.

Figure 3-10
EDC

Figure 3-11
Chloroform

Petroleum and the Food Supply

The Food-Hydrocarbon Mismatch

This textbook devotes a considerably number of pages to analysis of hydrocarbon compounds found in food. From a chemical standpoint, however, it is highly unusual to place hydrocarbons at the center of such an analysis. In its naturally-occurring state, food simply does not contain much hydrocarbon content. This absence of hydro-carbons from food appears to linked to the fact that hydrocarbons are composed exclusively of hydrogen and carbon, and this limited combination of elements is simply too inflexible to serve the needs of living organisms.

All major components of food have critical features that distinguish them from hydrocarbons. The largest chemical component of food is water (H_2O), a molecule containing no carbon. The second largest food component, carbohydrate, combines water with carbon. However, it is still not a hydrocarbon, since it always contains oxygen. The third and fourth most common components of food, namely fats and proteins, are still distinctly different from hydrocarbons in their chemical composition. Fats, although somewhat similar to hydrocarbons in structure, always include oxygen in their composition. Proteins always include not only oxygen, but also nitrogen.

From a chemical standpoint, the fact that hydrocarbons have become a routine part of the U.S. food supply is chemically unusual. This highlight examines underlying reasons for this unusualness by focusing on historical events that lead up to the introduction of hydrocarbons into the food supply. The highlight also finds these historical events to end up sharing a common denominator, namely, petroleum.

Petroleum and the Earth Sciences

In earth sciences (like geology, physical geography, or oceanography), "sediment" is defined as any mineral or organic (carbon-containing) material that is derived from erosion of rocks or decay of plants over long periods of time. Under certain types of environmental conditions (for example, conditions in which little oxygen is present), plants materials can accumulate (instead of completely decomposing) in select spots across the earth on a large-scale basis. When this accumulation happens over an extended period of time, plant deposits become compacted due to burial pressure and form unique organic substances. These organic substances can be solid (like peat and coal) or liquid (like petroleum) or gaseous (like natural gas).

Peat is the first organic solid to accumulate under the conditions described above. It is soft, fibrous, brown or black in color, and found predominantly in swampy lowlands where water prevents complete decomposition of plant parts. If the compaction process continues, peat gets transformed into lignite, also called "brown coal." ◗

Although lignite is the softest of all compacted hydrocarbon sediments referred to as "coals," lignite is still substantially more solid than peat and has significant industrial value. In the U.S., lignite has been found in coal fields throughout the south (including Arkansas, Alabama, Louisiana, Mississippi and Texas) and in the mid-West (including North Dakota and Montana).

Further burial pressure over time converts lignite into primary and secondary bituminous coal. This soft, black coal has the widest spectrum of industrial uses. In the continental United States, primary bituminous coal fields are located in Alabama, Illinois, Indiana, Ohio, Pennsylvania, Tennessee, and West Virginia, while secondary bituminous coal deposits are located primarily in the Rocky Mountain ranges and in the Mid-West.

When bituminous deposits become subjected to even greater pressure over vast periods of time, the soft black coals can undergo metamorphosis from their dull iron-black color into a brighter, vitreous and more hardened material. The end-stage products of this metamorphosis,

namely anthracite and graphite, are the hardest of the black coals. Hundreds of millions of years are required for completion of these sedimentary processes. A summary of these coal-forming stages is presented in *Table 3-3* below.

Sedimentary deposits can also evolve in liquid form. Petroleum, or crude oil, is one such liquid and it is most commonly derived from bituminous deposits. Petroleum, like coal, is composed predominantly of carbon (82%) and hydrogen (15%), and thus consists almost solely of hydrocarbon mixtures. When processed industrially, petroleum is described as being broken down into fractions. The liquid propane gas (or LPG) fraction is formed primarily of the alkanes propane (three carbons) and butane (four carbons). Naphthas (which include the liquid we commonly refer to as gasoline) consist of hydrocarbons ranging in length from 4–100 carbons. Gasoline includes not only alkanes, but other hydrocarbons including cycloalkanes and aromatics. Asphaltic crude oils, which we use to make asphalt, constitute yet another petroleum fraction. ▶

Table 3.3. **The coal forming process**

Sedimentary stage	Description	Mechanism of formation
Peat	Partially decomposed plant material	Rapid plant growth with minimum activity of microorganisms
Lignite	Soft, brown coal	Burial pressure
Bituminous	Soft, black coal	Burial pressure
Anthracite	Hard, black coal	Metamorphosis

HISTORICAL PERSPECTIVES: Petroleum and the Food Supply
CONTINUED

When industrial processing subjects coal to high heat and oxygen, yet another hydrocarbon mixture can be formed. This mixture is called coke. Coke can be used as a key components in the manufacturing of steel. Within the coal industry, coke remains one of the key products of coal distillation.

Petroleum and Food Production

Equally helpful in understanding the unnatural appearance of hydrocarbons in the food supply is a brief historical review of business relationships between the petroleum and food industries. Prior to the second world war, most increases in food production in the United States had been accomplished by increases in amount of land under cultivation.[40] Following the war, increases in yield began to be accomplished not by increasing land cultivation but by increasing "energy inputs." These "inputs" focused on petroleum-based chemicals and petroleum-driven machinery.[41] As agriculture became more dependent upon chemical technology and the technology of gas-driven machinery, food companies began to expand their boards of directors to include senior management members from corporations involved in petroleum extraction and refinement. A 1980s profile of boards of directors from the largest food companies in the United States (including Beatrice, Borden's, Campbell's, ConAgra, CPC International, General Foods, General Mills, Heinz, Kellogg, Kraft, PepsiCo, and Pillsbury) shows widespread board representation from gasoline companies like Amoco, Exxon, and Mobile, as well as chemical production companies like American Cyanamid, Dow Chemical, and 3M.

Overlapping corporate interest in food/chemical production has been more recently been illustrated by the emergence of companies like Novartis. Formed in 1996 by the merger of CIBA-Geigy and Sandoz, Novartis remains the largest pesticide-producing company in the world. (In 1997, agrochemical sales by Novartis totaled $4.2 billion.) Simultaneously, through its nutritional products like Resource™ , Novartis remains a central figure in the practice of professional dietetics. Novartis ranks annually among the top 10 advertisers in the *Journal of the American Dietetic Association*, and among the top 10 contributors to the National Center for Nutrition and Dietetics (a research and information organization founded by the American Dietetic Association).

Use of petroleum by-products in food processing can be viewed as a natural outcome of corporate interests that encompass production of industrial chemicals as well as production of food. The appearance of solvents like benzene, pesticides like dieldrin, and coal tar dyes like erythrosine in the U.S. food supply can be expected to continue alongside of these overlapping corporate interests. (For a closer look at coal tar dyes like erythrosine, see the section "Coal Tar Dyes" beginning on page 109 of this chapter.) ■

Figure 3-12
Ethene

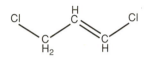

Figure 3-13
Dichloropropene

Unsaturated Hydrocarbons

Alkenes

In contrast with single, covalent bonds in which atoms share one pair of electrons, atoms can also decide to share two or more electron pairs. When two pairs are shared, the covalent bond is referred to as a double bond. Hydrocarbons containing at least one double bond are referred to as unsaturated hydrocarbons.

Alkenes are the simplest of the unsaturated hydrocarbons. A list of the seven simplest alkenes is presented in *Table 3-4*. *Figure 3-12* shows the structure of ethene, the simplest of the alkenes. When unsaturated hydrocarbons contain two double bonds, they are referred to as dienes. If the number of double bonds is three, the alkenes are designated as trienes.

While alkene-related toxicity from diets is most likely to involve the plastic packaging of foods, (see "Polymerized Alkenes" below), halogenated alkenes can also be directly incorporated into food through the use of alkene-based fumigants and pesticides. 1,3-dichloropropene is one such alkene. This soil fumigant is based on the three-carbon molecule propene, in which two chlorine atoms have been substituted for two hydrogen atoms at the first and third carbons. (*Figure 3-13*).

Polymerized Alkenes

"Polymerization" refers to the process of making polymers. A polymer (from the Greek *poly* + *meros*, or "many parts") is defined as any large molecule that was made by taking a single structural unit and repeating it. In the case of polymerized alkenes, the single structural unit is an alkene. If the simplest of the alkenes is chosen, the two-carbon molecule ethene becomes the structural unit to be repeated (*Figure 3-12*). In the plastic-making industry, ethene

Table 3.4. Alkenes

Name	Carbons	Hydrogens	Formula
Eth*ene*	2	4	C_2H_4
Prop*ene*	3	6	C_3H_6
But*ene*	4	8	C_4H_8
Pent*ene*	5	10	C_5H_{10}
Hex*ene*	6	12	C_6H_{12}
Hept*ene*	7	14	C_7H_{14}
Oct*ene*	8	16	C_8H_{16}

is more commonly referred to as ethylene. When hundreds of ethylene units are attached to form a long ethylene chain is formed, the resulting polymer is called *polyethylene* (*Figure 3-14*). During the process of polymerization the double-bond is lost. Number 2 plastic, frequently used to make milk jugs and other food containers, is typically referred to as "HDPE" or high density polyethylene. Number 4 plastic, commonly found in bread bags, food wraps, and grocery store produce bags, is designated as "LDPE" or low density polyethylene.

If, instead of a two-carbon alkene, a three-carbon alkene is chosen, the repeating structural unit becomes propene (*Figure 3-15*). When propene (also called propylene) is polymerized, the resulting molecule is referred to as polypropylene. Containers for margarine, syrup, and yogurt, as well as drinking straws, are frequently made out of polypropylene. Polypropylene or "PP" is also designated as Number 5 plastic. The six basic types of plastic, their alkene-based structural units, and their most-common uses in food packaging are summarized in *Table 3-5*. The symbols used on packaging to represent these types of plastics to consumers are shown in the first column of *Table 3-5*.

$$(-CH_2-CH_2-)_n$$

n = number of ethene molecules

Figure 3-14
Chemical formula for polyethylene

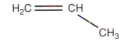

Figure 3-15
Propene

Table 3-5. **Plastic packaging**

Number	Abbreviation	Name	Uses
1	PET	Polyethylene terephthalate	Beverage bottles (like 2-liter pop bottles), frozen food boil-in-the-bag pouches and microwave food trays
2	HDPE	High density polyethylene	Milk jugs, trash bags, detergent bottles, base cups of large pop bottles
3	V	Vinyl	Cooking oil bottles, packaging around meat
4	LDPE	Low density polyethylene	Grocery store produce bags, bread bags, and film food wrap
5	PP	Polypropylene	Yogurt containers, shampoo bottles, straws, syrup bottles, and margarine tubs
6	PS	Polystyrene	(Better known as styrofoam™) hot beverage cups, fast food clamshell containers, egg cartons, and meat trays. Crystal version is used in clear plastic drinking cups and deli containers
7	Other		All other materials

Research studies have clearly shown migration of plastics into food across a wide range of temperatures and with a wide variety of foods. What is debated in the research literature is not whether these plastics migrate, but how much migration is needed before toxicity becomes a health risk. Later in this chapter (page 103, under "Phthalic acid") we will look at one example of packaging migrants that can compromise health, and in Chapter 5 (page 214, under "Toxic Induction of P450 Enzymes") we will review the role of several additional packaging migrants in compromising liver health through overactivation of liver enzymes.

In addition to being polymerized, alkenes may also be halogenated in order to construct certain packaging materials. Within the food industry, the most widely-used of the polymerized, halogenated alkenes is PVC, or polyvinyl chloride. In PVC, the repeating structural unit is vinyl chloride (*Figure 3-16*). This structural unit consists of an ethylene molecule in which one hydrogen has been replaced by one chlorine. PVC containers are used for a wide variety of foods, including drinking water, alcoholic beverages, and vinegars.

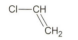

Figure 3-16
Vinyl chloride

Unsubstituted Monocyclic Aromatics

No group of hydrocarbons contributes more risk of toxicity to the food supply than the group of unsaturated hydrocarbons referred to as the aromatics. What this group of unsaturated hydrocarbons has in common is a benzene ring system of atoms (or a system very similar to it). *Figure 3-17* illustrates this benzene ring system of atoms. Although the term "aromatic" suggests that all hydrocarbons in this category have a definite smell or odor, many do not. The term "aromatic" is a left-over from the early history of organic chemistry. During that time, substances found in peppermint, thyme, and vanilla possessed distinctive fragrances and were the best-researched of the aromatic hydrocarbons. Today, however, there is an equal or even greater amount of research involving aromatic hydrocarbons like aspirin (acetylsalicylic acid) that have no fragrance.

The benzene system of atoms is molecularly unique. The electrons shared by carbon atoms in the benzene ring participate in what is called pi bonding. This unusual type of bonding allows electrons contained in the outermost shells of the carbon atoms to spread out and become more stable. The stability of benzene does not mean, however, than it cannot readily transform from a liquid to a gas, or that it cannot be subjected to a vast number of substitution reactions in which its hydrogen atoms get replaced by other atoms or chemical groups.

Earlier in this chapter (page 90, under "Halogenation of Alkanes") we

Figure 3-17
Benzene

reviewed the process of halogenation and described the ability of the halogens (fluorine, chlorine, bromine, and iodine) to replace hydrogen atoms in the structure of the alkane molecules. This substitution (of halogens for hydrogens) also takes place in benzene rings. The vast majority of aromatic food toxins have undergone substitution in their benzene ring structure. (These substituted aromatics are reviewed in the following section of this chapter.) However, several non-substituted monocyclic aromatics are also important contaminants in the food supply.

Benzene. Discovered in compressed oil gas by chemist Michael Faraday in 1825 and easily obtained from the coking of coal, benzene has achieved almost universal presence in the environment. Its vast array of industrial uses has earned it a ranking as the fifth most hazardous substance in the U.S., according to the 1997 CERCLA (Comprehensive Environmental Response, Compensation, and Liability Act) Priority List of Hazardous Substances (*see Appendix B*).[43] Part of the characteristic odor of unleaded gasoline at fuel pumps is provided by benzene, which can account for 3% of some unleaded fuels. A wide variety of oils and resins, paints and dyes, plastics and adhesives, and industrial and household cleaners are benzene-based since benzene contains outstanding solvent properties. Manufacture of asphalt, rubber, and detergents is also likely to involve use of benzene. (The chemical structure of benzene is illustrated in *Figure 3-17*).

Following its widespread industrial use, benzene has also emerged as a critical contaminant in the U.S. food supply. The USEPA has set a maximum contaminant level of 5 ppb (5 micrograms per liter) for drinking water. Benzene residues in excess of this amount have also been found in a wide variety of foods. These foods include a variety of fruits and vegetables,[44] salmon,[45] chicken, and eggs (following ingestion by the chickens of water previously determined to be contaminated with benzene).[46] Benzene has also been shown to migrate from non-stick cookware and microwave susceptors into food at a micrograms-per-square-decimeter level.[47]

Not appearing on the CERCLA Priority List of Hazardous Substances (*see Appendix B*), but also prevalent in the U.S. food supply is the substance benzoic acid (*Figure 3-22*). Benzoic acid consists of a single benzene ring in which one hydrogen has been replaced by a carboxylic acid group. Since benzoic acid is chemically classified as a substituted monocyclic aromatic hydrocarbon, it is discussed on the following page, under the heading "Substituted Moncyclic Aromatics."

Unsubstituted monocyclic aromatic hydrocarbons form a major part of a loosely-defined and vast category of organic substances generally known

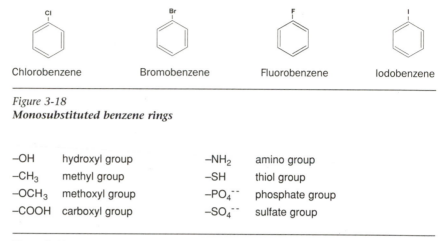

Figure 3-18
Monosubstituted benzene rings

−OH	hydroxyl group	−NH₂	amino group
−CH₃	methyl group	−SH	thiol group
−OCH₃	methoxyl group	−PO₄⁻⁻	phosphate group
−COOH	carboxyl group	−SO₄⁻⁻	sulfate group

Figure 3-19
Non-halogen functional groups

as VOCs, or volatile organic compounds. VOCs are carbon-containing molecules that readily evaporate and form gases at room temperature. Literally thousands of compounds can be classified as VOCs. Because of their gas-forming ability, VOCs are often chosen as a category for analysis in studying airborne pollutants, or pollutants that are measured in the exhaled breath of human subjects.

Substituted Monocyclic Aromatics

As described earlier, pi bonding in a benzene ring allows the molecule to become more stable and strongly resistant to disruption. It does not, however, prevent the molecule from reacting with other chemicals. Earlier in this chapter (page 90, under "Halogenation of Alkanes") we reviewed the process of halogenation and described the ability of the halogens (fluorine, chlorine, bromine, and iodine) to replace hydrogen atoms in the structure of the alkane molecules. This substitution (of halogens for hydrogens) also takes place in benzene rings. When a single hydrogen is replaced, the resulting benzene ring is referred to as a monosubstituted benzene. *(Figure 3-18)* are examples of monosubstituted (and halogenated) benzene rings.

Halogens are not the only elements that can substitute for hydrogen atoms on benzene rings. Nitrogen-containing groups, sulfur-containing groups, phosphorus-containing groups, oxygen-containing groups, and methyl groups are additional functional groups that commonly replace hydrogen in benzene rings. *Figure 3-19* illustrates several of the most common non-halogen functional groups.

When at least one hydrogen atom within a benzene ring has been replaced by a hydroxyl group, the resulting compound can be classified as a phenol. Phenols are simply benzene rings with hydroxyl groups attached. While many phenolic compounds are discussed in this text in relationship to their potential for toxicity, food naturally contains thousands of phenols that are indispensable to health. While not technically classified as phenols, the aromatic amino acids tyrosine, phenylalanine, and tryptophan either contain a phenolic residue or are precursors to other compounds (like the neurotransmitters epinephrine and serotonin) that contain such residues (*Figure 3-20*).

Many nutritive constituents of plants are classified as phenols. These constituents include substances found in the volatile oils of spices and seasonings. Examples of volatile oil components found in peppermint, thyme, and vanilla bean are illustrated in *Figure 3-21*. All flavonoids, including the citrus fruit flavonols, the soybean isoflavones, and select components of milk thistle (*Silybum marianum*), gingko (*Gingko biloba*), and literally hundreds of other medicinal herbs are also classified as phenols or polyphenols, (which contain at least two phenolic residues).

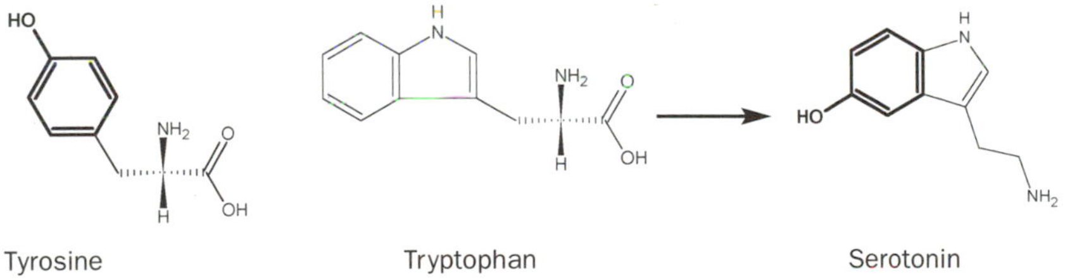

Tyrosine   Tryptophan   Serotonin

Figure 3-20
Phenolic residues in amino acids or their derivatives

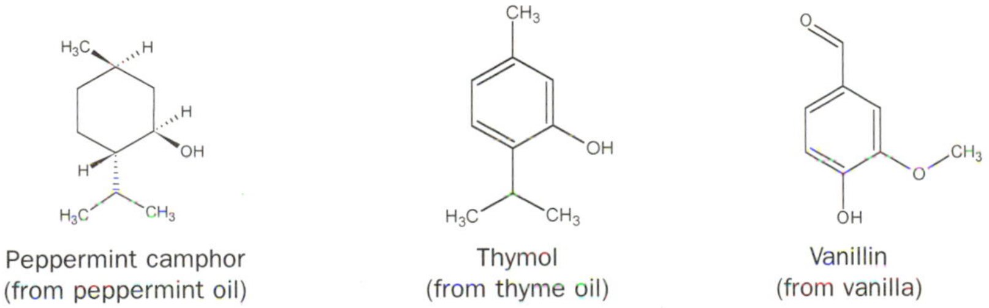

Peppermint camphor   Thymol   Vanillin
(from peppermint oil)   (from thyme oil)   (from vanilla)

Figure 3-21
Constituents of volatile oils classified as phenols

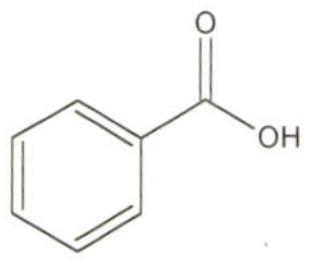

Figure 3-22
Benzoic acid

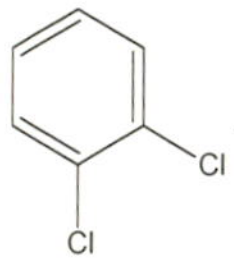

Figure 3-23
Dichlorobenzene

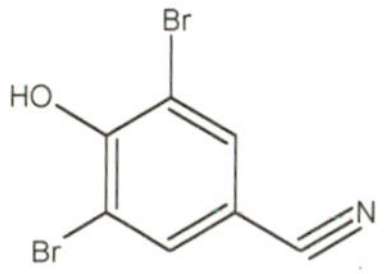

Figure 3-24
Bromoxynil

Benzoic Acid. The widely-used food preservative benzoic acid (*Figure 3-22*) is also classified as a substituted monocyclic aromatic hydrocarbon. As previously described, benzoic acid consists of a benzene ring in which one hydrogen atom has been replaced by a carboxylic acid group. Benzoic acid is commonly found in foods in the form of sodium benzoate, and was included along with 674 other substances on the original GRAS List established under the 1958 Food Additives Amendment to the Food, Drug and Cosmetic Act of 1938. Because of its ability to inhibit the growth of bacteria, yeasts, and molds, benzoic acid is commonly found in a wide variety of foods including sodas, fruit products (including jellies), margarines, syrups, sauces and salad dressings, cakes, chewing gum and candies. In a double-blind, placebo-controlled study, ingestion of benzoic acid by children has been associated with increased risk of urticaria.[48] Anaphylaxis and asthma have also been associated with ingestion of benzoic acid,[49] as well as with airborne exposure.[50]

It is also common for substitution to occur at several hydrogen sites on a benzene ring. When this happens, the benzene ring is described as *polysubstituted*. The common air deodorizer and moth repellent *p*-dichlorobenzene (or DCB, *Figure 3-23*) is a polysubstituted (and halogenated) benzene ring. It is a chemical that has also been found in the urine of 980 out of 1,000 adults living across the United States in concentrations reaching 8.7 milligrams per liter.[51] In fact, exposure of U.S. citizens to dichlorobenzene has been so common that the U.S. Centers for Disease Control in Atlanta, Georgia have set urinary reference ranges for dichlorobenzene for all U.S. adults.[52]

Halogenated and polysubstituted benzene systems are also common among pesticides. Included in this category are the insecticides hexachlorobenzene (HCB, also called lindane), and the pre-harvest defoliant and herbicide pentachlorophenol (PCP). In many instances, different hydrogens on a benzene ring get replaced by different types of chemical groups. The insecticide 2,4-dinitrophenol and the herbicide bromoxynil (*Figure 3-24*) are examples of differentially polysubstituted benzene rings. Like dichlorobenzene, these molecules have had more than one hydrogen replaced within their ring structure. However, unlike dichlorobenzene which has two hydrogens replaced by two chlorines, 2,4-dinitrophenol and bromoxynil have hydrogen atoms replaced by more than one type of chemical group.

BHA and BHT. The widely-used food preservatives BHA (butylated hydroxytoluene) and BHT (butylated hydroxyanisole) are also good examples of compounds containing differentially polysubstituted benzene rings. In both cases, hydrogens in the benzene system have been replaced by methyl, methoxyl, and hydroxyl groups (*Figure 3-25*). (The presence of these hydroxyl groups allows these molecules to be classified as phenols, as describe above). Foods most likely to include BHA as a preservative include flaked breakfast cereal, baked goods, cake icing, muffin mix, and dried meat. BHT is commonly found in the same products, along with potato flakes, enriched rice products, and shortening. Both the FAO/WHO (Food and Agricultural Organization/World Health Organization) and the EEC (European Economic Community) have set limits on the amount of BHA and BHT that they find acceptable in a daily diet. A Netherlands study has found these limits to be routinely exceeded for BHT in all age and sex groups, with particular excesses occurring in children ages 1–6.[53]

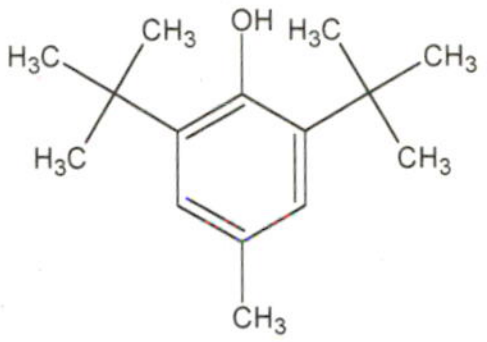

Coupled with their use as direct food additives is the use of BHA and BHT as packaging components. Rather than placing these preservatives directly in food, many companies have created packaging materials that contain BHT. When used in this way BHT may legally be classified as an "incidental" food additive and need not be reported on a list of ingredients.

Phthalic Acid. Phthalic acid is a final polysubstituted benzene system that deserves special mention in relationship to food. This aromatic hydrocarbon is a single benzene ring in which two hydrogens have been replaced by two carboxyl groups (*Figure 3-26*). Our most common exposure to phthalic acid comes in the form of Number 1 plastic, or PET (polyethylene terephthalate). Soda pop bottles, water bottles, boil-in-the-bag frozen food pouches, and microwave containers are commonly composed of PET. PET is also used on the interior surfaces of microwave packaging to heighten the absorption of microwave energy and allow quicker heating and browning. The gray or mirror-like surface on the inside of microwave pizza packaging is an example of PET used in this capacity. PET has been shown to migrate from plastic containers into carbonated soft drinks,[54] butters/margarines,[55] and french fries, waffles, popcorn, fish sticks, and pizza.[56]

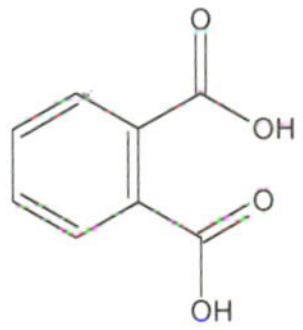

Halogenated Biphenyls. When a carbon atom from one benzene ring covalently bonds to a carbon atom from a second benzene ring, the resulting molecule is referred to as a biphenyl. (A second way for benzene rings to join together is by fusing. When benzenes fuse, two-carbon atoms are actually shared by both rings, the resulting molecules are referred to as polycyclic aromatic hydrocarbons, or PAHs. These molecules will be reviewed in the next section of this text. The difference between biphenyls and two-ring polycyclic aromatic compounds is illustrated in *Figures 3-27* and *3-28*.

If benzene rings get joined together by a carbon-to-carbon bond and also become halogenated, they are described as halogenated biphenyls. The

Figure 3-25
BHT

Figure 3-26
Phthalic acid

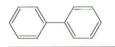

Figure 3-27
Basic structure of biphenyls

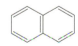

Figure 3-28
Basic structure of 2-ring polyclyclic aromatics

most famous of the halogenated biphenyls are the highly-toxic PCBs (poly-chlorinated biphenyls) and PBBs (polybrominated biphenyls).

PCBs and PBBs. Several decades ago, the low flammability of PCBs spawned their widespread industrial use as coolants for electrical and hydraulic equipment. During the 1960s and 1970s, they also found frequent use in the manufacturing of plastics, adhesives, inks, and dyes. When several regulatory organizations like the National Institute of Occupational Safety and Health (NIOSH) began to classify PCBs as occupational carcinogens, their widespread use in manufacturing rapidly decreased. However, they continue to be used in the manufacture of electrical equipment like transformers and capacitors, and persist in the environment in surprising amounts. During the past five years, PCBs have repeatedly been found in the fat cells and liver cells of adults,[57] in fetal fat stores,[58] and in the milk of nursing mothers.[59]

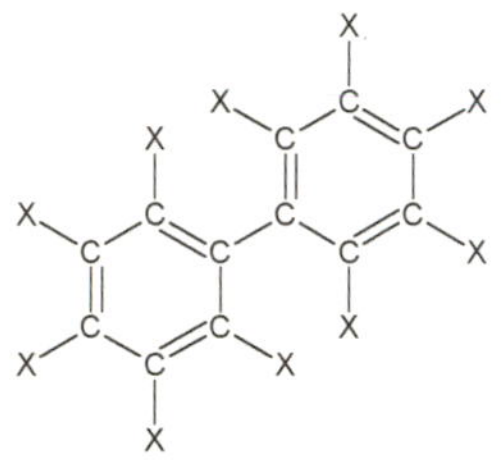

Figure 3-29
PCBs and PBBs

Like PCBs, PBBs *(figure 3-29)* have frequently been used for their fire-resistant quality. Use of PBBs has been especially common in the manufacturing of electronic equipment that contains plastic parts and is subject to overheating. The pervasive presence of PBBs has been evidenced by a study of Michigan residents. In the study, fat cells from 844 randomly-selected adults were analyzed. 97% of all samples were found to contain PBBs.[60] Additionally, highest PBB levels in these Michigan adults could be traced to areas of the state in which livestock and dairy products had previously been shown to have undergone the greatest contamination with PBBs.[61]

Halogenated Diphenyls

DDT. Dichlorodiphenyltrichloroethane (or DDT, and also often called chlorophenothane) has earned a unique place in the history of chlorinated hydrocarbons. DDT is usually considered together with its dechlorinated breakdown products, dichlorodiphenyldichloroethylene (or DDE) and dichlorodiphenyldichloroethane (or DDD).

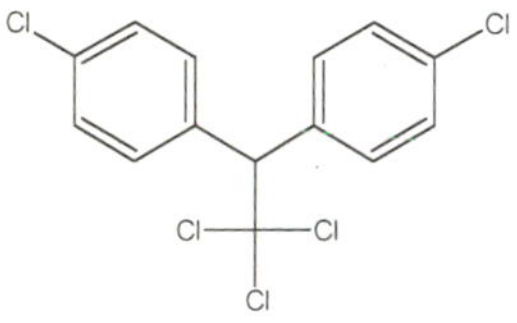

Figure 3-30
DDT

Although DDT is technically classified as an alkane because of its two-carbon ethane backbone, the molecule contains two non-fused benzene rings (like a biphenyl) and each of the benzene rings contains a halogen (chlorine) substitution *(Figure 3-30)*. Unlike the halogenated biphenyls whose benzene rings share a direct carbon-to-carbon bond, DDT is a diphenyl whose benzene rings are connected to a central ethane group. This combination of features, while leaving DDT technically classified as an alkane, gives it a commonality with substituted aromatic hydrocarbons, and with other organochlorines.

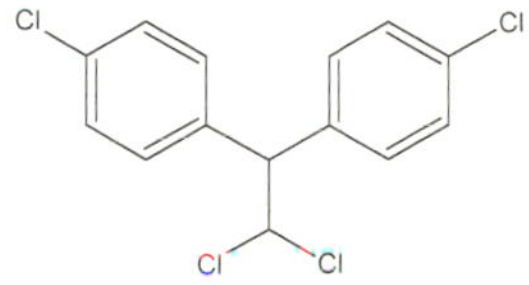

Through the activity of dechlorinating enzymes, DDT can be converted in the body to DDE *(Figure 3-31)*. During this process, one chlorine atom is stripped off. When further dechlorinated to DDD, two additional chlorines are removed, creating a water-soluble molecule that can be excreted in the urine. Unlike DDD and its routine excretion from the body, DDT and DDE are often stored for long periods of time in human tissue. All three molecules have been manufactured and sold as pesticides. DDD, while much less commonly used, has sometimes been designated as TDE, or tetrachlorodiphenylethane.

DDT was first produced on a large scale during the second world war to help control malaria by killing mosquitos. (The discovery that DDT could be produced by reacting chlorobenzene with trichloroacetaldehyde helped make this production possible.) In 1972, however, DDT was banned from production in the United States, following evidence of its unexpected accumulation within the environment, and particularly within the food supply. U.S. companies produced DDT for export until 1976.

Widespread use of DDT in the 1970s was reflected in data obtain from the Second National Health and Nutrition Examination Survey (NHANE-SII). This nationwide survey was based on a representative sample of the U.S. civilian population. In the study, 5,964 out of 5,994 subjects from whom blood samples were obtained were determined to have DDE in their serum.[62] But because DDT, and to an even greater extent DDE, can remain trapped inside fatty tissue for extended periods of time, presence of these chlorinated hydrocarbons within the food supply and risk of human toxicity continues to remain great even now, more than two decades later.

A 1993 study analyzing 806 pasteurized milk samples from 63 locations representing 80% of the U.S. milk supply showed about half of the samples to contain either DDE or dieldrin. Some of the samples contained DDE at the level of 19 ppb.[63] In Mexico, a 1996 study showed DDE in 304 out of 345 samples of butter available in Mexican supermarkets.[64] Consistent with these findings have been recent reports of DDT and DDE in the fatty tissue of human breasts[65] and in general subcutaneous fat stores.[66]

Figure 3-31
DDD

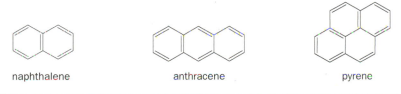

naphthalene   anthracene   pyrene

Figure 3-32
Unsubstituted PAHs

Unsubstituted Polycyclic Aromatics

Up until now, we have been reviewing aromatic hydrocarbons that contain only one or two benzene rings. It is common, however, for aromatics to contain more than two benzene rings, and compounds that contain two or more such rings are collectively referred to as polycyclic aromatic hydrocarbons (or PAHs). PAHs, like alkanes and alkenes, are naturally-occurring components of coal and coal tar. Naphthalene, anthracene, and pyrene *(Figure 3-32)* are the simplest of the PAHs, containing two, three, and four benzene rings respectively. (The term "anthracite" used to classify the hardest of the black coals is related to the three-ringed PAH anthracene contained in it). PAHs can also be found in by-products of coal processing. Soot produced by the burning of coal was one of the first substances to prompt research on PAHs as possible carcinogens. That research dates back to the late 1700s when public health officials noticed a higher incidence of scrotal cancer in chimney sweeps who had been exposed to unusually high levels of soot (and the PAHs contained in it).

PAHs enter the food supply indirectly. The burning of coal, wood, garbage, petroleum products, and tobacco releases PAHs into the atmosphere. In the food industry, manufacturing facilities where meat products are smoked are locations of high PAH release. Once released into the environment, natural processes distribute PAHs to soils, waters, plants, and livestock. The PAHs that are most abundant in the environment also turn up most consistently in foods and humans. For example, a 1991 study in Rome, Italy found anthracene and pyrene in all samples of olive oil procured for research, and estimated an annual yearly intake of PAHs at 560 micrograms per person based upon consumption of olive oil alone.[67]

Substituted Polycyclic Aromatics

A special subset of PAHs are the substituted PAHs. These molecules contain two or more fused benzene rings, and have hydrogens in their system replaced by other elements or chemical groups. The majority of substituted PAHs that come into contact with the food supply are pesticides, and the vast majority of substitutions involve halogenation, and more specifically, chlorination. The list of pesticides that fall into this chemical category of chlorinated PAHs includes captan, chlordane, dieldrin, eldrin, endrin, endosulfan, and heptachlor.

Because different pesticides are most effective on different crops, the presence of these halogenated PAHs in the food supply is often crop-specific. For example, captan is found predominantly on apples, grapes, peaches, strawberries, and watermelon. Dieldrin is commonly detected on corn, cucumbers, potatoes, and sweet potatoes. Endosulfan residues are routinely found in apples, bell peppers, cantaloupes, cauliflower, celery, cucumbers, peaches, pears, spinach, and strawberries.[68]

A substantial percentage of U.S. adults are estimated to have dietary intake of dieldrin above USEPA standards,[69] and as far back as the mid-1970s, dieldrin has been detected in the blood of a significant number of U.S. adults.[70] Serum concentrations of this pesticide have also been determined to vary seasonally in relationship with agricultural use, and to be significantly higher in farm residents.[71]

Dioxin. A final compound in the category of chlorinated polycyclic aromatic hydrocarbons that is surprisingly common in global food supplies is dioxin. Unfortunately, the term "dioxin" has been used in two somewhat confusing ways in the research literature.

In one context, the term has been used to refer to a broad family of compounds that includes many different types of molecules. For example, when the term "dioxin" is used in this way, one type of molecule can be identified by the presence of a chlorinated phenoxyl group. This chemical group has three features: a benzene ring, an attached hydroxyl group (allowing it to be classified as a phenol), and at least one site at which a hydrogen atom has been replaced by a chlorine. 2,4-dichlorophenoxyacetic acid (or "2,4-D") and 2,4,5-trichlorophenoxyacetic acid (or "2,4,5-T," *Figure 3-33*) are examples of chlorophenoxy compounds that can be classified as dioxins when the term is used in this broadest sense. In this first context, the term "dioxin" can also include chlorinated furan molecules. (A furan or tetrole ring is illustrated in *Figure 3-34*). When phenoxy and furan molecules are chlorinated at one or more sites, they can become highly toxic.

However, the term "dioxin" can also be used to refer to a single unique chemical compound. It is this single, identifiable "dioxin" that has been best re-searched in the toxicology literature, and it is classified as a poly-substituted polycyclic aromatic hydrocarbon called TCDD (2,3,6,7-tetra-chlorodibenzo-p-dioxin). TCDD (*Figure 3-35*) contains a triple benzene ring system with four halogen (chlorine) substitutions. (Because there are several molecules virtually identical to TCDD except for the number of chlorine atoms they contain, TCDD is also frequently described as being a member of the PCDD (polychlorinated dibenzo-*p*-dioxin) group.

In order to provide a broad overview of dioxins during the remainder of this section, we will use the term "dioxin" to refer to the first of these two options, i.e., a diverse group of molecules that includes, but is not limited to TCDD.

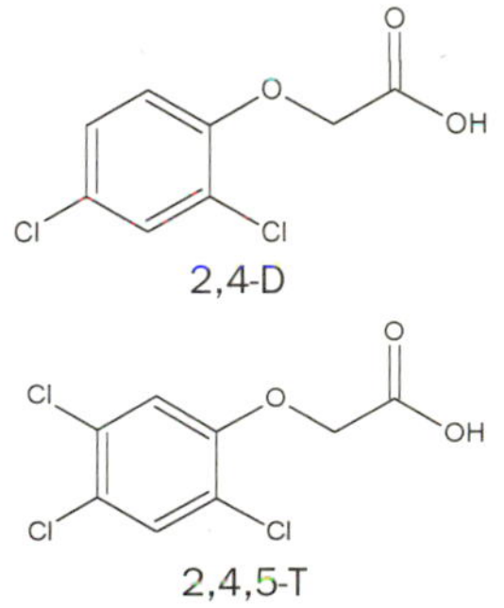

Figure 3-33
2,4-D and 2,4,5--T ("dioxins")

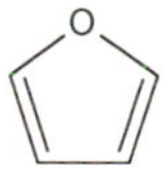

Figure 3-34
Furan ring

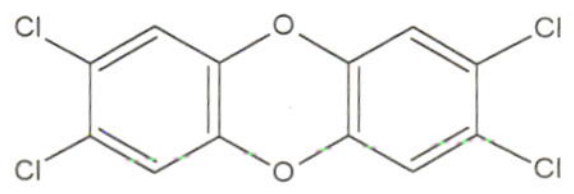

Figure 3-35
TCDD ("dioxin")

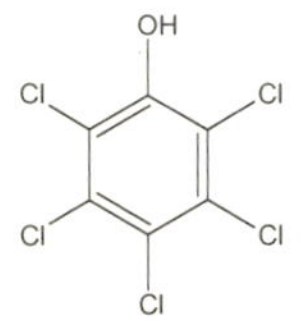

Figure 3-36
PCP

Dioxins are produced in a wide variety of ways. Bleaching of paper, incineration of waste, incineration of sewage sludge, forest fires, burning of coal, smoking of tobacco, combustion of leaded gasoline, combustion of tires, firing in cement kilns, secondary copper smelting, secondary lead smelting, and manufacture or use of pentachlorophenol (or PCP, *Figure 3-36*) all result in production of dioxins. Release of PCP into the environment, for example, has been shown to be a critical source of dioxin exposure and food supply contamination. Over 50 billion pounds are produced annually in the U.S. The uses of PCP are diverse and include termite control, preharvest defoliation of crops, general herbicidal use on crops, wood preservation, and leather protection (including shoe leather). A 1984 study within the U.S. showed PCP to be present in all 1,072 samples of chicken liver and all 723 samples of chicken fat analyzed in the study.[72]

It was herbicidal use of dioxin during the Vietnam war that initially brought widespread attention to this family of toxic compounds. During the Vietnam period 12 million gallons of 2,4-D and 2,4,5-T were mixed in a 1:1 ratio and sprayed in forests as a defoliant to kill underlying brush. The compound was named (after the color of its storage bins) "Agent Orange." Physician contact with Vietnam veterans after the war lead to a recognition of the severe illness that could be caused by dioxin exposure. Liver damage, decreased testosterone levels, porphyria, immune dysfunction, and psychiatric disturbance were included among the symptoms of dioxin exposure.[73]

Because dioxins are highly insoluble in water, most dioxins in the food supply exist in fat-based foods. Animal foods in particular have been the subject of ongoing dioxin research. As recounted in the introduction to this textbook, it was dioxin contamination of chickens and eggs in the summer of 1997 led the federal government to impose its first restriction on dioxin in food, limiting its presence to one part per trillion. (This USEPA restriction was not stated as a legally binding limit but only as a "level of concern.") As early as 1992, the USEPA had estimated that the average U.S. adult was likely to be consuming 300 to 600 times the acceptable daily dose of dioxin. At that time, this acceptable amount had been identified as 0.7 picograms.[74] In addition to poultry and eggs, milk, cream, cheese, ice cream, red meat, fish, and pork are common sources of dioxin exposure.[75] The dioxins found in these fat-containing animal products appear to originate in air-based release from the industrial and agricultural practices described above. For example, up to 80% of dioxin found in beef has been traced to vapor-phase transfer from contaminated air above pasture soils.[76] The storage of fat-containing dairy products in bleached cartons has also been identified as a important source of dioxin contamination.[77]

Coal Tar Dyes

The appearance of hydrocarbons in the food supply has never been more prominent than in coloration of food products with dyes obtained from coal tar. Coal tar, like coke, is a by-product of coal distillation. (For a complete description of coal formation and processing, see this chapter, page 93, under "Historical Perspectives: Petroleum and the Food Supply.") Like coal itself, coal tar is a hydrocarbon mixture, although most of its hydrocarbons are aromatic hydrocarbons rather than alkanes or unsaturated aliphatics.

As early as 1900, 695 coal tar dyes had been introduced into the U.S. marketplace, and many were being routinely added to the food supply.[42] At this time, use of coal tar dyes was totally unregulated. The Food and Drug Act of 1906 vastly transformed this situation by authorizing only seven dyes for use in the U.S. food supply. With respect to these seven dyes, however, no limits were set on the amount that could be added to food. Several decades later, Congress passed the Food, Drug and Cosmetic Act of 1938, authorizing the use of eight additional coal tar dyes for use in food, and once again stipulating no maximum amount. It was not until the Color Additives Amendment of 1960 that Congress placed limits on the amount of coal tar dyes in food products.

Nine color additives are currently permitted in the U.S. food supply. In 1984, 3,200 tons of these additives were put into foods. These certifiable colors included: FD&C (Food, Dye & Coloring) Blue No. 1 (brilliant blue FCF), added to beverages, dairy products, desserts, jellies, confections, condiments, baked goods, icings, syrups, and extracts; Blue No. 2 (indigotine or indigo carmine) added to baked goods, cereals, snack foods, ice cream, confections, and cherries); Green No. 3 (fast green FCF), added to beverages, puddings, ice cream, sherbet, cherries, confections, baked foods, and dairy products); Red No. 3 (erythrosine), added to cherries, fruit cocktail, canned fruit salad, confections, baked goods, dairy products, and snack foods; Red No. 40 (Allura red AC), added to gelatin, puddings, dairy products, confections, beverages, and condiments; Yellow No. 5 (tartrazine), added to cereals, confections, preserves, custards, beverages, and ice cream; Yellow No. 6 (sunset yellow FCF), added to cereals, baked goods, ice cream, confections, snack foods, beverages, and dessert powders; Orange B (added to sausage casings), and Citrus Red No. 2 (added to orange skins).

Between 1938 and 1998, several coal tar dyes were removed from the Congressionally-authorized list of color additives due to research showing increased cancer risk. These dyes included Red No. 2, Red No. 4, Violet No. 1, Orange No. 1, and Carbon Black.

POPs

Hydrocarbons, and especially aromatic hydrocarbons, can remain intact within ecosystems and individual organisms for extended periods of time. The long-term potential risk posed by such compounds is often used as a criterion for grouping them together and studying their toxicity. In the language of many regulatory agencies, long-lived toxic compounds are referred to as bioaccumulative chemicals of concern (BCCs). For members of the chemical manufacturing industry, a common designation is persistent toxins that bioaccumulate (PTBs). Among ecologists and environmentalists, a more common term is persistent organic pollutants (POPs).

Several categories of aromatic compounds reviewed in this chapter are typically classified as POPs. These compounds include the polycyclic aromatic hydrocarbons (PAHs), PCBs (polychlorinated biphenyls), polychlorinated dibenzo-p-dioxins (PCDDs), polychlorinated dibenzo-*p*-furans (PCDFs), and numerous pesticides (including DDT, DDE, and DDD).

In addition to their long-term presence, POPs are capable of extensive migration and concentration. High concentrations of DDT in unhatched petrel bird eggs on the island of Bermuda have been traced to ocean runoff from the Atlantic coast 600 miles away.[78] (For other types of toxins, this migration can be even more extensive. Particulates like sulfates release from manufacturing plants in Europe have been traced over 3,000 miles to the Arctic,[79] and radioactive gasses released into the air from the nuclear power station at Three Mile Island near Pittsburgh, Pennsylvania reached Albany, New York (over 300 miles away) in 18 hours.[80]

Biomagnification

The ability of POPs to concentrate as they move through food webs is called biomagnification. For example, although DDD levels in the waters of Clear Lake, California have been measured at only 0.02ppm, this concentration has been found to increase to 5.3ppm when measured in plankton living in the lake.[81] When measured in small fish that eat plankton, the concentration has been found to double (to 10ppm); in larger fish that eat smaller fish, DDD concentrations have been magnified over 100-fold (to 1500ppm); in grebe, (the birds that dive for fish in the lake, DDD concentrations reach 1600ppm.[82]

Given their longevity, ability to migrate, and tendency to become concentrated as they pass through a food web, several researchers have argued that POPs can only be understood on an ecological and global basis.[83] Accepting this argument would further complicate analysis of toxicity in the U.S. food supply since routine import of foods from neighboring countries and routine transport of food across thousands of miles within the U.S. would amplify the number of origination points for toxic contamination from long-lived, migratory POPs.

Summary

Up until this point in the chapter, we have been looking exclusively at organic food toxins, that is, food contaminants containing carbon atoms (and falling into the general category of hydrocarbons). A summary of these food-related organic toxins according to their chemical classification is presented in *Table 3-6*. At this point we will shift gears and review some of the inorganic substances that pose a risk of toxicity in the food supply.

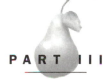

PART III

Classification of Toxins by Chemical Group: Inorganic Molecules and Compounds

Chemical Overview

In a chemical context, the term "inorganic" simply means "without any carbon atoms." This clear but very general definition of "inorganic" allows a wide range of food toxins to be classified as inorganic, even though they fall into different chemical divisions. These divisions include: 1) elements, 2) acids, 3) bases, and 4) salts. While inorganic food toxins can be found in each of these four divisions , the best-researched and most prevalent of the inorganic toxins are the heavy metal elements. This final section of the chapter provides a detailed review of three heavy metal elements (cadmium, lead, and mercury) frequently found in the U.S. food supply.

Elements

At present, the International Union of Pure and Applied Chemistry (IUPAC) recognizes 105 elements. For chemists, an element constitutes the simplest type of matter. (Matter is defined as anything possessing mass,

Table 3-6. *Food-related organic toxins*

Chemical category	Subcategory	Food toxin	Food-related use
Saturated hydrocarbons	Alkanes	*n*-hexane	Oil extraction
	Alkanes (halogenated)	Methyl bromide	Fumigant
		EDB, EDC	fumigants
		Dichloromethane	Decaffeination
		Carbon tetrachloride	Propellants
		Chloroform	Solvent
		DDT, DDE	(None currently)
Unsaturated hydrocarbons	Aliphatic/ alkenes	Polyethylene	Packaging
		(HDPE)	Packaging
		(LDPE)	Packaging
		Polypropylene	Packaging
		Vinyl	Packaging
	Halogenated alkenes	Vinyl chloride	Packaging
		Trichloroethylene	Solvent
		Teflon™	Cookware
	Aromatic (general)	(VOCs)	Varied
	Substituted monocyclic aromatics	Toluene	Solvent
		Phthalic acid	Packaging
		PET	Packaging
		Benzoic acid	Preservative
		Xylene	Solvent
		Styrene	Packaging
		Hexachlorobenzene	Pesticide
		Lindane	Pesticide
		Pentachlorophenol	Pesticide
		2,4-dinitrophenol	Pesticide
		Bromoxynil	Herbicide
		BHA	Preservative
		BHT	Preservative
	Halogenated biphenyls	PCBs	(None currently)
		PCCs	(None currently)
	Polycyclic aromatic (PAHs)	Anthracene	Coal tar dyes
		Naphthalene	Coal tar dyes
		Pyrene	Coal tar dyes
	Halogenated PAHs	Captan	Pesticide
		Chlordane	Pesticide
		Dieldrin	Pesticide
		Eldrin	Pesticide
		Endrin	Pesticide
		Endosulfan	Pesticide
		Heptachlor	Pesticide
		Dioxins/PCP	Herbicides, packaging

occupying space, and able to exist as a solid, liquid, and gas.) The "simplicity" of elements refers to the notion that elements are stable, have an identity, and cannot be broken down into anything simpler without losing some of that stability and identity. The 105 elements recognized by IUPAC range in molecular weight from 1 (hydrogen) to 260 (hahnium), and all elements identified as essential for living organisms have molecular weights under 53 (iodine).

When a chemist speaks about elements in an abstract sense, refering to an "atom" of carbon or an "atom" of nitrogen, the elements are regarded as being electrically neutral (possessing no electrical charge). However, in the life world, where most elements are found in a water-based medium (like cells, blood, or extracellular fluid) elements often become electrically charged. When an element carries with it an electrical charge, that element is no longer referred to as an "atom," but rather as an ion. To a chemist, a chlorine atom becomes a chlorine ion when it takes on an electrical charge.

Ions

Atoms take on electrical charges by losing or gaining electrons from their outer shells. Positive ions (also called cations) are atoms that have given up electrons. Negative ions (also called anions) are atoms that have taken on additional electrons. An atom of chlorine, for example, contains seven electrons in its outer shell when non-dissolved and existing in its neutral atomic state. Once in solution, this same chlorine atom can take on an additional electron and become a negative ion. In this anionic state, chlorine is symbolized by its standard abbreviation (Cl) followed by a superscripted hyphen (i.e., Cl^-) to indicate its additional electron charge.

Elements can be found in most body fluids in both ionized and non-ionized forms. About half of the calcium in the bloodstream, for example, is ionized and found in the divalent cationic form (Ca^{++}). When producing toxicity in the body, many metals are also in ionized form. For example, aresnic, cadmium, and mercury in their trivalent and divalent cationic forms (i.e., As^{+++} Cd^{++} and Hg^{++}) are recognized to trigger apoptosis (programmed cell death) in leukemia cells, and have been used in treatment of acute promyelocytic leukemia for this reason.[84] The divalent cationic form of mercury (Hg^{++}) has also been shown to upset metabolic balances involving other divalent cations inside of cells, particularly nerve cells.[85]

Acids and Bases

One specific ion is particularly important in understanding the second and third categories of inorganic substances, namely, the categories of acids and bases. This unique ion is the hydrogen ion. When the element hydrogen ionizes, it loses one electron from its outermost shell and becomes a mono-valent cation (H^+). However, because hydrogen contains only one electron to begin with, the loss of this electron leaves hydrogen with no electrons at all, and nothing more than a single proton inside of its nucleus (provided that we are talking about hydrogen in its non-isotope form where no neutrons are involved). Because the hydrogen ion is essentially a bare proton, it is often referred to as just that: a proton. Substances that give off protons (hydrogen ions) in water are called *acids*. Substances that accept protons are called *bases*.

Nitric (HNO_3) and nitrous (HNO_2) acid; sulfuric (H_2SO_4) and sulfurous (H_2SO_3) acid; and phosphoric (H_3PO_4) and carbonic (H_2CO_3) acid are examples of common acids. Potassium (KOH), calcium [$Ca(OH)_2$], and magnesium [$Mg(OH)_2$] hydroxide are examples of common bases.

Salts

Salts are formed when a cation (positively charged ion) and anion (negatively charged ion) meet to form an ionic compound. This definition of a salt applies to all cations and anions except for hydrogen ions (H^+). and hydroxide ions (OH^-). Between 5–10% of the calcium in blood, for example, is found in salt form. In the case of calcium these salts include calcium sulfate ($CaSO_4$) and calcium phosphate [$(CaPO_4)_2$].

Elements acting as toxins within the body can also be found in salt form. For example, mercuric chloride ($HgCl_4$) is the salt formed by a mercury cation and a chlorine anion. This salt has been shown to produce neural toxicity by disrupting ionic balances within the membrane of astrocyte cells.[86] (Astrocytes are cells within the brain that connect neurons to capillaries and allow exchange of nutrients and information between the circulatory and nervous system.)

This brief review of inorganic substances and the primary categories of ions, acids, bases, and salts brings us to the inorganic substances of primary interest in understanding food toxicity. These substances are the heavy metals. In the following section, we will review basic factors in the understanding of heavy metals, and focus attention on three members of the heavy metal family, namely cadmium, lead, and mercury.

Metals and Heavy Metals

Metals constitute an important division within the elements. Metals are defined as elements that are shiny, conduct electricity, and can be formed into wires and sheets. The vast majority of elements identified in the human body are metals. These 13 metals include calcium, potassium, sodium, magnesium, iron, zinc, copper, manganese, cobalt, chromium, molybdenum, nickel and vanadium. The 10 non-metals found in humans include oxygen, carbon, hydrogen, nitrogen, sulfur, phosphorus, chlorine, selenium, fluorine, iodine and boron. Three elements found within the body, silicon, arsenic, and germanium, are not classified as metals or non-metals. Instead, these elements are classified as metalloids. Metalloids are elements that have the appearance and physical properties of metals but behave chemically like non-metals. Despite the greater number of metals in the body, non-metals contribute far more to body weight (*Table 3-7*).

Alkali and Alkaline Earth Metals

The IUPAC further divides metals into groups based on their chemical behavior. Alkali metals are elements that react with water to create a high pH (alkaline) solution. The alkali metals include sodium and potassium (*Table 3-8*, on the following page). Alkaline earth metals bring about the same result, but consist of metals commonly found in the earth's crust. The

Table 3-7. Metals, non-metals, and metalloids as a percentage of body weight

Non-metals[a]	% TBW[d]	Metals[b]	% TBW	Metalloids[c]	% TBW[d]
O	62.8	Ca	1.6	Si	0.03
C	19.4	K	0.2	As	<0.0001
H	9.3	Na	0.14	Ge	<0.0001
N	2.9	Mg	0.05		
P	1.0				
S	0.25	Fe	0.005		
Cl	0.14	Zn	0.003		
		Cu	0.0001		
Se	<0.0001	Mn	<0.0001		
F	<0.0001				
I	<0.0001	Co	<0.0001		
		Cr	<0.0001		
Bo	<0.0001	Mo	<0.0001		
		Ni	<0.0001		
		V	<0.0001		

[a] Non-metals are substances that do not conduct electricity, do not have a metallic luster, and cannot be formed into wires and sheets.
[b] Metals are substance that conduct electricity, have a metallic luster, can be formed into wires and sheets, and have basic oxides.
[c] Metalloids are substances that have the physical appearance and properties of metals but behave chemically like non-metals.
[d] Total body weight.

Table 3-8. **The alkali metals**

Number	Symbol	Name	k	l	m	n	o	p
3	Li	Lithium	2	1				
11	Na	Sodium	2	8	1			
19	K	Potassium	2	8	8	1		
37	Rb	Rubidium	2	8	18	8	1	
55	Cs	Cesium	2	8	18	32	8	1
87	Fr	Francium	2	8	18	32	18	8

Table 3-9. **The alkaline earth metals**

Number	Symbol	Name	k	l	m	n	o	p
4	Be	Beryllium	2	2				
12	Mg	Magnesium	2	8	2			
20	Ca	Calcium	2	8	8	2		
38	Sr	Strontium	2	8	18	8	2	
56	Ba	Barium	2	8	18	32	8	2
88	Ra	Radium	2	8	18	32	18	8

alkaline metals include calcium and magnesium (*Table 3-9*). In addition to the halogen family of elements (previously discussed, see *Table 3-2*), several other families are helpful in understanding metals, non-metals, and metalloids. The carbon family (*Table 3-10*) includes the non-metal carbon, the metals tin and lead, and the metalloids silicon and germanium. The nitrogen family (*Table 3-11*) includes the non-metals nitrogen and phosphorus, the metal bismuth, and the metalloids arsenic and antimony. The oxygen family (*Table 3-12*) includes the non-metals oxygen, sulfur, and selenium, and the metalloids tellurium and polonium.

Heavy Metals

Heavy metals are defined as metals with a density at least five times as great as water. Density is the ratio of mass to volume. Although density changes with temperature, the density of water remains close to 1.0 from freezing (when the density is 0.99987) to boiling (when the density is 0.95838). For a metal to be classified as a heavy metal, a density of approximately 5.0 or greater is therefore required. Metals meeting this requirement include cadmium, lead, and mercury, as well as zinc, copper, iron, cobalt, nickel, tin, manganese and molybdenum. Thus, while the term "heavy metal" may have the popular connotation "primarily toxic," many heavy metals like zinc and copper are in fact essential nutrients. Conversely, metals do not need to be heavy in order to pose a toxic risk. Aluminum, for example, can increase formation of lipofuscin (an aging-related pigment) in heart muscle cells,[87] promote accumulation of tau protein in neurons (a protein whose accumulation has been associated with symptoms of Alzheimer's disease),[88] and prevent the kidneys from synthesizing vitamin D.[89] These effects occur despite the fact that the density of aluminum is only two and one half times that of water and disqualifies it as a heavy metal.

The density of heavy metals like cadmium (approximately 8), lead (approximately 11) and mercury (approximately 14) is strikingly high in comparison to the density of most matter in the body. For example, the densities of sodium, potassium, magnesium, and calcium are all less than 2.0. Bone, which we think of as one of the more dense and heavily mineralized

Table 3-10. **The carbon family**

Number	Symbol	Name	*k*	*l*	*m*	*n*	*o*	*p*
6	C	Carbon	2	4				
14	Si	Silicon	2	8	4			
32	Ge	Germanium	2	8	18	4		
50	Sn	Tin	2	8	18	18	4	
82	Pb	Lead	2	8	18	32	18	4

Table 3-11. **The nitrogen family**

Number	Symbol	Name	*k*	*l*	*m*	*n*	*o*	*p*
7	N	Nitrogen	2	5				
15	P	Phosphorus	2	8	5			
33	As	Arsenic	2	8	18	5		
51	Sb	Antimony	2	8	18	18	5	
83	Bi	Bismuth	2	8	18	32	18	5

Table 3-12. **The oxygen family**

Number	Symbol	Name	*k*	*l*	*m*	*n*	*o*	*p*
8	O	Oxygen	2	6				
16	S	Sulfur	2	8	6			
34	Se	Selenium	2	8	18	6		
52	Te	Tellurium	2	8	18	18	6	
84	Po	Polonium	2	8	18	32	18	6

body tissues, has a density of approximately 1.75. This juxtaposition of high density metals in a low density body has its counterpart in the environment, where human activities like mining and manufacturing have dramatically relocated high density metals within the earth's crust which is formed primarily from lower density metals. As we will review in the next section, it is not possible for a low density living organism to contain toxic amounts of high density metals unless the earth's crust has been disrupted by non-natural events.

Metals, Mining, and Earth's Crust

Table 3-13, opposite, presents 46 elements and their relative contribution to the earth's crust. A small number of elements contribute disproportionately to the total composition of the crust. Within the group of 11 elements contributing 1,000 parts per million (ppm) or more to the composition of the crust, only 3 are non-metals (oxygen, hydrogen, and phosphorus). Of the remaining 8 metals or metalloids, most contribute to the crust's composition at the level of 10,000ppm. These metallic elements include aluminum, iron, calcium, sodium, magnesium, and potassium. The metalloid silicon contributes to the crust's composition at a level of 100,000ppm.

Excluded from the previously-described list are many key elements in human nutrition. These elements include manganese, sulfur, chlorine, vanadium, chromium (contributing to the earth's crust at the 100ppm level); nickel, zinc, copper, cobalt, and nitrogen (contributing at 10ppm); molybdenum and arsenic (contributing at 1ppm level); iodine (contributing at 100 parts per billion, or ppb); and selenium (contributing at 10ppb). The key heavy metals for review in this chapter (cadmium, lead, and mercury) all contribute to the earth's crust at these lower concentration. For lead, the contribution is 14ppm; for cadmium, 100ppb; and for mercury, only 10ppb. Human exposure to concentrations greater than these typically requires human intervention. For example, mercury is present in the crust at only 10ppb, and virtually all of this mercury comes in the form of mercury sulfide (cinnabar). Mining inside of the U.S. in Arkansas, California, Idaho, Oregon, Nevada, Texas, and Utah, and outside of the U.S. in Italy, Peru, Spain, and Yugoslavia has made it possible, however, for mercury to become more available than would be predicted from its low concentration in the earth's crust.

After being mined, mercury has been refined and incorporated into a wide variety of manufactured products. Batteries, vapor lamps, light switches, thermostats, dental amalgams, thermometers, fungicides, insecticides, and anti-mildew treated paints (manufactured outside of the U.S.)

can all contain mercury. Release of mercury into the environment can be associated with these products in a variety of different ways. In the case of fungicides, this release is immediate and intentional: methylmercury is intentionally brought into direct contact with soil, plants, and air. In the case of vapor lamps or anti-mildew paints, this release is less immediate and unintentional: over time, mercury vapors are inadvertently released into the air, even though the products were not designed to have this effect. In the case of batteries or thermometers, release occurs unintentionally and may not be significant until the life of the product has ended. Discard of

Table 3-13. **Elements in the earth's crust**

PPM[a]	Element	Multiplier[b]	PPM[a]	Element	Multiplier[b]
10^5 (100,000ppm)	O	4.61	10^1 continued	Zn	7.00
	Si	2.82		Ce	6.65
10^4 (10,000ppm)	Al	8.23		Cu	6.00
	Fe	5.63		Nd	4.15
	Ca	4.15		Y	3.30
	Na	2.36		Co	2.50
	Mg	2.33		Sc	2.20
	K	2.09		Nb	2.00
10^3 (1,000ppm)	Ti	5.65		N	1.90
	H	1.40		Ga	1.90
	P	1.05		Pb	1.40
10^2 (100ppm or	Mn	9.50		B	1.00
100,000ppb)	F	5.85	10^{-1} (1ppm or	Tl	8.5
	Ba	4.25	1,000ppb)	Lu	8.0
	Sr	3.70		Tm	5.2
	S	3.50		I	4.5
	C	2.00		In	2.5
	Zr	1.65		Sb	2.0
	Cl	1.45		Cd	1.5
	V	1.20		Pd	1.5
	Cr	1.02		Se	5.0
10^1 (10ppm or	Rb	9.00		Ag	7.5
10,000ppb)	Ni	8.40		Hg	8.5

[a] Parts per million. Example: 10^5=10 X 10 X 10 X 10 X10 =100,000 parts per million
[b] Multiplier. Example: O (oxygen) = 4.61 X 10^5 or 461,000 parts per million.

batteries into municipal landfills and incineration of industrial wastes are examples of this type of release.

The extent to which mercury mining and manufacturing can alter exposure to this geologically rare heavy metal was demonstrated in Iraq in the 1970s. Use of methylmercury fungicides on grain crops in that country were shown to result in human hair concentrations of mercury greater than 1,000,000ppb.[90] In other words, human hair became 100,000 times more concentrated with mercury than would naturally occur in the earth's crust.

Mercury is one of three heavy metals particularly well-researched in environmental toxicology. The other two heavy metals are cadmium and lead. Because each of the three is also a common contaminant in the U.S. food supply, we will now look in greater detail at their profile and effects.

Heavy Metals in the Food Supply

Cadmium

Geology. Cadmium is a soft, silvery-white metal that does not often occur naturally in its elemental form. Within the earth's crust, the only real mineral ore to contain cadmium is greenockite. This ore contains cadmium in its sulfide form (cadmium sulfide, or CdS). Minable greenockite deposits are also relatively rare, occurring worldwide in Scotland and Bolivia, and within the U.S. in Arkansas, Illinois, Kentucky, Missouri, and New Jersey. So rare is cadmium as a naturally-occurring substance within the earth's crust that it ranks 65th out of all 82 detectable elements. In oceans, cadmium is most often present as cadmium chloride (or $CdCl$, its most water-soluble form), and in the atmosphere, as cadmium oxide (or CdO).

Industrial and Commercial Use. Because of cadmium's infrequent solo appearance as a mineral ore, most cadmium used in manufacturing is obtained as a by-product of zinc smelting and refining. (At one time, lead smelting was also a significant source of domestic production). Electric furnace dust produced by the U.S. steel industry is also harvested for its cadmium content.

Because of its anti-corrosive properties, cadmium became extremely popular during World War II as a metal plating agent. During the war, cadmium became a standard requirement in the coating of metal parts at risk of corrosion, including sea-going aircraft and sailing vessels. Coatings and platings continue to be a significant application for cadmium, although battery manufacturing accounts for a greater percentage of cadmium use. Nickel-cadmium batteries are expected to create an even greater demand for cadmium production in the future given the intention of countries like

France to produce as many as 100,000 electronic vehicles in the next three years that will use cadmium batteries to store electrical energy.

Other applications of cadmium include the production of cadmium pigments based on cadmium sulfate and cadmium sulfoselenide (e.g., cadmium red). Although these pigments are still used to produce colors in print media, including food packaging, their use has decreased alongside of stricter governmental regulation and greater availability of alternative pigments (like cerous sulfide). Manufacture of solders, electroplating, and stabilized plastics also serve as industrial uses of cadmium.

Exposure. According to the Environmental Health Center Division of the National Safety Council in the U.S., almost 250,000 pounds of cadmium or cadmium-containing compounds were released into the air in 1987. Once airborne, cadmium can produce toxic effects at relatively low concentrations. Risk of carcinogenicity has been shown at air vapor concentrations as low as 50 micrograms per cubic meter.[91] In addition to cancer risk, exposure to cadmium has been related to increased risk of anemia, hypertension, emphysema, liver damage, teratogenesis, pulmonary edema, testicular necrosis, placental necrosis, renal tubular damage, osteomalacia, and deficiency of other minerals including iron, copper, and zinc.[92]

Food Contamination. Once airborne, cadmium can move downward into water and soil and become bioconcentrated in both plant and animal foods. As many as 200 micrograms per kilogram of cadmium have been found in shellfish;[93] over 739 micrograms per kilogram in poppy seed;[94] over 42 micrograms per kilogram in wheat-based breakfast cereals;[95] and up to 192 micrograms per kilogram in pasta products.[96] In the Netherlands, average lifelong cadmium intake from food has been estimated at 435,000 micrograms.[97]

In addition to the migration of cadmium from air to soil to food, U.S. regulations currently place no limit on the amount of cadmium that can be present in fertilizer. (In Canada, by contrast, the legal limit is 20ppm). Because incinerator ash, coal ash, and hazardous waste produced by steel mills are legal soil amendments and can be used as raw material for fertilizer, cadmium also gets introduced into the food supply from these sources.

The USEPA has currently placed a limit of 5 micrograms per liter on the permissible amount of cadmium in public drinking water, and the U.S. Agency for Toxic Substances and Disease Registry (ATSDR), as required under the 1997 Comprehensive Environmental Response, Compensation, and Liability Act (CERCLA), ranks cadmium as the seventh most hazardous substance to which U.S. citizens are exposed (*see Appendix B*).

Lead

Out of 275 substances included on the ATSDR priority list of hazardous substances (see Appendix B), lead is ranked five places above cadmium as the second most significant health hazard facing U.S. citizens. (Arsenic is ranked first as the single most hazardous substance).

Geology. Lead is a whitish gray, soft metal that does not tend to form crystals and therefore does not usually occur as an isolated mineral. When lead is present in the earth's crust it is typically concentrated in other mineral ores including anglesite, cerussite, galena, and minium. Even when considered in all of its geologic forms, lead only contributes about 13ppb to the earth's crust.

Industrial and Commercial Use. The U.S. is the world's leading producer of lead, and within the U.S., Missouri serves as the key production state. Lead remains the primary component in lead-acid storage batteries, including the batteries used in vehicles, ships, and aircraft. Commercial suppliers of electrical power also use lead-acid systems to meet peak voltage demands or to assure emergency back-up power. In addition to its use in batteries, lead is also used as a component in the manufacture of soundproofing materials, piping and conduit, radiation shields, ammunition, gasoline, and pencils.

Exposure. The presence of lead in drinking water is related directly or indirectly to virtually all manufacturing uses of lead, both past and present. For example, in the case of lead solder for water piping, the U.S. Congress in 1986 restricted the concentration of lead in solder to 0.2%. For faucets, pipes, and other plumbing materials, the maximum allowable concentration was set at 8.0%. Despite these restrictions, however, levels of lead in public drinking water routinely reach the 100–500ppb level.[98] The USEPA has set a National Drinking Water Standard of 20ppb for lead.

Direct use of lead in plumbing is only one pathway of drinking water contamination. Despite the fact that paint and gasoline manufacturers have largely eliminated use of lead in these products, significant amounts of lead originating from these products remain in the environment and filter down into drinking water. In the Seattle, Washington area, for example, soils near homes built before 1950 often contain lead at concentrations of 500–1,000ppm.[99] (These soil concentrations correspond to 500,000–1,000,000ppb and would qualify such sites as hazardous waste clean-up sites). Residue from leaded paints and leaded gasoline emissions often create concentrations of lead in city soils in the range of 150–300ppm (or 150,000–300,000ppb).[100]

Food Contamination. Like cadmium, lead is unregulated in the U.S. as a component in agricultural fertilizers. (In Canada, the maximum allowable level of lead in fertilizers is 500ppm). Use of incinerator ash, steel mill dusts, and coal ash bring lead into soil and plants when these wastes are used as raw material for fertilizer. Analysis of animal products in the U.S. food supply (including milk, eggs, meat, fish, and shellfish) show an average of 20–400ppb lead.[101] A 1993 study by the World Health Organization has shown average weekly adult intake of lead to be between 70 micrograms and 4.4 milligrams.[102] Some of this lead can be traced to the continued use of lead in the canning of foods, particularly in the form of lead solder used to complete sealing of the cans.[103]

Packaging materials for food and kitchenware are legally allowed to contain lead according to a variety of different standards. Most of these standards involve the amount of lead that is allowed to leach from materials when exposed to a 4% solution of acetic acid. For example, ceramic plates and saucers containing lead glazing are allowed to leach lead at the rate of 7ppm; coffee, tea, and juice cups at 5ppm; and pitchers at 2.5ppm.[104]

A surprising source of lead exposure from food involves migration of lead-containing inks from plastic packaging. Labeling on plastic bread bags may involve the use of lead-containing inks, and total bag content of lead can reach the 32,000 microgram level.[105] Researchers have estimated that exposure to weak acids such as vinegar can easily cause leaching of lead from the bags at the 100 microgram level.[106] Such leaching would most likely take place if plastic bags were reused, turned inside out, and used to store food leftovers.

Mercury

Geology. A geological profile of mercury was presented earlier in this section (page 118, under "Metals, Mining, and the Earth's Crust"). Cinnabar (mercuric sulfide) is one of the few naturally-occurring mercuric compounds in the earth's crust. Total mercury deposits contribute to the composition of the earth's crust at a 10 parts per billion level.

Industrial and Commercial Use. Industrial and commercial use of mercury are also reviewed earlier in this chapter (pages 118–120). Mercury is commonly found in batteries, vapor lamps, light switches, thermostats, dental amalgams, thermometers, fungicides, insecticides, and anti-mildew treated paints (manufactured outside of the U.S.).

Exposure. Mercury is ranked third on the ATSDR priority list of hazardous substances (*see Appendix B*) because of its many routes of exposure. These numerous routes of exposure are also routes of access to the food supply.

As described earlier, methylmercury fungicides have been used on grain crops worldwide, and once introduced into food webs, can become greatly biomagnified and toxic. In the 1950s, for example, when a chemical plant in Minamata, Japan dumped large amounts of methylmercury-containing compounds into Minamata Bay, passage of mercury through the aquatic food web led to human deaths following consumption of fish that lived in the bay.[107]

Food Contamination. Fish constitute a major source of mercury in the diet. In the Minamata Bay example described above, concentration of mercury in fish reached levels as high as 35,700ppb.[108] A 1991 study of 220 cans of water-packed tuna in the U.S. showed an average methylmercury content of 170ppb with concentrations ranging as high as 750ppb.[109] In Japan, where fish constitute the major source of dietary exposure to mercury, average daily intake of mercury has been estimated at approximately 10 micrograms.[110]

Several routes of access converge to make grains a second major source of mercury in the diet. One route, as described earlier in this chapter, involves direct use of methylmercury fungicides on grain crops. These compounds help prevent growth of fungi and mildew on grains, but persist long after harvest and show up in grain products appearing on the store shelf. Under extreme circumstances, mercury that originated from use of fungicide on grain can reach levels as high as 900ppb in a grain product like bread.[111] Use of sewage sludge to fertilize grain crops is a second route of mercury contamination. Between 80–100% of the mercury contained in sewage sludge may remain in crop soils up to 25 years later.[112] Disposal or incineration of municipal wastes, the burning of coal and petroleum products, and the disposal of medical wastes (including dental amalgams) also create pathways for mercury contamination of food.

1. Hodgson E. (1987). Introduction to toxicology. Chapter one. In: Hodgson and Levi PE. A textbook of modern toxicology, Elsevier, New York, p.1.

2. Nielsen FH. (1990). Other trace elements. Chapter 34. In: Present knowledge in nutrition. Sixth edition. International Life Sciences Institute, Washington, D.C., p. 295.

3. *Ibid.*

4. Environmental Protection Agency. (1982). An exposure and risk assessment for arsenic. EPA-440/4-85-005. Springfield, VA. National Technical Information Service (NTIS), U.S. Department of Commerce.

5. Harte J, Holdren C, Schneider R et al. (1991). Toxics A to Z. University of California Press, Berkeley, CA, p. 217.

6. Smith AH, Hopenhayn-Rich C, Bates MN et al. (1992). Cancer risks from arsenic in drinking water. Environ Health Perspect 97:259–267.

7. Environmental Protection Agency, *op. cit. (see reference 4).*

8. *Ibid.*

9. Smith AH, Hopenhayn-Rich C, Bates MN et al, *op. cit (see reference 6).*

10. Engel RR and Smith AH. (1994). Arsenic in drinking water and mortality from vascular disease: an ecologic analysis in 30 counties in the United States. Arch Environ Health 49(5):418–427.

11. Branen AL, Davidson MP, and Salminen S. (Eds). (1989). Food additives. Food science and technology series 35. Marcel Dekker, New York.

12. Saladino AJ, Willey JC, Lechner JF et al. (1985). Effects of formaldehyde, acetaldehyde, benzoyl peroxide, and hydrogen peroxide on cultured normal human bronchial cells. Canc Res 45(6):2522–2526.

13. Babich H, Zuckerbraum HL, Wuzburger BJ et al. (1996). Benzoyl peroxide cytotoxicity evaluated in vitro with the human keratinocyte cell line, RHEK-1. Toxicol 106(1-3):187-196.

14. Guyton KZ, Gorospe M, Kensler TW et al. (1996). Mitogen-activated protein kinase (MAPK) activation by butylated hydroxytoluene hydroperoxide: implications for cellular survival and tumor promotion. Canc Res 56(15):3480-3485.

15. Pereira CM and Oliveira CR. (1997). Glutamate toxicity on a PC12 cell line involves glutathione (GSH) depletion and oxidative stress. Free Rad Biol Med 23(4):637-647.

16. Johansen KS and Berger EM. (1983). Effect of sodium benzoate on polymorphonuclear leukocyte function. Acta Pathol Microbiol Immunol Scand 91(6):361-365.

17. Montano G and Orea M. (1989). Frequency of urticaria and angioedema induced by food additives. Rev Alerg Mex 36(1):15–18.

18. Meng Z and Zhang L. (1992). Cytogenic damage induced in human lymphocytes by sodium bisulfite. Mutat Res 298(2):63–69.

19. Mott L and Snyder K. (1987). Pesticide alert. Sierra Club Books, San Francisco, p.8.

20. Rea WJ. (1996). Pesticides. J Nutr Environ Med 6:55.

21. Hill RH, Head SL, Baker S et al. (1995). Pesticide residues in urine of adults living in the United States: reference range concentrations. Environ Res 71(2):99–108.

22. Environmental Working Group. (1996). Executive Summary: Tough To Swallow. Washington, D.C.

23. Breuning JC. (1989). Seeking a cure for sick building syndrome. Occup Haz 18:85.

24. Thomas KW, Pellizzari ED, Perritt RL et al. (1991). Effect of dry-cleaned clothes on tetrachloroethylene levels in indoor air, personal air, and breath for residents of several New Jersey homes. J Expo Anal Environ Epidemiol 1(4):475–490.

25. Wickstrom K, Pyysalo H, Plaami-Heikkila S et al. (1986). Polycyclic aromatic compounds (PAC) in leaf lettuce. Z Lebensm Unters Forsch 183(3):182–185.

26. Lorber M, Cleverly D, Schaum J et al. (1994). Development and validation of an air-to-beef food chain model for dioxin-like compounds. Sci Total Environ 156(1):39–65.

27. Environmental Working Group. (1996). Executive Summary: Tough To Swallow. Washington, D.C.

28. Smith AH, Hopenhayn-Rich C, Bates MN et al. (1992). Cancer risks from arsenic in drinking water. Environ Health Perspect 97:259–267.

29. Millette JR, Clark PJ, Stober J et al. (1983). Asbestos in water supplies of the United States. Environ Health Perspect 53:45–48.

30. Aschengrau A, Zierler S, and Cohen A. (1989). Quality of community drinking water and the occurrence of spontaneous abortion. Arch Environ Health 44(5):283–290.

31. *Ibid.*

32. *Ibid.*

33. Vogtmann H and Biedermann R. (1985). The nitrate story—no end in sight. Nutr Health 3(4):217–239.

34. Fagliano J, Berry M, Bove F et al. (1990). Drinking water contamination and the incidence of leukemia: an ecologic study. Am J Publ Health 80(10):1209–1212.

35. Savitz DA, Andrews KW and Pastore LM. (1995). Drinking water and pregnancy outcome in central North Carolina: source, amount, and tri-halomethane levels. Environ Health Perspect 103(6):592–596.

36. Cheftel JC, Cuq J-L, and Lorient D. (1985). Amino acids, peptides, and proteins. Chapter 5 in: Fennema OR. (Ed.). Food chemistry. Second edition. Marcel Dekker, New York, p.327.

37. WHO Working Group. (1991). *n*-hexane. Environ Health Criteria 122:133.

38. Takeuchi Y. (1993). *n*-hexane polyneuropathy in Japan: a review of *n*-hexane poisoning and its preventive measures. Environ Res 62(1):76–80.

39. Min KS, Terano Y, Onosaka S et al. (1991). Induction of hepatic metallothionein by nonmetallic compounds associated with acute-phase response in inflammation. Toxicol Appl Pharmacol 111(1):152–162.

40. Brown LR. (1981). Building a sustainable society. W.W. Norton and Company, New York, p.90.

41. Powledge F. (1984). The fat of the land. Touchstone Books, Simon & Schuster, New York, p.27.

42. Francis FJ. (1985). Pigments and other colorants. Chapter 8 in: Fennema OR. (Ed.). Food chemistry. Second edition. Marcel Dekker, New York, p.576.

43. Agency for Toxic Substances and Disease Registry (ATSDR). (1997). 1997 CERCLA priority list of hazardous substances. ATSDR Information Center, Division of Toxicology, Atlanta, Georgia.

44. Gorna-Binkul A, Keymeulen R, Van Langenhove H et al. (1996). Determination of monocyclic aromatic hydrocarbons in fruit and vegetables by gas chromatography-mass spectrometry. J Chromatography 734(2):297–302.

45. Isigigur A, Heras A, and Ackman RG. (1996). An improved method for the recovery of petroleum hydrocarbons from fish muscle tissue. Food Chem 57(3):457–462.

46. Vodela JK, Lenz SD, Renden JA et al. (1997). Drinking water contaminants (arsenic, cadmium, Lead, benzene, and trichloroethylene): 2. Effects on reproductive performance, egg quality, and embryo toxicity in broiler breeders. Poultry Sci 76(11):1493–1500.

47. Jickells SM, Philo MR, Gilbert J et al. (1993). Gas chromatographic/mass spectrometric determination of benzene in nonstick cookware and microwave susceptors and its migration into foods on cooking. J AOAC Internatl 76(4):760–764.

48. Supramanium G and Warner JO. (1986). Artificial food additive intolerance in patients with angio-oedema and urticaria. Lancet 2:907–909.

49. Tarlo SM and Sussman GL. (1993). Asthma and anaphylactoid reactions to food additives. Can Fam Phys 39:1119–1123.

50. Nethercott JR, Lawrence MJ, Roy AM et al. (1984). Airborne contact urticaria due to sodium benzoate in a pharmaceutical manufacturing plant. J Occup Med 26(10):734–736.

51. Hill RH, Ashley DL, Head Sl et al. (1995). *P*-dichlorobenzene exposure among 1,000 adults in the United States. Arch Environ Health 50(4):277–280.

52. Hill RH, Head SL, Baker S, et al. (1995). Pesticide residues in urine of adults living in the United States: reference range concentrations. Environ Res 71(2):99–108.

53. Verhagen H, Deerenberg I, Marx A et al. (1990). Estimate of the maximal daily dietary intake of butylated hydroxyanisole and butylated hyddroxytoluene in the Netherlands. Food Chem Toxicol 28(4):215–220.

54. Eberhartinger S, Steiner I, Washuttl J et al. (1990). The migration of acetaldehyde from polyethylene terephlhalate bottles for fresh beverages containing carbonic acid. Z Lebensm Unters Forsch 191(4–5):286–289.

55. Page BD and Lacroix GM. (1992). Studies into the transfer and migration of phthalate esters from aluminum foil-paper laminates to butter and margarine. Food Addit Contamin 9(3):197–212.

56. Begley TH, Dennison JL and Hollifield HC. (1990). Migration into food of polyethylene terephthalate (PET) cyclic oligomers from PET microwave susceptor packaging. Food Addit Contamin 7(6):797–803.

57. Weistrand C and Noren K. (1997). Methylsulfonyl metabolites of PCBs and DDE in human tissues. Environ Health Perspect 105(6):644–649.

58. Bosse U, Bannert N, Niessn KH et al. (1996). Chlorinated carbohydrate content of fetal and pediatric organs and tissues. Zentralbl Hyg Umweltmed 198(4):331–339.

59. Gajduskova V, Ulrich R, Ledvinova J et al. (1996). Concentrations of polychlorinated biphenyls and chlorinated pesticides in human breast milk—a case study. Cent Eur J Publ Health 4(2):110–114.

60. Wolff MS, Anderson HA, and Selikoff IJ. (1982). Human tissue burdens of halogenated aromatic chemicals in Michigan. JAMA 247(15):2112–2116.

61. *Ibid.*

62. Stehr-Green PA. (1989). Demographic and seasonal influences on human serum pesticide residue levels. J Toxicol Environ Health 27(4):405–421.

63. Trotter WJ and Dickerson R. (1993). Pesticide residues in composited milk collected through the U.S. Pasteurized Milk Network. J AOAC Int 76(6):1220–1225.

64. Waliszewski SM, Pardio VT, Waliszewski KN et al. Organochlorine pesticides in Mexican butter. J AOAC Int 79(3):784–786.

65. Archibeque-Engle SL, Tessari JD, Winn DT et al. (1997). Comparison of organochlorine pesticide and polychlorinated biphenyl residues in human adipose breast tissue and serum. J Toxicol Environ Health 52(4):285–293.

66. Lordo RA, Dinh KT, and Schwemberger JG. (1996). Semivolatile organic compounds in adipose tissue: estimated averages for the US population and selected subpopulations. Am J Publ Health 86(9):1253–1259.

67. Menichini E, Bocca A, Merli F et al. (1991). Polycyclic aromatic hydrocarbons in olive oils on the Italian market. Food Addit Contamin 8(3):363–369.

68. Mott L and Snyder K. (1987). Pesticide alert. Sierra Club Books, San Francisco,pp.12–15.

69. MacIntosh DL, Spengler JD, Ozkaynak H et al. (1996). Dietary exposures to selected metals and pesticides. Environ Health Perspect 104(2):202–209.

70. Stehr-Green PA, *op. cit. (see reference 62).*

71. *Ibid.*

72. Neidert E, Saschenbrecker PW, and Patterson JR. (1984). Detection and occurrence of pentachlorophenol residues in chicken liver and fat. J Environ Sci Health 19(7):579–592.

73. Rea WJ. (1996). Pesticides. J Nutr Environ Med 6:55–124.

74. U.S. Environmental Protection Agency. (1995). Estimating exposure to dioxin-like compounds. Vol II. Properties, sources, occurrence and background exposures. EPA/600/6–88/005Cb. USEPA, Washington, D.C.

75. *Ibid.*

76. Lorber M, Cleverly D, Schaum J et al. (1994). Development and validation of an air-to-beef food chain model for dioxin-like compounds. Sci Total Environ 156(1):39–65.

77. Harte J, Holdren C, Schneider R, et al. (1991). *Op.cit. (see reference 5),* p. 297.

78. Wurster CF. (1968). DDT residues and declining reproduction in the Bermuda petrel. Sci 159:979–981.

79. Kerr RA. (1981). Pollution of the Arctic atmosphere confirmed. Sci 212:371–374.

80. Whalen M. Kunz CO, Matuszek JM et al. (1980). Radioactive plume from the Three Mile Island accident: xenon-133 in air at a distance of 375 kilometers. Sci 207:638–639.

81. Flint ML and van den Bosch R. (1981). Introduction to integrated pest management. Plenum Press, New York.

82. *Ibid.*

83. Wania F and Mackay D. (1996). Tracking the distribution of persistent organic pollutants. Environ Sci Technol 30(9):390A–396A.

84. Kitamura K, Yoshida H, Ohno R et al. (1997). Toxic effects of arsenic (As3+) and other metal ionis on acute promyelocytic leukemia cells. Int J Hematol 65(2):179–185.

85. Denny MF and Atchinson WD. (1996). Mercurial-induced alterations in neuronal divalent cation homeostasis. Neurotoxicol 17:47–61.

86. Aschner M, Rising L, and Mullaney KJ. (1996). Differential sensitivity of neonatal rat astrocyte cultures to mercuric chloride (MC) and methylmercury (MeHg): studies on K+ and amino acid transport and metallothionein (MT) induction. Neurotoxicol 17:107–116.

87. Marzabadi MR and Jones CB. (1992). A study on myocardial cells cultured under varying oxidative stress. Mech Ageing Dev 66(2):159–171.

88. Mesco ER, Kachen C, and Timiras PS. (1991). Effects of aluminum on tau proteins in human neuroblastoma cells. Mol Chem Neuropathol 14:199–212.

89. Moon J. (1994). The role of vitamin D in toxic metal absorption: a review. J Am Coll Nutr 13(6):559–569.

90. Bakir F, DamlujiSF, Amin-Zaki L et al. (1973). Methylmercury poisoning in Iraq. Sci 181:230–241.

91. Szymczak W. (1997). A qualitative evaluation of health risk associated with occupational inhalation exposure to cadmium in production plants in Poland. Med Pr 48(1):35–43.

92. Ragan HA and Mast TJ. (1990). Cadmium inhalation and male reproductive toxicity. Rev Environ Contam Toxicol 114:1–22.

93. Galal-Gorchev H. (1993). Dietary intake, levels in food and estimated intake of lead, cadmium, and mercury. Food Addit Contamin 10(1):115–128.

94. Hoffmann J and Blasenbrei P. (1986). Cadmium in blue poppy seeds and poppy seed-containing products. Z Lebensm Unters Forsch 182(2):121–122.

95. Tahvonen R and Kumpulainen J. (1993). Lead and cadmium in some cereal products on the Finnish market 1990–91. Food Addit Contamin 10(2):245–255.

96. *Ibid.*

97. Kreis IA, Wijga A, and van Wijnen JH. (1992). Assessment of the lifetime accumulated cadmium intake from food in Kempenland. Sci Total Environ 127(3):281–292.

98. Anonymous. (1993). EPA finds high lead levels across nation. Nutr Week 19:6.

99. Roberts JW, Camann DE, and Spittler TM. (1990). Monitoring and controlling lead in house dust in older homes. Proceedings of the Fifth International Conference on Indoor Air, Indoor Air 90, Toronto, Canada.

100. Davidson CL and Elias R. (1986). Environmental concentrations and potential pathways to human exposure. Air quality criteria for lead. USEPA, Research Triangle Park, North Carolina.

101. Jelinek CF. (1982). Levels of lead in the United States food supply. J Assoc Off Anal Chem 65(4):942–946.

102. Galal-Gorchev H, *op. cit. (see reference 93).*

103. National Center for Environmental Health. (1997). Facts on lead. Centers for Disease Control and Prevention, Atlanta, GA.

104. Lecos CW. (1987). Pretty poison: lead and ceramic ware. U.S. Department of Health and Human Services, HHS Publication No. (FDA) 87–1139, Rockville, MD.

105. Weisel C, Demak M, and Goldstein BD. (1991). Soft plastic bread packaging: lead content and reuse by families. Am J Publ Health 81(6):756–758.

106. *Ibid.*

107. Tsubaki T and Irukayama K. (Eds). (1977). Minamata disease. Kodansha, Tokyo.

108. *Ibid.*

109. Yess NJ. (1993). U.S. Food and Drug Administration survey of methyl mercury in canned tuna. J AOAC Int 76(1):36–38.

110. Tsuda T, Inoue T, Kojima M et al. (1995). Market basket and duplicate portion estimation of dietary intakes of cadmium, mercury, arsenic, copper, manganese, and zinc by Japanese adults. J AOAC Int 78(6):1363–1368.

111. Bakir F, Damluji SF, Amin-Zaki L et al., *op. cit. (see reference 90).*

112. Granato TC, Pietz RI, Gschwind J et al. (1995). Mercury in soils and crops from fields receiving high cumulative sewage sludge applications: validation of the U.S. EPA's risk assessment for human ingestion, Water Soil and Air Pollut 80(1–4):1119–1127.

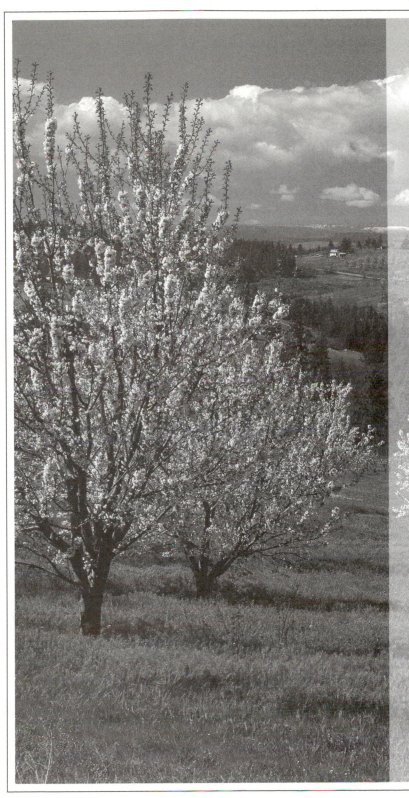

CHAPTER 4

Toxins in the U.S. Food Supply

PART I
Regulation

PART II
Levels of Toxicity

CONTENTS

Chapter 4: **Toxins in the U.S. Food Supply**

Toxins in the U.S. Food Supply

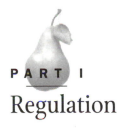

PART I

Regulation

In this chapter we will review two aspects of the U.S. food supply: its regulation and level of toxicity. Toxins in the U.S. food supply are regulated and surveyed at a variety of levels. The majority of this regulation and surveillance is conducted by government agencies at the instruction of the U.S. Congress. However, non-governmental organizations in both the public and private sectors also play an important role in the surveillance of food toxins.

Government Agencies

The United States Environmental Protection Agency (EPA), the United States Department of Agriculture (USDA), and the Food and Drug Administration (FDA), housed within the Department of Health and Human Services (HHS) constitute the three major government agencies directly involved in regulation of the U.S. food supply. In this section we will look more closely at each of these organizations and its role in regulating food toxins.

EPA

Following passage of the National Environment Policy Act (NEPA) in 1969, the United States Environmental Protection Agency was created through Congressional legislation in December 1970 to develop and enforce standards for environmental protection. The EPA currently oversees implementation of two pieces of legislation controlling food quality.

Safe Drinking Water Act (SDWA)

The first and oldest of these legislative acts is the Safe Drinking Water Act (SDWA) of 1974. Under this act, the EPA is charged with assurance of safe water at the tap. In order to provide this assurance, the EPA monitors groundwater throughout the United States, and has special enforcement powers to protect areas in which a single underground aquifer serves as the primary source of drinking water. Under SDWA, the EPA monitors levels of approximately one hundred potential toxins in drinking water. Examples of safe drinking water standards are presented in *Table 4-1.*

Table 4-1. Examples of EPA safe drinking water standards

Inorganic

Element	Maximum allowable level
Arsenic	50mcg/L
Barium	1000mcg/L
Cadmium	10mcg/L
Lead	50mcg/L
Mercury	2mcg/L
Silver	50mcg/L
Fluoride	4000mcg/L

Organics

Substance	Maximum allowable level
Endrin	.2mcg/L
Lindane	4mcg/L
Methoxychlor	100mcg/L
Benzene	5mcg/L
Carbon tetrachloride	5mcg/L
p-Dichlorobenzene	75mcg/L
Vinyl chloride	2mcg/L
1,2 dichloroethane	5mcg/L
Trichloroethylene	5mcg/L
Total trihalomethanes	100mcg/L

Also under SWDA, the EPA is required to maintain Offices of Water Enforcement and Permits, Water Regulations and Standards, Water Programs Operations, Drinking Water, and Groundwater. An Office of Pollution Prevention and Toxics is required under the Toxic Substances Control Act (TSCA) of 1976.

Several other pieces of national legislation affect EPA regulation of water. These acts include the Federal Insecticide, Fungicide and Rodenticide Act (FIFRA) of 1947; the Clean Air Act (CAA) of 1970; the Clean Water Act (CWA) of 1972; the Lead-Based Paint Poisoning Prevention Act (LBPPPA) of 1973; the Resource Conservation and Recovery Act (RCRA) of 1976; the Toxic Substances Control Act (TSCA) of 1976, the Surface Mining Control and Reclamation Act (SMCRA) of 1977; the Hazardous Liquid Pipeline Safety Act (HLPSA) of 1979; the Comprehensive Environmental Response, Compensation and Liability Act (CERCLA) of 1980; and the Asbestos Hazard Emergency Response Act (AHERA) of 1986.

Food Quality Protection Act (FQPA)

The second piece of legislation whose implementation falls under EPA jurisdiction is the Food Quality Protection Act (FQPA) of 1996. Under FQPA, the EPA is required to perform a combined risk assessment for substances in food that produce adverse affects through a common mechanism of toxicity. The phrase "common mechanism of toxicity" allows the EPA to combine risks associated with different chemicals in food whenever the mechanism of injury from these chemicals is expected to be the same. It also allows EPA to treat the effects of different food chemicals as additive.[1]

Under FQPA, the EPA is also instructed to follow major revisions made by Congress in the Federal Food, Drug and Cosmetic Act (FFDCA) of 1938. The most significant of these revisions is repeal of the Delaney Clause for pesticides. Perhaps the best known aspect of food legislation over the past fifty years, the Delaney Clause was a key provision of the Food Additives Amendment of 1958 to the FFDCA. This provision, named after Congressman James Delaney (the former Democrat from New York), stated:

> "Provided, that no additive shall be deemed safe if it is
> found to induce cancer when ingested by man or animal,
> or if it is found, after tests which are appropriate for the
> evaluation of the safety of food additives, to induce cancer
> in man or animals...."

The standard set by the Delaney Clause was a standard of "zero tolerance." In other words, once a substance was shown to have cancer-inducing effects, it was not permitted in the food supply in any amount. The history

of the Delaney Clause, its repeal in 1996 under the FQPA, and ongoing toxicology debates over units of measurement are vitally important in understanding current debates over toxins in the food supply. For this reason, we
will look more closely at this history and its significance for food regulation.

The Delaney Clause and Units of Measurement

At the time of Delaney, food laboratories throughout the country were able
to measure potential toxins at the level of 100 parts per billion (ppb). To
understand this unit of measurement more concretely, imagine a container
holding exactly one liter, or 33.8 ounces of water. Now think about dividing up this liter of water into thousands of smaller portions. You could
divide it up into single drops, in which case you would end up with about
30,000 one-drop portions. Or you could divide it up more arbitrarily into
1,000 equal portions. Each of these portions would be one milliliter containing about 30 drops of water. These one drop and thirty drop portions
are still much larger than ppb units of measurement.

In order to visualize the ppb units of measurement used at the time of
Delaney to assess toxic risk, imagine taking the 30,000 drops of water and
dividing each one into a thousand mini-droplets. In this case, the container
would contain not 30,000, but 30,000,000 (30 million) mini-droplets, and it
would take 1,000 of these droplets to equal one drop. At the time of Delaney,
a food could be withdrawn from the marketplace if 3 out of these 30,000,000
mini-droplets (or approximately 3/100ths of one drop) contained within it
could be determined to cause cancer. Detecting 3 out of 30,000,000 droplets
is the same as detecting 1 out of 10,000,000, and also the same as detecting
100 out of 1,000,000,000 (one billion). At the time of the Delaney Clause,
that was exactly the level of toxin that could be detected in food labs: 100
ppb. Nothing smaller (for example, 1ppb) could be detected.

To detect a toxin at the level of 1ppb, or at an even smaller level like
1 ppt (one part per trillion), an imaginary container of water would have
to be divided up into smaller units. Instead of being 3/100ths of a drop in
size, these new units would have to be closer to 3/100,000ths of one drop.
It was precisely this jump in precision that took place in toxic assessment
between the original passage of the Delaney Clause in 1958 and the passage
of the FQPA in 1996. During this period of time, food labs gained the ability to detect toxic substances at the ppt level. *Table 4-2* summarizes the
basic relationship between parts per million, parts per billion, and parts per
trillion measurement.

As more and more time passed following the passage of Delaney, many
government officials, including officials within the EPA, began to argue
that changes in laboratory capability were changing the meaning of "zero

TOXINS IN THE U.S. FOOD SUPPLY **137**

Table 4-2. Levels of measurement

Level	Abbreviation	Detection based on a per-kilogram equivalent	Absolute level of detection	Order of magnitude
Parts per million	ppm	1 milligram/kilogram	micrograms	10^{-6}
Parts per billion	ppb	1 microgram/kilogram	nanograms	10^{-9}
Parts per trillion	ppt	1 nanogram/kilogram	picograms	10^{-12}

tolerance." Since laboratory measurements in 1958 could not detect the presence of toxins below 100 ppb, "zero" in 1958 meant anything less than one hundred out of one billion. However, undetectable quantities of toxins labeled "zero" in 1958 had become fully detectable by 1980, and "zero" had to be redefined as anything less than one hundred out of one trillion.

By the mid 1980s, these new measurement capabilities created a regulatory dilemma for organizations like the EPA. On the one hand, the EPA was required under Delaney to prohibit carcinogens in food in any amount. On the other hand, pervasive presence of carcinogens in the environment had left carcinogenic residues throughout the food supply at this newly-detectable, ppt level. Although this dilemma involved many types of food carcinogens, no type posed more problems for EPA regulators than pesticides. (While pesticides also posed problems for the United States Food and Drug Administration, the agency responsible for monitoring presence of pesticides in food, their impact was greater upon the EPA since it was responsible for regulating use and sale.)

As early as the 1960s, exposure to pesticides had been linked to increased risk of tumors.[2] By the early 1970s, specific links had been made between the magnitude of pesticide exposure and the risk of leukemia[3] as well as breast cancer.[4] By the early 1990s, the cancer-pesticide connection list had been expanded to include brain cancer,[5] non-Hodgkin's lymphoma,[6] testicular cancer,[7] and liver cancer.[8] Alongside of this mounting evidence about the carcinogenicity of pesticides was their increasing presence in the food supply. By the end of the 1960s, farmers were buying over one billion dollars' worth of pesticides per year, over five times the amount purchased at the time of Delaney.[9] The increasing agricultural use of pesticides continued through the 1970s and 1980s, so that by 1988, almost 850 million pounds of pesticides were used by U.S. farmers.[10] As of 1992, 73 pesticides authorized for agricultural use were classified as potential carcinogens by the EPA.[11] As of 1996, almost three fourths (71.8%) of all fruits and vegetables analyzed by the USDA's Pesticide Data Program were determined to contain pesticide residues.[12]

The EPA's initial response to this cancer-pesticide detection dilemma was to ignore the Delaney Clause and in 1986 to announce a new approach to food carcinogens. This new approach was based on the doctrine of *de minimis*.[13] Under this doctrine, the EPA argued that many carcinogenic substances clearly forbidden under Delaney could actually be permitted in the food supply at ppt levels, provided that intake of these food carcinogens did not increase lifelong risk of cancer development by more than one chance in one million. Although particularly helpful with respect to pesticides, the *de minimis* doctrine was subsequently applied to all potential food carcinogens.

In 1996 under FQPA, Congress ended the need for a *de minimis* approach to pesticides by officially repealing the Delaney Clause with respect to food-use pesticides. The 1996 law stated that residues from pesticides would be permitted in food, even when these pesticides had been shown to be carcinogenic, provided that there existed "a reasonable certainty that no harm will result." As a result of FQPA, numerous pesticide manufacturers, including Bayer AG (based in Germany), Novartis (based in Switzerland), and Dow Chemical (based in Midland, Michigan, USA) began to immediately increase experimentation on pesticide effects in human subjects.[14]

USDA

The United States Department of Agriculture (USDA) was a direct outgrowth of the National Board of Agriculture established by the first president of the United States in 1796. Since that time, the USDA has evolved into a multi-service operation that oversees the quality of the U.S. food supply through a variety of intradepartmental services.

Animal and Plant Health Inspection Service (APHIS)

The USDA's Animal and Plant Health Inspection Service (APHIS) is empowered to negotiate legislation, intercept food shipments, and sample products in an effort to help reduce food supply problems caused by organisms like salmonella, weevils, fruit flies and screwworm.

Federal Grain and Inspection Service (FGIS)

The Federal Grain and Inspection Service (FGIS) publishes procedures for fumigation of grains, and inspects grain shipments that travel by ground, primarily by railway. Inspection of grain manufacturing and storage facilities also falls under FGIS jurisdiction. FGIS is empowered to help revise standards applied to food. For example, in 1990, the service subdivided white wheat into hard and soft classifications in response to marketplace requests.

Food Safety and Inspection Service (FSIS)

The Food Safety and Inspection Service (FSIS) is USDA's meat and poultry inspection service. About 50 billion pounds of animal products are inspected annually, and onsite inspections follow the Hazard Analysis and Critical Control Point (HACCP) system. In this system, a "critical control point" is defined as any step or procedure in which biological contaminants can be killed or controlled. Steps like rapid cooling of foods to 40° Fahrenheit, total time in "danger zone" temperatures, and handwashing are emphasized in HACCP. FSIS also samples approximately 500,000 animal products from production plants across the country and analyzes approximately 150 chemical residues on an annual basis. Non-biological contaminants like hormonal or antibiotic residues are not monitored through HACCP.

HACCP is actually one aspect of a broader, umbrella-like set of governmental regulations that are designed to promote safety of the food supply. This broad set of regulations is referred to as GMP, or Good Manufacturing Practice. GMP for the food industry undergoes continual government revision and has a broad scope that includes activities as diverse as bacterial testing of food, use of chemical sanitizers in manufacturing plants, and installation of plumbing.

Since 1917, when the first grading standards were established for potatoes, the USDA has also been responsible for classification of foods based on non-nutritional standards to facilitate commercial transactions in the marketplace. Standards were initially designed to provide a fair basis for establishing price, and also to assist in determination of loan values for products in storage. Grades were established for virtually all categories of food by the mid-1930s.

FDA

History

Originally established in 1862 as the Chemical Division of the USDA, the United States Food and Drug Administration (FDA) has undergone several reincarnations during its statutory and institutional history. Renamed the Division of Chemistry in 1890, and the Bureau of Chemistry in 1901, the organization was involved in enforcement of the Biologics Act of 1902, a Congressional response to tetanus-triggered deaths of children in St. Louis, Missouri following innoculation for diphtheria with tetanus-infected antitoxin.[15] Also carried out within the Division of Chemistry was a 1990 study of food additives by 12 USDA employees. These employees themselves became subjects in a dietary intake study analyzing the effect of boron-containing additives, salicylates, sulfur-containing additives (including sulfites), and benzoic acid derivatives in food.[16]

The name "Food, Drug and Insecticide Administration" was chosen in 1927 to reflect the increased responsibility of the organization in this area. Three years later, the present-day name was adopted, although in 1953, jurisdiction over the FDA was transferred from the USDA to the United States Department of Health, Education and Welfare (HEW). That agency was itself renamed in 1979 as the United States Department of Health and Human Services (HHS) and still provides the FDA with its current home. At present, the FDA employs approximately 9,000 persons, including 1,100 inspectors in food and non-food areas. Just under 100,000 U.S. businesses have practices that fall under FDA jurisdiction, and approximately 15,000 facilities receive on-site inspections each year.

General Legal Jurisdiction

FDA is charged with enforcement of a wide variety of federal laws. *Table 4-3* lists these laws and their dates of passage.

Specific Jurisdiction Over Food Irradiation

A final food-related area of FDA jurisdiction is irradiation. Because this area of oversight is both complex and rapidly expanding in the regulation of food safety, we will look closely at its status.

Overview. Food irradiation involves short-term exposure of food, often in packaged form on ready-to-send shipping pallets, to electromagnetic radiation in the rage of 10–10 to 10–14 meters wavelength (million trillionths of a meter) and 1019 to 1022 frequency (one trillion trillion cycles per second). These extremely high-frequency and short wavelength forces are called *gamma rays*, and the type of radiation is called *gamma radiation*. Unlike other forms of radiation, including alpha radiation (in which rays have a positive electrical charge and consist of a stream of helium nuclei) or beta radiation (in which rays have a negative charge and consist of a stream of electrons), gamma rays have no charge at all and consist of a stream of photons. Gamma rays also operate at exponentially shorter wavelengths and exponentially quicker frequencies than either microwaves or X-rays.

Regulatory History. Irradiation of food has been legal in the United States for over 35 years, and its regulation primarily involves two government agencies. The FDA is responsible for setting irradiation policy, and since 1963, has issued rulings for 9 separate categories of food and their authorized treatment by irradiation. The USDA, through APHIS, can order irradiation as a quarantine treatment for food being imported into the United States. Through FSIS, it can order irradiation following inspection of meat and poultry.

Approved Uses. Table 4-4, on the following page, summarizes FDA rulings on food irradiation since August 1963. As presented in this table, food irradiation has been approved for use in controlling insects, parasites, and bacteria that can contaminate food, and also for altering the natural life cycles of plants. For example, delaying the ripening of fruit and delaying sprouting of potatoes are approved uses of food irradiation.

Approved Doses. The doses of radiation listed in *Table 4-4* are extremely high in comparison to doses received by living organisms. In order to understand the difference in magnitude between these doses, it is helpful

Table 4-3. *Federal laws enforced by the FDA*

Law	Date of Passage
Federal Food and Drug Act of 1906	1906
Food, Drug and Cosmetic Act of 1938	1938
Public Health Service Act	1944
Miller Pesticides Amendment	1954
Poultry Products Inspection Act (PPIA)	1957
Food Additives Amendment of 1958	1958
Color Additives Amendment of 1960	1960
Fair Packaging and Labeling Act (FPLA)	1966
Federal Meat Inspection Act	1967
Radiation Control for Health and Safety Act (RCHSA)	1968
Controlled Substances Act	1970
Controlled Substances Import and Export Act (CSIEA)	1970
Egg Products Inspection Act (EPIA)	1970
Lead-Based Paint Poisoning Prevention Act (LBPPPA)	1971
Toxic Substances Control Act (TSCA)	1976
Medical Device Amendments of 1976	1976
Federal Pesticide Act of 1978	1978
Infant Formula Amendment of 1980	1980
Federal Anti-Tampering Act	1983
Drug Price Competition and Patent Restoration Act of 1984	1984
Nutrition Labeling and Education Act (NLEA)	1990
Safe Medical Devices Act	1990
Dietary Supplement and Health Education Act (DSHEA)	1994

Table 4-4. FDA-approved uses of food irradiation

Food	Date of Approval	Dose Permitted (RADS)	Approved Purpose
Wheat/wheat powder	1963	20,000-50,000	Insect decontamination
White potatoes	1965	5,000-15,000	Prevention of sprouting
Spices/seasonings	1983	3,000,000	Insect decontamination
Dehydrated enzymes	1985	1,000,000	Insect decontamination
Pork	1985	30,000-100,000	Parasite decontamination
Fresh fruit	1986	100,000	Delayed ripening
Dry vegetable substances	1986	3,000,000	Microbe decontamination
Poultry	1990	300,000	Microbe decontamination
Beef, lamb	1997	450,000 (fresh) 700,000 (frozen)	Microbe decontamination

Table 4-5. Units of measurement in radiation assessment

Unit	Definition
Rad	Radiation absorbed dose
Millirad	0.001 rad
Kilorad	1,000 rads (also equal to 10 Gy)
Megarad	1,000,000 rads (also equal to 10 kGy)
Gray (Gy)	100 rads
Kilogray (kGy)	1,000 Gy (also equal to 100,000 rads)

to know basic measurement units used by radiologists to study radiation. These basic measurement units are summarized in *Table 4-5*.

An average chest x-ray exposes the human body to approximately 10 millirads of radiation. This level is the same as 1/100th of one rad, or 300 million times smaller than the allowable dose applied to spices in the marketplace. While most scientists believe that a single chest x-ray can be conducted without significant harm to the individual, tissue tolerances to radiation in living organisms are relatively low. Major health compromise can occur from exposure to radiation in the range of 1,000s or even 100s of rads. Some examples of tissue tolerance are listed in *Table 4-6*, on page 145.

Supporters of food irradiation have downplayed the difference in magnitude between medical and food irradiation by focusing upon the difference between living (human) and dead (food) organisms. Research findings suggest that this difference may not be as large as irradiation supporters

BACK TO BASIC CONCEPTS

Irradiated Beef and Forgotten Wholeness

Most objections to food irradiation have focused on the issue of food quality. These objections cite the failure of irradiation to address the underlying, root-level causes of food contamination in the U.S. food supply. As an example of this failure, critics have pointed to the story of Hudson Foods, and the most recent FDA expansion of food irradiation to include beef.

The Hudson Foods Recall

On December 3, 1997, in response to a petition by the Hudson Foods Company based in Rogers, Arkansas, the FDA announced its decision to allow irradiation of beef at 4.5–7.0 kGy. The decision came after a six-month series of events that began in early June 1997 when one of Hudson's meat packing facilities in Columbus, Nebraska unknowingly began to pack beef contaminated with the *E. coli* bacterium 0157:H7. The $16 million dollar beef packing facility had been opened by Hudson in 1995 to process beef for the Burger King fast food chain. Each week it produced approximately 2.5 million pounds of beef.

On August 12, 1997, Hudson voluntarily recalled 20,000 pounds of beef following reports received by the Colorado Department of Public Health and Environment linking *E. coli* poisoning to Hudson-packed meat. By August 15, 1.2 million pounds had been recalled. By August 20, following reports of illness in Gainsville, Florida also linked to Hudson, all 25 million pounds of beef packed since June 5, 1997 were recalled and the

Nebraska plant was shut down. On August 23, Burger King announced that it would stop buying meat from Hudson Foods. On August 28, the Columbus, Nebraska packing facility was sold by Hudson to IBP, the Dakota City, Nebraska meat-packing company (and the largest meat packer in the United States).

Critics of food irradiation like Least Cost Formulations, Ltd. in Virginia Beach, Virginia have argued that while irradiation of the Hudson beef would likely have prevented these *E. coli* 0157:H7 outbreaks, and in this respect, would have been a life-saving public health step, it would, in the long run, only have placed consumers and the food supply in further jeopardy by leaving the real source of the problem untouched. This reasoning of Least Cost Formulations is parallel to the reasoning about environmental nutrition presented in the first chapter of this book. Chapter 1 argued that over the past hundred years, nutritionists limited their research focus to the *association* between food and nutrients, rather than exploring the underlying interactions that made this association possible. According to the reasoning presented in Chapter 1, if these *underlying interactions* had been explored, nutritionists would have found themselves looking further into the environment and would have recognized environmental standards as the real source of nourishment. Similarly, nutritionists looking at underlying inteactions would have recognized environmental disruption as the true source of malnourishment and health problems. ◗

suggest. For example, just as radiation therapy has been shown to deplete vitamin B-12[23] and vitamin D[24] in cancer subjects, so has food irradiation been shown to deplete B vitamins[25, 26] as well as fat-soluble vitamins like A and E.[27] Similarly, both human radiation therapy and food irradiation have been shown to alter cell structures and intracellular activity. Increased free

---

BACK TO BASIC CONCEPTS: Irradiated Beef and Forgotten Wholeness

CONTINUED

Origins of *E. Coli* Contamination

Critics of the FDA decision to prevent future Hudson Foods episodes by irradiating beef have argued that the *association* between *E. coli* 0157:H7 and beef is not nearly as important as the underlying interactions that made this association possible. The real issue, they-have argued, is how *E. coli* 0157:H7 got into the beef in the first place. Least Cost Formulations has proposed a number of factors as being responsible for the presence of *E. coli* in Hudson Foods beef. These factors include the failure of ranchers to wash manure off cattle before sending them to market; the failure of ranchers to stop feeding animals at least half a day before slaughter, thus reducing their intestinal contents and lessening the chance of bursting at slaughter; the practice of packagers like Hudson to reuse "rework" (broken or poorly formed meat patties) two and three days after initial processing, thus extending the risk of contamination by reusing product over several days; the failure of food servers at fast food restaurants to cook ground beef at 160 degrees Fahrenheit; the lack of *E. coli* testing at multiple points along the beef production process; and the failure of governmental agencies like the USDA and FDA to set and enforce regulations preventing all of the failures described above.[17]

From the point of view of this book, each of these failures can also be classified as an example of forgotten wholeness. Once cattle have been separated from their natural environment and ranchers have been separated from their natural instinct to care for animals, there is no way for irradiation to gallop in and save the day. Once the underlying dynamics of contamination have been ignored, there is no way to avoid a response that is targeted exclusively at the presence of the bacteria. Such a response exchanges the good of the whole for the good of one part at the present moment, and it reduces the overall capacity of the food supply to provide nourishment.

The Future of Irradiation

Ongoing disregard for underlying environmental dynamics will most likely encourage increasing use of food irradiation. With 346 million bushels of wheat being produced annually in the U.S.,[18] over 500,000 tons of poultry meat and processed poultry products,[19] and total animal protein consumption reaching 224 pounds per person per year,[20] the potential for increase is high. About 65 million pounds of spices and dried or dehydrated vegetable products are irradiated annually in the U.S.[21] Worldwide, total food irradiation has been estimated at 500,000 tons, or 500 million pounds per year.[22] ■

radical production has been demonstrated in corn starch irradiated at 20kGy,[28] in fruit irradiated at 5kGy,[29] and in egg yolk irradiated at 10 kGy.[30] Similarly, in humans, ionizing radiation has been shown to generate increased free radical production,[31] and through this process, to cause increased oxidation of unsaturated lipids in cell membranes.[32] Damage to cellular structures in both food and humans may also occur through other mechanisms. Double- and single-stranded breaks in DNA[33] and changes in plasma membrane permeability to non-electrolytes[34] have been shown in humans, while changes in plasma membrane permeability to electrolytes[35] have been shown in food.

Consumption-Related Health Risks. Much less clear than the above similarities between food irradiation and human radiation therapy are the consequences of human consumption of irradiated foods. Perhaps the highest-risk consequence that remains the subject of an unresolved debate is the consequence of genetic polyploidy.

Polyploidy refers to a condition in which two or more sets of chromosomes are created within the cells of an organism. Human cells, for example, ordinarily contain a single set of 46 chromosomes. A polyploid human cell might contain two sets (92 chromosomes), three sets (138 chromosomes), or even more sets of chromosomes. The mechanism for polyploidy in humans can be relatively simple, including events like dispermy (the penetration of two sperm into a single ovum). However, despite this relative simplicity, polyploidy in humans is relatively rare, and particularly in comparison to other organisms like plants, where polyploidy can occur almost 50% of the time.[36]

While polyploidy has yet to be definitively connected to adverse health effects in humans, several organizations, including the European Centre for Ecotoxicology and Toxicology of Chemicals (ECETOC) in Brussels, Belgium

*Table 4-6. **Tolerances to radiation in living tissue**[37]*

Type of tissue	Problematic effects	Dose of occurrence (rads)
Bone marrow	Aplasia	250
Kidney	Nephrosclerosis	2,000
Lung	Pneumonitis, fibrosis	2,500
Liver	Hepatitis	3,000
Intestine	Ulceration, fibrosis	4,500
Heart	Pericarditis	4,500
Skin	Sclerosis, dermatitis	5,000
Brain	Infarct, necrosis	6,000

have recommended routine testing for polyploidy in humans.[38] Polyploidy has been associated with adverse postnatal life expectancy when occurring in pregnancy,[39] uterine adenomyomas in mid-life,[40] embryonal renal neoplasms,[41] use of antiparasitic drugs like flubendazole,[42] and tumorigenesis in the head and neck regions.[43]

In their outstanding review of ionizing radiation, polyploidy, and cell function,[44] researchers at the Institute of Medicine Research Center in Julich, Germany have divided the potential impact of radiation-induced polyploidy into two basic categories. In the first category is the effect of radiation-induced polyploidy on cells that are undergoing active mitosis. In the absence of any restriction upon cytoplasmic growth, these cells are harmed by radiation-induced polyploidy since amplification divisions (normally passed through by cells before terminal differentiation) are eliminated and the total number of differentiated cells produced through mitosis is reduced. In a second category are terminally differentiated cells, not passing through mitosis. These cells are protected by radiation-induced polyploidy, since extra identical chromosomal sets can help offset the impact of genetic lesions created by radiation and the remaining life span of the cells can be lengthened. Also falling into this second category are cells that are undergoing mitosis, but with a concurrent restriction on cytoplasmic growth during this mitosis period. In this case, radiated cells are also protected by induction of polyploidy. Because cells in foods under going irradiation are presumably not engaged in mitosis, these distinctions made by the Institute of Medicine researchers may apply much more directly to human oncotherapy than to food irradiation. However, they may also give us a helpful conceptual framework for trying to understand the research controversy over food irradiation and polyploidy which saw the induction of polyploidy in both human and animal subjects following consumption of irradiated foods.

The controversy over food irradiation and polyploidy began in the mid 1970s when studies on animals and humans showed increased polyploidy following consumption of irradiated wheat. In the animal studies, rats[45] and hamsters[46] were fed diets containing wheat irradiated at very low doses in the rage of 5–10 rads. In both studies, however, questions were raised about the nature of the association between polyploidy and irradiated food, since the incidence of polyploidy did not appear to increase when doses of radiation applied to wheat were increased, and since chromosomal breaks and deletions were also observed to occur in association with other dietary parameters like protein deficiency.

Rather than providing clear anwers, a 1975 study on consumption of irradiated wheat in humans raised similar questions. In this study, increased polyploidy was observed in children fed diets containing irradiated wheat.[47] Firm conclusions about the relationship between irradiation and polyploidy could not be made however, since overall malnourishment and protein deficiency in some children were also viewed as possible causes of polyploidy.

Radioactivity in Science and Industry

Physics and Chemistry

It was the work of French physicists Henri Becquerel and Marie and Pierre Curie in the late 1800s that led to the present-day understanding of radioactivity. These researchers determined that energy levels differed not only in the electron structure of atoms, but also within their nuclear structure. Their experiments uncovered a connection between energetic changes within the two structures. When electrons fell to lower energy levels within the electron structure of an element, they noted that nucleons (either protons or neutrons) in an unstable nucleus could fall to lower energy levels as well and in this process could emit (and eject) photons (quantum units of light). Elements undergoing these changes were described as radioactive (and in this case, to be emitting gamma radiation). The ejection of electrons from an unstable nucleus, causing an element to emit beta radiation, is now known to occur in a similar fashion. Also similar is the ejection of helium nuclei (containing two protons and two neutrons, and therefore positively charged) from an unstable nucleus. Elements undergoing this process are alpha reactive.

All elements have isotopes whose total neutron number and total proton number are different and thus create nuclear instability. Moreover, about 50 elements have more radioactive, unstable isotopes than stable ones, and are therefore net natural emitters of radiation. Given this natural occurrence of radioactivity across a wide range of elements, it might be expected that our human exposure to radiation would be naturally high. However, this exposure turns out to be quite low for two reasons. First, many radioactive isotopes rapidly decay (that is, quickly transmute into non-radioactive elements). Sodium 24, for example, decays within 15 hours, and magnesium 28 in 21 hours. Second, even though many elements decay exceptionally slowly (over billions of years), they remain locked inside of natural rock formations where they remain distant and shielded from human beings. For example, uranium 238 is a natural component of uraninite, a pitch-like, submetallic mineral found in hydrothermal replacement deposits not normally in striking distance of human beings. It takes 4.5 billion years for this uranium 238 to decay into lead 206 (its non-radioactive, ▶

stable transmutate), but unless uraninite is deliberately mined for its uranium content, these 4.5 billion years can pass harmlessly. In addition to uranium 235 and 238, naturally-occurring emitters of gamma radiation in our environment include potassium 40, radium 226, and thorium 230.

In addition to these naturally-occurring radioisotopes are artificial radioisotopes created through the use of nuclear reactors. These artificial isotopes are created by bombardment of a specific element with some form of high-energy radiation including alpha, beta, or gamma radiation. By far the most common element to get bombarded in man-made nuclear reactors is uranium.

Nuclear Fission

Throughout the 1930s, 1940s, and 1950s, scientists worldwide began to experiment with nuclear reactions involving two basic types of processes. Some of these experiments involved nuclear fission, that is, the process described above in which the nucleus of an atom could be split into smaller parts by raising the energy level of electron-based repulsive forces above the energy level of nuclear-based attractive forces. The splitting of atoms was found to work best with the element uranium, particularly if this element was first purified into one of its isotopes, uranium 235 (^{235}U). (Symbols for isotopes use the chemical symbol, in this case "U" for uranium, preceded by a numerical superscript indicating the mass number, i.e., the total number of neutrons plus protons in the

isotope). Once purified, this ^{235}U could be bombarded with a neutron, split into smaller parts, and forced to release an enormous amount of energy in the process. This enormous energy release was demonstrated on August 6, 1945 when a uranium-based fission bomb the size of a baseball was dropped onto Hiroshima, Japan killing more than 60,000 persons. (A further demonstration occurred three days later when a plutonium (^{239}Pu) fission bomb was dropped on Nagasaki, Japan killing 36,000 more persons.)

Fission Fragments

In the process of fissioning uranium, other isotopes called fission fragments are created. In other words, some of the uranium is actually transmuted into other elements. These fission fragments are themselves radioactive isotopes with highly unstable nuclei. Today, we know that it can take hundreds of thousands of years for all of the fission fragments created in a nuclear reaction to return to a stable energy state. The most important fission fragments created by neutron bombardment of uranium in nuclear reactors are iodine 131 (^{131}I), strontium 90 (^{90}Sr), cesium 134 and 137 (^{134}Cs and ^{137}Cs) and cobalt 60 (^{60}Co).

Both ^{137}Cs and ^{60}Co are used as sources of gamma rays for irradiation of food. The vast majority of food irradiation facilities use ^{60}Co. Approximately 85% of all ^{60}Co used worldwide, both for food irradiation and for cancer radiation therapy and sterilization of medical equipment, comes from Canada. Canadian scientists provide this large supply ◗

of ^{60}Co not by fissioning more uranium, but by creating conditions inside their nuclear reactors in which other materials besides uranium can be inserted into the reactor core once uranium has been fissioned, thus allowing these other materials to become bombarded by the large supply of neutrons that have already been created inside.

Nuclear Fusion

During this same 1930s to 1950s period of time, a second type of nuclear process, called nuclear fusion, was also the subject of much experimentation. In the fusion process, nuclei of smaller atoms are joined together into single, heavier nuclei. Like fission, the fusion process releases an enormous amount of energy. A hydrogen fusion bomb, based on deuterium (the single neutron, single proton isotope of hydrogen) was first exploded in 1954. [60]Co was also involved in this second type of nuclear process, because scientists quickly learned that the hydrogen fusion bomb could be improved by encapsulating it within a cobalt shell. Explosion of these "cobalt bombs" during the 1950s were found to produce [60]Co.

Nuclear Reactors and Military Applications

The fissioning of uranium quickly escalated during the 1960s and 1970s alongside of the production of nuclear warheads within the U.S. In 1960, only three nuclear reactors had been built, and they supplied only one tenth of one percent of the total electricity produced in the U.S.[48] By 1976, the number of operable reactors had risen to 61[49], and by 1999, to 112.[50] (These 112 reactorsΔ160 produced 21% of all electricity in the U.S.[51]) They also provided the plutonium needed to produce 12,000 nuclear warheads including land-based intercontinental ballistic missiles (ICBMs), submarine-launched ballistic missiles (SLBMs), and cruise missiles on long-range bombers.[52]

Unfortunately, the process of fissioning uranium to create plutonium for a nuclear warhead produces as a by-product approximately the same amount of radioactivity as if the warhead itself had been exploded. So over this same period of time, the U.S. Department of Energy not only oversaw the production of plutonium for military use, but also created a stockpile of uranium fission fragments, including 200 megacuries of cesium 137 (^{137}Cs).[53] Like ^{60}Co, ^{137}Cs is a gamma ray emitter. Unlike ^{60}Co, however, which has a half-life of 5.5 years, ^{137}Cs has a half-life of 30 years.[54] (A "half-life" is defined as the period of time it takes for half of the atoms in a sample of isotopes to undergo radioactive decay to a stable state.)

This detailed historical review of radioactivity and gamma-producing isotopes provides a context in which the use of ^{60}Co and ^{137}Cs to irradiate food can be viewed not as a forward-looking step in the desire to improve food safety and food quality, but as a backward-looking step designed to provide an economically viable and politically acceptable use for nuclear "waste" products. ∎

Subsequent studies in 1983[55] on mice and 1993[56] on rats continued to leave most questions unanswered. While consumption of irradiated wheat was determined to increase polyploidy in the 1993 study, the timing of the increase and the pattern of cellular alterations suggested a hypothesis to the researchers involving undernutrition rather than irradiation per se. The researchers hypothesized that feeding of irradiated wheat acted in a similar fashion to dietary restriction, and that irradiation might have altered the fatty acid composition of the wheat in such a way as to trigger a adaptive response not unlike the body's response to dietary restriction.[57]

Congressional Legislation Affecting Multiple Agencies

Although there are several dozen pieces of legislation that directly regulate levels of toxins in food, there are also numerous acts of Congress that indirectly regulate food toxins by establishing guidelines for levels of toxins in the environment. The Clean Air Act of 1990 (reauthorization of the original 1970 Act) and The Clean Water Act of 1987 (reauthorization of the original 1972 Act) are examples of governmental regulations that do not specifically target the food supply but greatly affect its quality. The Poultry Products Inspection Act of 1957, the Federal Meat Inspection Act of 1967, and the Egg Products Inspection Act of 1970 are examples of legislation directly regulating food contaminants.

Non-Governmental Organizations (NGOs)

Non-governmental organizations, or NGOs, serve as both formal and informal participants in food monitoring and food regulation process. At the most formal level, NGOs officially collaborate with governmental organizations in the creation of legal agreements related to food quality and food production. In 1997 and 1998, for example, a broad coalition of NGOs helped carve out the Rotterdam Convention on the Prior Informed Consent Procedure for Certain Hazardous Chemicals and Pesticides in International Trade. NGOs involved in the negotiations included Consumers International, the Pesticides Trust, and the International Union of Food, Agricultural, Hotel, Restaurant, Catering, Tobacco and Allied Workers Association. Government officials from 100 countries signed the agreement in September 1998.[58] Once formally ratified by 50 governments, the agreement will become law.

NGOs also take legal action to ensure that food-related legislation is upheld and enforced. For example, the National Resources Defense Council (NRDC) in New York City, New York lobbies on an ongoing basis to win cleanup funds for nuclear production sites and chemical contamination sites. It also brings lawsuits against governmental agencies to force compliance with hazardous waste disposal laws and ensure consequences for hazardous waste violations. A brief list of NGOs working in the United States in the area of environmental nutrition is presented in *Table 4-7*, on the following page.

PART II

Levels of Toxicity

Despite the work of legislators, governmental agencies and NGOs, toxins have become routine components of the U.S. food supply. The range of toxins is as broad as the categories for chemical classification described in Chapter 3. Alkanes, substituted and non-substituted alkenes, aliphatics, monocyclic and polycyclic aromatics, and inorganics have all been identified in all categories of food, including grains; fruits and vegetables; oils, nuts and seeds; eggs and dairy; meat and poultry; fish; beverages; and drinking water. Amounts range from a few parts per trillion (ppt) to hundreds of parts per million (ppm). In some instances, the packaging of food appears to play a greater role in its toxicity than its agricultural production or industrial processing. In this section we will review recent studies evaluating the magnitude of toxicity in the U.S. food supply.

When thinking about toxins in food, it can be helpful to consider three separate stages in the food delivery process: 1) agricultural production; 2) food processing and packaging; and 3) food preparation and home storage by the consumer. Toxins can be introduced into food at any or all of these three stages. For example, an organically-grown food might escape toxic contamination by pesticides, heavy metals, and other sewage sludge components, only to be packaged in thin-film plastics that subsequently migrate into the food. Similarly, a consumer might store an organically-grown food in aluminum foil and then cook it in an aluminum pot, causing migration of the metal into the food.

*Table 4-7. **Non-governmental organizations (NGOs) involved in
environmental nutrition***

NGO	Headquarters	Primary activities
Americans for Safe Food (ASF)	Washington, D.C.	Consumer advocacy
Citizens for Health	Tacoma, WA	Lobbying, advocacy
Citizens United for Food Safety (CUFFS)	Bellevue, WA	Lobbying, publication
Clean Water Action Project (CWAP)	Washington, D.C.	Consumer advocacy
Community Nutrition Institute	Washington, D.C.	Publication, advocacy
Council for Responsible Nutrition (CRN)	Washington, D.C.	Lobbying, publication
Environmental Defense Fund	New York, NY	Litigation, lobbying
Environmental Research Foundation	Annapolis, MD	Research, publication
Food First—Institute for Food Development and Policy	San Francisco, CA	Lobbying, publication, advocacy
Food & Water, Inc.	Walden, VT	Lobbying, advocacy
Human Society of the United States	Washington, D.C.	Publications, advocacy, litigation, lobbying
International Federation of Organic Agriculture Movements (IFOAM)	Buenos Aires, Argentina	Lobbying, advocacy, publication
The Land Institute	Salina, KS	Publication, advocacy
National Coalition Against Misuse of Pesticides	Washington, D.C.	Lobbying, publication
National Coalition for Alternatives to Pesticides	Eugene, OR	Publication, advocacy
National Coalition to Stop Food Irradiation (NCSFI)	San Francisco, CA	Lobbying, advocacy
National Environmental Law Center (NELC)	Boston, MA	Litigation
National Resources Defense Council (NRDC)	New York, NY	Lobbying, litigation, publications
National Toxics Coalition (NTC)	Boston, MA	Consumer advocacy, lobbying
Organic Farming Research Foundation (OFRF)	Santa Cruz, CA	Research, publication
Pesticide Action Network of North America (PANNA)	San Francisco, CA	Publication, lobbying, advocacy
World Resources Institute	Boston, MA	Publication
Worldwatch Institute	Washington, D.C.	Publication, advocacy

Toxins in Grains, Flours and Pastas

Agriculturally-Related Contaminants

Although not proportionally represented in *Table 4-8* below, fumigants are the most likely toxins to be found in grains and grain products like breads and pastas. These fumigants include ethylene dibromide (EDB) and ethylene dichloride (EDC) commonly used to prevent insect contamination of grains stored in elevators, warehouses, and silos. Hexachlorocyclohexane (HCH) and one of its eight stereoisomers, lindane, are also frequently-found fumigant residues. Among the grains, rice and rice-based products are particularly likely to contain HCH residues.

Like fumigants, pesticides are also commonly used on grain crops. The carbamate pesticides commonly referred to as EBDCs (ethylenebisdithio-carbamates) frequently appear as grain contaminants. The EBDCs include the pesticides zineb, maneb, metiram, and mancozeb. The organochlorine pesticide alachlor is a common contaminant of corn and corn products. Corn is often lower in pesticide residues than might be expected, however, due to the partial protection afforded by the plant's husks.

The heavy metal content of grains depends primarily upon fertilizer use and soil conditions. In Canada, for example, fertilizer concentrations of cadmium (20ppm) and lead (500ppm) are restricted, but no such fertilizer restrictions exist in the U.S. Use of sewage sludge as a fertilizer is a common source of heavy metal contamination. Runoff from industrially-polluted waters and use of methylmercury-containing fungicides are also common sources of heavy metal contamination. Although not technically a heavy metal, grain products are also frequently contaminated with the metal aluminum. This metal is deliberately introduced as a food additive when leavening agents are added to cake mixes, pancake mixes, self-rising flours, and frozen doughs.

Processing and Packaging-Related Contaminants

Processing of grains can also introduce a wide variety of toxins into grain products. Most products manufactured from white flour contain residues of the bleaching agent benzoyl peroxide. Butylated hydroxytoluene (BHT) and butylated hydroxyanisole (BHA) are commonly added to cereals, breads, rolls, and cake products to extend shelf life and prevent oxidative damage. Polysorbates 60, 65, and 80 are another category of shelf-life extenders which also help maintain tenderness of baked products. (Although still controversial in the research literature, polysorbates

Table 4-8. Toxins detected in grains, flours, and pastas

Food	Toxin	Amount detected	Place of study	Year of study
Wheat seedlings[a]	Terbufos	7.4–10.6 ppm	Canada	1988[59]
Wheat seedlings[b]	Terbufos	320–580 ppb	Canada	1988[60]
Barley seedlings[a]	Terbufos	4.44–7.0 ppm	Canada	1988[61]
Barley seedlings[b]	Terbufos	210–340 ppb	Canada	1988[62]
Rye flour	Cadmium	9 ppb	Finland	1993[63]
	Lead	16 ppb	Finland	1993[64]
Rye-based cereal	Cadmium	19 ppb	Finland	1993[65]
	Lead	26 ppb	Finland	1993[66]
Wheat-based cereal	Cadmium	22 ppb	Finland	1993[67]
	Lead	42 ppb	Finland	1993[68]
Oat-based cereal	Cadmium	17 ppb	Finland	1993[69]
	Lead	2 ppb	Finland	1993[70]
Rice-based cereal	Cadmium	31 ppb	Finland	1993[71]
	Lead	10 ppb	Finland	1993[72]
Maize-based cereal	Cadmium	11 ppb	Finland	1993[73]
	Lead	18 ppb	Finland	1993[74]
Muesli	Cadmium	27 ppb	Finland	1993[75]
	Lead	34 ppb	Finland	1993[76]
Pasta	Cadmium	79 ppb	Finland	1993[77]
	Lead	18 ppb	Finland	1993[78]
Egg noodles	Methyl bromide	40 ppm	U.S.	1986[79]
Baked prods w/poppy sd.	Cadmium	107 ppb	Germany	1986[80]
Wheat flour	HCH[c]	4.42 ppm	India	1990[81]
	DDT[d]	120 ppb	India	1990[82]
	EDB[e]	8 ppb–4 ppm	U.S.	1981[83]
Biscuits	EDB[e]	500 ppt–260 ppb	U.S.	1981[84]
Corn	DDT[d]	9.6 ppb	U.S.	1998[85]
	Chlordane	1.4 ppb	U.S.	1998[86]
	Dieldrin	1.0 ppb	U.S.	1998[87]
Bread[f]	Wax	50 ppm	U.K.	1994[88]
Crackers[f]	Wax	185 ppm	U.K.	1994[89]
Bread[f]	Mineral oil	550 ppm	U.K.	1994[90]
Cake[g]	Polyisobutylene	1–5 ppm	U.K.	1992[91]
Pies[h]	DEP[i]	1.8 ppm	Canada	1995[92]

[a] measurements taken at 10 days postseedling; treatment of acreage with terbufos varied from 1.5kg/hectare to 3.0kg/hectare
[b] measurements taken at 52 days postseedling; treatment of acreage with terbufos varied from 1.5kg/hectare to 3.0kg/hectare
[c] hexachlorohexane
[d] dichlorodiphenyltrichloroethane
[e] ethylene dibromide
[f] packaged in wax paper
[g] wrapped in polyethylene/polyisobutylene plastic food film
[h] stored in cartons with plastic windows containing diethyl phthalate
[i] diethyl phthalate

may outgas ethylene oxide into foods containing them.) In cake mixes and other desert-like grain products, Yellow #5 (tartrazine) is also a common contaminant.

Summary

In *Table 4-8* is an abbreviated list of toxins that have been detected in grains.

Toxins in Oils, Nuts and Seeds

Agriculturally-Related Contaminants

A variety of pesticides and fumigants are used on nut and seed crops. Peanuts, for example, are frequently treated with the organochlorine pesticide aldicarb. Another pesticide, chlordane, is often used on oil seed crops. Because the organochlorine pesticide alachlor is commonly used on soybeans, it has also been detected as a contaminant in soy oils.

Processing and Packaging-Related Contaminants

Processing of oils, nuts and seeds can also introduce a variety of toxins. Margarines, for example, are almost always protected from mold growth through the addition of benzoic acid or sodium benzoate. BHA and BHT are added to many oils to prevent rancidity and extend shelf-life. Like grains, vegetable oils may also contain trace amounts of polysorbates that have been added to maintain consistency, especially following hydrogenation.

As illustrated in *Table 4-9*, packaging migrants are also frequent contaminants of oils that have been stored in plastic, shatter-proof bottles. In addition to polyvinyl chloride (PVC) and the plasticizers dioctyladipate (DOA) and acetyltributylcitrate (ATBC) listed below, di-(2-ethylhexyl) phthalate (DEHP) is also a common contaminant of oils packaged in plastic. Soft "squeeze bottled" margarines, and margarines packaged in plastic tubs are also likely to contain these packaging contaminants.

Summary

A brief list of toxins related to food grade oils, nuts and seeds is presented in *Table 4-9*, on the following page.

Toxins in Vegetables

Agriculturally-Related Contaminants

Vegetables represent a mixed category of foods in which agricultural inputs and processing measures contribute in equal measure to toxic risk. From an agricultural standpoint, use of pesticides can vary widely depending on

Table 4-9. Toxins detected in oils, nuts, and seeds

Food	Toxin	Amount detected	Place of study	Year of study
Olive oil[a]	DOA[b]	302.8 mg/L	Greece	1995[93]
Olive oil[c]	ATBC[d]	3.3 mg/L	Greece	1995[94]
Olive oil[e]	ATBC[d]	5.1 mg/L	Greece	1995[95]
Poppy seed	Cadmium	739 ppb	Germany	1986[96]
Mustard oil	HCH[f]	1.26 ppm	India	1990[97]
	DDT[g]	2.42 ppm	India	1990[98]

[a] stored in food-grade polyvinyl chloride films containing dioctyladipate (28.3%) and actytributylcitrate (5.0%), irradiated at 8-10 degrees Centigrade and then stored for 47 hours at 4-5 degrees Centigrade
[b] dioctyladipate
[c] stored in food-grade polyvinyl chloride films containing dioctyladipate (28.3%) and acetyltributylcitrate (5.0%) and then stored for 29 hours at 20 degrees Centigrade
[d] acetyltributylcitrate
[e] stored in food-grade polyvinyl chloride films containing dioctyladipate (28.3%) and acetyltributylcitrate (5.0%) and then stored for 94 hours at 20 degrees Centigrade
[f] hexachlorohexane
[g] dichlorodiphenyltrichloroethane

locale, proximity of food to the soil, and protection provided by the natural design of the plant. Leaves surrounding cauliflower florets, for example, often reduce pesticide residues in that vegetable. Ethylenebisdithiocarbamates (EBDCs) are nitrogen and sulfur-containing pesticides commonly used on root vegetables including potato and onion. Also common on both potatoes and sweet potatoes is the organochlorine pesticide aldicarb. Other root vegetables like celery and carrot typically contain a variety of pesticide residues, since over 50 different chemicals are approved for use on these plants. As might be expected, greater concentrations of pesticides are present in the outer surfaces and skins of root vegetables, since these surfaces come into direct contact with the soil. (Skins also contain greater concentrations of essential nutrients.)

As in grains, the heavy metal content of vegetables depends primarily upon fertilizer use and soil conditions. Sewage sludge is once again a common source for heavy metal contamination of vegetable crops, and among the heavy metals, cadmium is the most common contaminant.

Processing and Packaging-Related Contaminants

Processing introduces vegetables to a wide variety of potential contaminants. Dehydrated vegetables and spices are particularly subject to contamination, since virtually all dehydrated vegetable products are either irradiated, sulfited, or fumigated with ethylene oxide. Potato flakes and dehydrated potato products are also a special cause for concern, since sulfites, BHT, and irradiation are all possible treatments during processing.

The waxing of vegetables to prevent bruising during shipment and dehydration during storage has also been a topic of ongoing debate. From a strict chemical standpoint, waxes are esters of alcohols and fatty acids. The core of a wax molecule is essentially a long chain saturated hydrocarbon, often having 50 or more carbons. Myricyl cerotate, for example, the main component of carnauba wax obtained from Brazilian carnauba palm trees, contains 56 carbons (and 92 hydrogens). Myricyl palmitate, the main component of beeswax, has a similar composition.

Waxes can be obtained from plants, insects, animals, or petroleum. The most common plant source is the carnauba palm described above, although other wood rosins are also used. From insects, the most common sources are beeswax (secreted from glands on the underside of a bee's abdomen) and shellac (obtained from the lacca secretion of the lac beetle, native to Pakistan and India). Petroleum-based waxes typically contain residues of petroleum solvents used to extract the wax, and may also contain chemicals related to petroleum processing like o-benzyl-p-chlorophenol. Solvents like ethyl alcohol or ethanol are usually added to waxes to promote consistency, and "film formers" like milk casein (a milk protein commonly implicated in dairy allergy) are also widely used. Soaps (sodium or potassium salts of fatty acids) are also commonly added to waxes as flowing agents that will soften the waxes for vegetable applications.

Summary

A brief list of toxins detected in vegetables is presented in *Table 4-10*.

*Table 4-10. **Toxins detected in vegetables***

Food	Toxin	Amount detected	Place of study	Year of study
Leek	Cadmium	13 ppb	Finland	1995[109]
Turnip greens	Permethrin	2–6 ppm	U.S.	1985[100]
Turnip roots	Permethrin	50 ppb	U.S.	1985[101]
Chili peppers	HCH[a]	480 ppb	India	1990[102]
Carrots	Disulfoton	>1 ppm	U.S.	1986[103]
	Phorate	>1 ppm	U.S.	1986[104]
Leaf lettuce	PAHs	4.8–94 ppb	Finland	1986[105]
Tomato sauce[b]	Aluminum	10–15 ppb	Switzerland	1993[106]

[a] hexachlorohexane
[b] cooked for 60 minutes in a non-coated aluminum pan

Toxins in Fruits

Agriculturally-Related Contaminants

As a general rule, the greatest risk of toxicity related to fruit intake involves pesticide and metal content. Like vegetables, fruits whose edible portions make contact with the soil are typically higher in pesticides than their fellow fruits. Strawberries are a good example of this principle, since their levels of the organochlorine pesticide captan can rise into the parts per million range. Even when they do not make contact with the soil, fruits with skins are likely to concentrate toxins in this outermost part. Skins of fruits are also common recipients of food additives.

Processing and Packaging-Related Contaminants

Like vegetables, fruits are commonly waxed, but in addition, may be artificially colored for cosmetic appearance. Up to 2 parts per million of the dye Citrus Red Number 2, for example, can be injected into orange peels for uniform appearance. For cherries, the dye is Red Number 3 (erythrosine, which does not have a parts per million restriction). When skins of fruits (like bananas) are not typically eaten by the consumer, however, pesticide and additive exposure can be greatly reduced. As a general rule of thumb, fruits that are "required" by consumers and the food industry to have the most uniform and non-individual cosmetic look are fruits that pose the greatest risk of toxicity.

Table 4-11. Toxins detected in fruits

Food	Toxin	Amount detected	Place of study	Year of study
Strawberries	Captan	10–150 ppb	U.S.	1986[107]
	Folpet	40 ppb	U.S.	1986[108]
Grapes	Captan	10–80 ppb	U.S.	1986[109]
	Folpet	10–50 ppb	U.S.	1986[110]
Mixed fruits	Captan	>5 ppm	Canada	1990[111]
Mixed fruits	EBDCs[a]	>7 ppm	Canada	1990[112]
Mixed fruit juices[b]	Aluminum	2.9–35 ppm	Finland	1992[113]
Juices for infants	Lead	200–250 ppb	U.S.	1982[114]
Currant berries[c]	Aluminum	19–77 ppm	Finland	1992[115]
Rhubarb juice[c]	Aluminum	170 ppm	Finland	1992[116]

[a] ethylenebisdithiocarbamates
[b] cooked for 60 minutes in a non-coated aluminum pan
[c] steamed in a covered aluminum pot

Preservation of dried fruit is often accomplished through sulfiting. In addition to commonly recognized dried fruits like raisins, cranberries, figs, and dates, shredded coconut can also be a concentrated source of sulfites. In the vast majority of fruit products that bear the names of fruits but actually contain little of the food, artificial colors and flavors are added. This rule of thumb also applies to most products bearing the names "fruit punch" or "fruit drink."

Many fruits are aseptically packaged in containers that include aluminum foil liners. Because of their relatively high acidity, fruits are better at leaching metals, including aluminum, from packaging and cookware. Levels of metals in fruits packaged in this manner can reach the 100ppm level.

Summary

A brief list of fruit-contained toxins is presented opposite, in *Table 4-11*.

Toxins in Soft Drinks and Other Beverages

Processing and Packaging

Although aluminum canning and plastic bottling of soft drinks account for a large percentage of the toxins found in soft drinks, toxins are also introduced into these beverages during the food processing stage of their development. Most non-transparent sodas contain Caramel Color III. Chemically, this coloring agent is classified as an imidazole and named 2-acetyl-4(5)-tetrahydroxybutylimidazole, or THI. Concentrations of THI in caramel-colored products may reach into the 10ppm level.[117] An equally common additive in both transparent and opaque sodas is benzoic acid to retard the growth of mold. Chloroform from tap water used as the liquid base of the sodas is also a common soft drink contaminant.

Several specific beverages also deserve mention in relation to commonly-detected residues. Decaffeinated coffee, when decaffeinated through the use of methylene chloride, will contain ppb- and ppm-level residues. Aluminum is another common coffee contaminant, and can originate through the storage of coffee beans in aluminum canisters. Beer may contain residues of ethylene oxide polymer used in fumigation of hops and other grain constituents, as well as residues of ethylenediamine tetraacetic acid (EDTA) used to remove metal ions that have migrated into the product during brewing.

Table 4-12. Toxins detected in soft drinks and other beverages

Food	Toxin	Amount detected	Place of study	Year of study
All carbonated	Aniline	190 ppt–12.6 ppb	Canada	1992[118]
All carbonated	Naphthylamine[a]	1.45–9.37 ppb	Canada	1992[119]
Carbonated cola in cans	Aluminum	24.4 μmol/L[b]	New S. Wales	1992[120]
Carbonated non-colas[c]	Aluminum	33.4 μmol/L[b]	New S. Wales	1992[121]
Carbonated cola[d]	Aluminum	250 ppb	Switzerland	1993[122]
All carbonated[e]	Acetaldehyde	200 mcg/L	Germany	1990[123]
All carbonated[e]	DEP[f]	65 ppb	Canada	1995[124]
Teabags[g]	Cadmium	300 ppb	U.K.	1997[125]

[a] includes both 1-naphthylamine and 2-naphthylamine
[b] micromoles per liter
[c] in aluminum cans
[d] in an internally lacquered aluminum can
[e] beverages stored in plastic bottles or bottles with plasticized caps or lid seals
[f] diethyl phthalate
[g] unbleached paper teabags

Summary

A list illustrating residue levels in soft drinks and other beverages is presented above, in *Table 4-12*.

Toxins in Eggs and Dairy

Three factors converge to make egg and dairy products frequent carriers of high-ppb and low-ppm levels of toxins. First, eggs and dairy products represent end-stage events in the food chain, and can biomagnify toxic concentrations that started out at low-ppb levels. Second, the processing of dairy products often involves a variety of food additives. Third, the naturally high fat content of dairy products makes a natural home for lipophilic (fat-loving) toxins.

Agriculturally-Related Contaminants

Pesticides originally sprayed on feed crops are common contaminants of dairy foods. These pesticides include persistent organic pollutants (POPs) like DDT that have not been used on U.S. crops for over two decades. Also common are residues of growth hormones and antibiotics used to maximize yield of product obtained from feedlot-raised animals. The role of toxins introduced early in the food chain is also exemplified by the organochlorine pesticide heptachlor. In one well-publicized episode involving Hawaiian pineapples, milk obtained from cows fed leftover pineapple tops and post-processing parts was found to contain high-ppb levels of the heptachlor used early in the pineapple-growing process.

Processing and Packaging-Related Contaminants

Packaging of dairy products often involves plastic tubs for soft butters, and wax-coated cardboard cartons or plastic jugs (typically 2-HDPE, or high density polyethylene) for liquid milk. Liquid milks may also be pasteurized in plastic containers, increasing the possibility of toxic migration from the container. Di-2-ethylhexyl phthalate, or DEHP, is a common plastic packaging migrant into dairy products including both liquid milks and butters. Cheeses are typically shrink-wrapped in a wrapped in a lower-density polyethylene or polyisobutylene plastic film. The plastic packaging migrant di-2-ethylhexyl adipate, or DEHA, can be found in plastic-wrapped cheeses at levels as high as 310ppm.[126] When examining dairy foods for packaging migrants, researchers often review a variety of phthalate-derived substances, including not only DEHP (di-2-ethylhexyl phthalate), but also dibutyl phthalate (DBP), butylbenzyl phthalate (BBP), and DEP (diethyl phthalate). Cheeses, including white and non-white cheeses, are often bleached during processing. Residues from benzoyl peroxide used in the bleaching process may also be found in these foods.

Also worth mentioning with respect to cheese are the additives used to produce "cheese foods." These softer, often individually-wrapped products typically require the use of emulsifiers for smoothness. Many of these emulsifiers are aluminum-containing. In addition, individual packaging of these cheese foods brings a higher volume of product into direct contact with packaging migrants.

A final category of toxins related to dairy products are hormonal residues. In the early 1990s, companies like Monsanto were granted permission by the U.S. Food and Drug Administration to inject genetically-engineered hormones into cattle to increase milk production. This practice has been the subject of ongoing controversy, particularly since feeding of bovine growth hormone (rBGH) to rats has been shown to trigger antibody response[127] and to elevate levels of insulin-like growth factor-1 (IGF-I).[128] The issue of hormonal residues in animal products is further reviewed on the following page, under "Toxins in Meat and Poultry."

Summary

Table 4-13, on the following page, illustrates levels of toxins that have been detected in eggs and dairy products.

Table 4-13. Toxins detected in egg and dairy

Food	Toxin	Amount detected	Place of study	Year of study
Pasteurized milk	DDE[a]	19 ppb	U.S.	1993[129]
Raw milk	DEHP[b]	120–280 ppb	U.K.	1994[130]
Low fat milk	DEHP[b]	10–70 ppb	U.K.	1994[131]
Milk, boiled[g]	Aluminum	200–800 ppb	Finland	1992[132]
Milk, sterilized[h]	Naphthalene	100–300 ppb	Hong Kong	1994[133]
Cream	DEHP[b]	200 ppb–2.7 ppm	U.K.	1994[134]
	Total phthalate	1.8–19.0 ppm	U.K.	1994[135]
Butter	HCH[c]	930 ppb	Mexico	1996[136]
	DDT[d]	560 ppb	Mexico	1996[137]
	DBP[e]	10.6 ppm	Canada	1992[138]
	BBP[f]	47.8 ppm	Canada	1992[139]
	DEHP[b]	11.9 ppm	Canada	1992[140]
Eggs (chicken)	DDT[d]	680 ppb	Kenya	1988[141]
Cheese	DEHP[b]	17 ppm	U.K.	1994[142]
	Total phthalate	114 ppm	U.K.	1994[143]
	polyisobutylene[i]	8–10 ppm	U.K.	1992[144]
	DEHA[k]	310 ppm	Canada	1995[145]

[a] dichlorodiphenyldichloroethylene
[b] di-2-ethylhexyl phthalate
[c] hexachorohexane
[d] dichorodiphenyltrichloroethane
[e] dibutyl phthalate
[f] butyl benzyl phthalate
[g] boiled in a non-coated aluminum pan
[h] sterilized in plastic low density polyethylene (LDPE) containers
[i] wrapped in a polyethylene/polyisobutylene plastic food film
[k] di-2-ethylhexyl adipate

Toxins in Meat and Poultry

Agriculturally-Related Contaminants

What holds true for eggs and dairy products naturally holds true for the animals that provide them, namely cattle and chickens. Pesticides introduced early in the food chain can biomagnify in these foods, and sewage sludge residues entering into animal feed can also be present in meats.

Livestock Handling-Related Contaminants

The toxicity of meats differs from the toxicity of eggs and milk in several important respects. First, higher levels of antibiotic residues are typically seen in meats versus egg or dairy products. Over 90% of commercially raised feedlot cattle in the U.S. are given hormonal implants to alter growth processes.[146] These implants are designed to allow matrix diffusion-controlled release of hormones and other anabolic agents into animals at particular stages of their development. Hormones and agents released include 17-beta estradiol,[147] gonadotropin releasing hormone (gonadorelin),[148] zeranol and trenbolone.[149] These implants have been shown to increase rate of calving in animals.[150] They have also been determined to increase thyroxine levels,[151] and to increase incidence of prepubertal estrus.[152] Implant residues in meats are difficult to detect, however, since naturally-occurring hormones released by implants combine with hormones produced by the animals' own organ systems. This difficulty of detection contrasts with the relative ease of detection twenty years ago, when synthetic agents like diethylstilbestrol (DES) were commonly used as growth-promoting agents. The use of DES was prohibited in 1979, however, after long-standing evidence of carcinogenicity.

In addition to hormonal residues, antibiotic residues are also common components of meat. Studies between 1991 and 1993 found 3,249 residues of antibiotics in 2,734 carcass samples obtained from 12 different states within the U.S.[153] In another study, approximately half of all chicken and beef samples were found to contain at least two different antibiotic residues.[154] Antibiotic residues present in the chicken included neomycin, tetracycline, gentamicin, oxytetracycline, penicillin, streptomycin, and chloramphenical.

Processing and Packaging-Related Contaminants

The greater perishability of meats in comparison to milks and eggs, and the greater risk posed by microbial contamination can also leave meats as the target of more preservative use within the food industry. (The history of irradiation in relationship to beef production is reviewed in this chapter, page 143, under "Historical Perspectives: Irradiated Beef and Forgotten Wholeness"). Nitrites are common components of cured meats and are designed to prevent occurrence of botulism from meat consumption. Meats preserved by smoking typically contain benzopyrenes, typically at the ppt level. BHT (butylated hydroxytoluene) is a common component of sausage, and is used to prevent rancidity.

Summary

Examples of meats and their toxic components are presented on the following page, in *Table 4-14*.

Table 4-14. *Toxins detected in meat and poultry*

Food	Toxin	Amount detected	Place of study	Year of study
Beef	dioxins	0.48 ppt	U.S.	1994[155]
Beef	dioxins	0.89 ppt	U.S.	1996[156]
Meat and poultry	HCB[a]	10–100 ppb	U.S.	1986[157]
Chicken liver/fat	PCP[b]	10 ppb	U.S.	1984[158]
Fresh beef[c]	ESBO[d]	1–4 ppm	U.K.	1990[159]
Cooked beef[c]	ESBO[d]	22 ppm	U.K.	1990[160]
Meat sandwiches[c]	ESBO[d]	1–27 ppm	U.K.	1990[161]
Meat sandwiches[e]	ESBO[d]	5–85 ppm	U.K.	1990[162]

[a] hexachlorobenzene
[b] pentachlorophenol
[c] wrapped in polyvinyl chloride film packaging containing epoxidised soya bean oil
[d] epoxidised soya bean oil
[e] wrapped in polyvinyl chloride film packaging containing epoxidised soya bean oil and then microwaved to re-heat

Toxins in Drinking Water

As reviewed in Chapter 3, water pollution can originate from a wide variety of sources. These sources include municipal wastewater-treatment plants, land-based disposal of treated sewage sludge, agricultural use of treated sewage sludge as a fertilizer, sewage sludge incineration, open lagoon treatment of toxic waste, municipal waste incineration, and other manufacturing and agricultural practices. In the Mississippi River (the longest river in the U.S.), for example, ppb-level release of cadmium, mercury and lead occurs daily from a single source, namely, a large wastewater-treatment facility in St. Paul, Minnesota.[163] In the U.S. Great Lakes (the largest freshwater reserve on earth), these heavy metal contaminants are also common, although a large amount of some concentrations, like mercury, may come from natural versus human-derived sources.[164]

Freshwater regions like the Great Lakes have also been found to contain a wide variety of organic contaminants. These include asbestos,[165] dioxins,[166] pesticides and PCBs.[167] Of particular concern are PCB levels, which have been determined to exceed international agreements for the Great Lakes region.[168]

Although water purification plants that process water for human consumption take steps to minimize chemical pollutants, ppb-level contaminants have routinely been found in municipal water supplies throughout the U.S. Over 1,100 compounds have been identified in drinking water across the U.S.[169] The U.S. Environmental Protection Agency address levels of 8 volatile organics, 16 inorganics, and 45 organics including pesticides, fumigants, solvents, and packaging migrants in its National Primary Drinking Water Standards (*Appendix A*). Many of these standards allow for routine presence of ppb-level contaminants in drinking water.

A brief summary of toxins detected in tap and well waters throughout the U.S. is presented below, in *Table 4-16*.

Toxins in Fish

Like the waters that provide their habitat, fish are subject to toxic contamination from a wide variety of inputs. The most studied of these inputs, however, are the human activities involving sewage sludge and industrial waste disposal and their contribution of heavy metals to the ecosystem and

Table 4-16. Toxins detected in drinking water

Site used for sampling	Toxin	Amount detected	Place of study	Year of study
Municipal tap	Asbestos	1–10million fibers/L	U.S.	1983[170]
Municipal tap	Atrazine	3.66–38.73 ppb	U.S.	1997[171]
Municipal tap	Cyanazine	2.10 ppb	U.S.	1997[172]
Municipal tap	Simazine	260 ppt	U.S.	1997[173]
Municipal tap	Acetachlor	190 ppt	U.S.	1997[174]
Municipal tap	Alachlor	3.65 ppb	U.S.	1997[175]
Municipal tap	Metachlor	4.34 ppb	U.S.	1997[176]
Municipal tap	Metribuzin	90 ppt	U.S.	1997[177]
Municipal tap	Arsenic	5.4–91.5mcg/L	U.S.	1994[178]
	Arsenic	>50mcg/L	U.S.	1992[179]
	Aluminum[a]	2.6 ppm	Switzerland	1993[180]
	Aluminum[a]	0.54–17.0 mg/L	Finland	1992[181]
Well	Xylenes	0.2–0.9 mcg/L	U.S.	1991[182]
Well	Arsenic	1.5–5.4mcg/L	U.S.	1991[183]
Well	1,2-DCP[b]	0.2mcg/L	U.S.	1991[184]
Well	EDB[c]	0.17mcg/L	U.S.	1991[185]
Well	Nitrate+nitrite	0.7–4.2mg/L	U.S.	1991[186]

[a] tap water boiled for 15 minutes in a non-coated aluminum pan
[b] 1,2 dichloropropane
[c] ethylene dibromide

Table 4-15. Toxins detected in fish

Food	Toxin	Amount detected	Place of study	Year of study
Shellfish	Cadmium	200 ppb	U.S.	1993[187]
Tuna	Mercury	100–750 ppb	U.S.	1993[188]

Table 4-17. Average intake of select dietary toxins

Toxin/food source	Time period	Amount consumed	Place of study	Year of study
Aluminum/wheat flour	Daily	9–12 mg	China	1994[189]
PAHs/olive oil	Annually	560 mcg	Italy	1991[190]
Styrene/total diet	Daily	9 mcg	U.S.	1995[191]
Lead/total diet	Weekly	1–63 ppb	U.S.	1993[192]
Cadmium/total diet	Lifetime	435 mg	Netherlands	1992[193]
Cadmium/total diet	Daily	35 mcg	Japan	1995[194]
Mercury/total diet	Daily	9.9 mcg	Japan	1995[195]
Vinyl chloride/water	Daily	>100ng	Italy	1991[196]
DEHA[a]/total diet	Daily	2.7–8.2 mg	U.K.	1994[197]

[a] di-2-(ethylhexyl) adipate, a plasticizer present in food-contact films

its aquatic components. The ppb-level consequences of these endeavors for cadmium and mercury concentrations in fish are presented above, in *Table 4-15*. Also of strong concern are PCB levels in North Atlantic fish, given the high PCB levels that have been associated with industrial activities surrounding the North Atlantic Ocean.

Estimated Total Intake of Dietary Toxins

Few studies have tried to quantify the cumulative dosage of toxins received on a daily, weekly, or annual basis by individuals living in a particular region of the country and eating foods from the national food supply. (Chapter 2 hypothesized what an individual's typical daily exposure might look like.) Any such attempt to quantify total daily food toxin exposure would undoubtedly find hundreds of toxins ranging from ppt to ppm concentrations.

Included in the list would be food toxins from all chemical categories, including alkanes, substituted and non-substituted alkenes, aliphatics, monocyclic and polycyclic aromatics, and inorganics. A brief list of research estimates involving daily, weekly, yearly, or lifelong intake of food-derived toxins is presented opposite, in *Table 4-17*.

1. Environmental Protection Agency. (1997). Guidelines for establishing a common mechanism of toxicity. Office of Pesticide Programs (7501C). Washington, D.C.

2. Innes JRM, Ulland BM, Valerio MG et al. (1969). Bioassay of pesticides and industrial chemicals for tumorigenicity in mice: a preliminary note. J Natl Canc Instit 42:1101–1114.

3. Milham S. (1971). Leukemia and multiple myeloma in farmers. Am J Epidemiol 91:307–310.

4. Reuber MD. (1978). Carcinogenicity of kepone. J Toxicol Environ Health 4(5–6):895–911.

5. Davis JR, Brownsor RC, Garcia R et al. (1993). Family pesticide use and childhood brain cancer. Arch Environ Contamin Toxicol 24(1):87–92.

6. Cantor KP, Blair A, Brown LM et al. (1992). Pesticides and other agricultural risk factors for non-Hodgkin's lymphoma among men in Iowa and Minnesota. Canc Res 52(9):2447–2455.

7. Wiklund K. (1986). Testicular cancer among agricultural workers and licensed pesticide applicators in Sweden. Scand J Work, Environ Health 12:630–631.

8. Stemhagen J, Slade J, Altman R et al. (1983). Occupational risk factors and liver cancer. Am J Epidemiol 117:443–454.

9. Murphy SD. (1986). Toxic effects of pesticides. In: Klassen CD, Amdur Mo, and Doull J. (Eds). Casarett and Doull's toxicology: the basic science of poisons. Third edition. Macmillan, New York.

10. National Coalition Against the Misuse of Pesticides. (1990). Index to pesticide statistics. NCAMP, Washington, D.C., p.3.

11. United States Environmental Protection Agency. (1992). Environmental Protection Agency list of food use pesticides evaluated for carcinogenicity. Chem Regul Reporter, EPA, Washington, D.C., Aug 28.

12. United States Department of Agriculture Pesticide Data Program. (1998). Pesticide data program: annual summary calendar year 1996, 1998. USDA-PDP, Washington, D.C.

13. Lowe MF. (1989). Risk assessment and the credibility of federal regulatory policy: an FDA perspective. Regul Toxicol Pharmacol 9(2):131–140.

14. Stecklow S. (1998). New food-quality act has pesticide makers doing human testing. Wall Street Journal, September 28, A1, A12.

15. Hutt PB and Merrill RA. (1991). Food and drug law. The Foundation Press, Westbury, New York, Chapter 1, p.8.

16. *Ibid*, p.9.

17. LaBudde RA. (1997). The facts of the matter: the Hudson Foods E. coli outbreak. Least Cost Formulations, Ltd. 824 Timberlake Drive, Virginia Beach, Virginia 23464–3239.

18. United States Department of Agriculture. (1997). Wheat yearbook 1997. United States Department of Agriculture, Washington, D.C.

19. American Meat Institute (AMI). (1997). Meat and poultry facts. American Meat Institute, Washington, D.C.

20. *Ibid*.

21. Marcotte M. (1998). Effects of irradiation on spices, herbs, and seasonings—comparison with ethylene oxide fumigation. Foundation for Food Irradiation Education, Washington, D.C.

22. International Consultative Group on Food Irradiation (ICGFI). (1991). Fact Series No. 14. Joint FAO/IAEA Division of Nuclear Techniques in Food and Agriculture, Vienna, Austria.

23. Bandy LC, Clarke-Pearson DL, and Creasman WT. (1984). Vitamin B12 deficiency following therapy in gynecologic oncology. Gynecol Oncol 17(3):370–374.

24. Jahnsen J and Vatn MH. (1989). Radiation injury of the intestine. Tidsskr Nor Laegeforen 109(25):2557–2558.

25. Raica N Jr, Scott J and Nielsen W. (1972). The nutritional quality of irradiated foods. Radiat Res Revs 3:447.

26. Fox JB, Lakritz L, and Thayer DW. (1993). Effect of reductant level in skeletal muscle and liver on the rate of loss of thiamin due to gamma-radiation. Int J Radiat Biol 64(3):305–309.

27. Elias PS and Cohen AJ. (1983). Recent advances in food irradiation. Elsevier Biomedical Press, Amsterdam.

28. Sokhey AS and Chinnaswamy R. (1993). Chemical and molecular properties of irradiated starch extrudates. Cereal Chem 70(3):260–268.

29. Kovacs E. (1997). Effect of chilling and irradiation on the ultrastructure of the membranes and mitochondria of fruits and vegetables. Acta Alimentaria 26(4):359–381.

30. Katusin-Razem B, Razem D, Matic S et al. (1989). Chemical and organoleptic properties of irradiated dried whole egg and egg yolk. J Food Prot 52(11):781–786.

31. Martinez JD, Pennington ME, Craven MT et al. (1997). Free radicals generated by ionizing radiation signal nuclear translocation of p53. Cell Growth Differ 8(9):941–949.

32. Sportelli L, Rosi A, Bonincontro A et al. (1987). Effect of gamma irradiation on membranes of normal and pathological erythrocytes (beta-thalassemia). Radiat Environ Biophys 26(1):81–84.

33. Nygren J and Ahnstrom G. (1996). DNA double- and single-strand breaks induced by accelerated He2+ and N6+ ions in human cells; relative biological effectiveness is dependent on the relative contribution of the direct and indirect effects. Int J Radiat Biol 70(4):421–427.

34. Sportelli L, Rosi A, Bonincontro A et al, *op. cit. (see reference 27).*

35. Kovacs E, *op. cit. (see reference 24).*

36. Ayala FJ and Kiger JA Jr. (1984). Modern genetics. Second edition. Benjamin/Cummings Publishing, Menlo Park, CA, p.725.

37. Directly adapted from Becker FF. (Ed.). (1977). Cancer—a comprehensive treatise. Vol. VI. Plenum, New York.

38. Aardema MJ, Albertini S, Arni P et al. (1998). Aneuploidy: a report of an ECE-TOC task force. Mutat Res 410(1):3–79.

39. Jambon AC, Tillouche N, Valat AS et al. (1998). Les triploidies. J Gynecol Obstet Biol Reprod (Paris) 27(1):35–43.

40. Fukunaga M, Endo Y, Ushigome S et al. (1995). Atypical polyploid adenomyomas of the uterus. Histopathol 27(1):35–42.

41. Beckwith JB. (1997). New developments in the pathology of Wilms tumor. Canc Invest 15(2):153–162.

42. Nianjun H, Cerepnalkoski L, Nwankwo JO et al. (1994). Induction of chromosomal aberrations, cytotoxicity, and morphological transformation in mammalian cells by the antiparasitic drug flubendazole and the antineoplastic drug harring-tonine. Fundamen Appl Toxicol 22(2):304–313.

43. Voravud N, Shun DM, Ro JY et al. (1993). Increased polysomies of chromosomes 7 and 17 during head and neck multistage tumorigenesis. Canc Res 53(12):2874–2883.

44. Von Wanghein KH, Peterson HP and Schwenke K. (1995). Review: a major component of radiation action: interference with intracellular control of differentiation. Int J Radiat Biol 68(4):369–388.

45. Vijayalaxmi SG. (1975). Chromosomal aberrations in rats fed irradiated wheat. (1975). Int J Radiat Biol Relat Stud Phys Chem Med 27(2):135–142.

46. Renner HW. (1977). Chromosome studies on bone marrow cells of Chinese hamsters fed a radiosterilized diet. Toxicol 8(2):213–222.

47. Bhaskaram C and Sadasivian G. (1975). Effects of feeding irradiated wheat to malnourished children. Am J Clin Nutr 28(2):130–135.

48. World Resources Institute. (1992). Environmental almanac. Houghton Mifflin, Boston, p.71.

49. Hoffman M. (Ed). (1990). World almanac and book of facts. 1990. World Almanac, New York, p.153.

50. World Resources Institute, *op. cit. (see reference 51),* p.71.

51. *Ibid.*

52. Hoffman M. (Ed), *op. cit. (see reference 52),* p.790.

53. Picconi R. (1987). Food irradiation. Excerpts of testimony before the Subcommittee on Health and the Environment of the U.S. House Committee on Energy and Commerce. Accord Research and Educational Associates, New York, p.2.

54. Bertell R. (1987). No immediate danger—prognosis for a radioactive earth. Book Publishing Co., Summertown, Tennessee.

55. Delcour-Firquet MP. (1983). Effects of irradiated wheat flour in the AKR mouse. I. Effects on longevity, morbidity, and pathology. Toxicol Eur Res 5(1):7–15.

56. Maier P, Wenk-Siefert I, Schwalder HP et al. (1993). Cell-cycle and ploidy analysis in bone marrow and liver cells of rats after long-term consumption of irradiated wheat. Food Chem Toxicol 31(6):395–405.

57. *Ibid.*

58. Pesticide Action Network of North America. (1998). NGOs call for rapid implementation of informed consent. September 14, 1998. Pesticide Action Network of North American Update Service (PANUPS), San Francisco, California.

59. Westcott ND. (1988). Terbufos residues in wheat and barley. J Environ Health Sci 23(4):317–330.

60. *Ibid.*

61. *Ibid.*

62. *Ibid.*

63. Tahvonen R and Kumpulanainen J. (1993). Lead and calcium in some cereal products on the Finnish market 1990–91. Food Addit Contam 10(2):245–255.

64. *Ibid.*

65. *Ibid.*

66. *Ibid.*

67. *Ibid.*

68. *Ibid.*

69. *Ibid.*

70. *Ibid.*

71. *Ibid.*

72. *Ibid.*

73. *Ibid.*

74. *Ibid.*

75. *Ibid.*

76. *Ibid.*

77. *Ibid.*

78. *Ibid.*

79. Cova D, Molinari GP, and Rossini L. (1986). Residues after fumigation with methyl bromide: bromide ion and methyl bromide in middlings and final cereal foodstuffs. Food Addit Contam 3(3):235–240.

80. Hoffmann J and Blasenbrei P. (1986). Cadmium in blue poppy seeds and poppy seed-containing products. Z Lebensm Unters Forsch 182(2):121–122.

81. Kaphalia BS, Takroo R, Mehrota S et al. (1990). Organochlorine pesticide residues in different Indian cereals, pulses, spices, vegetables, fruits, milk, butter, Deshi ghee, and edible oils. J Assoc Off Anal Chem 73(4):509–512.

82. *Ibid.*

83. Rains DM and Holder JW. (1981). Ethylene dibromide residues in biscuits and commercial flour. J Assoc Off Anal Chem 64(5):1252–1254.

84. *Ibid.*

85. Aigner EJ, Leone AD, and Falconer RL. (1998). Concentrations and enantio-meric ratios of organochlorine pesticides in soils from the U.S. corn belt. Environ Sci Tech 32(9):1162–1168.

86. *Ibid.*

87. *Ibid.*

88. Castle L, Nichol J, and Gilbert J. (1994). Migration of mineral hydrocarbons into foods. 4. Waxed paper for packaging dry goods including bread, confectionery and for domestic use including microwave cooking. Food Addit Contam 11(1):79–89.

89. *Ibid.*

90. *Ibid.*

91. Castle L, Nichol J, and Gilbert J. (1992). Migration of polyisobutylene from polyethylene/ployisobutylene films into foods during domestic and microwave oven use. Food Addit Contam 9(4):315–330.

92. Page BD and Lacroix GM. (1995). The occurrence of phthalate ester and di-2-ethylhexyl adipate plasticizers in Canadian packaging and food sampled in 1985–1989: a survey. Food Addit Contam 12(1):129–151.

93. Goulas AE, Kokkinos A, and Kontominas MG. (1995). Effect of gamma-radiation on migration behaviour of dioctyladipate and acetyltributylcitrate plasticizers from food-grade PVC and PVDC/PVC films into olive oil. Z Lebensm Unters Forsch 201(1):74–78.

94. *Ibid.*

95. *Ibid.*

96. Hoffmann J and Blasenbrei P, *op. cit. (see reference 80).*

97. Kaphalia BS, Takroo R, Mehrota S et al, *op. cit. (see reference 81).*

98. *Ibid.*

99. Tahvonen R and Kumpulainen J. (1995). Lead and calcium in some berries and vegetables on the Finnish market in 1991–1993. Food Addit Contam 12(2):263–279.

100. George DA. (1985). Permethrin and its two metabolite residues in seven agricultural crops. J Assoc Off Anal Chem 68(6):1160–1163.

101. *Ibid.*

102. Kaphalia BS, Takroo R, Mehrota S et al, *op. cit. (see reference 81).*

103. Suett DL. (1986). Insecticide residues in commercially-grown-quick-maturing carrots. Food Addit Contam 3(4):371–376.

104. *Ibid.*

105. Wickstrom K, Pyysalo H, Plaami-Heikkila S et al. (1986). Polycyclic aro-matic compounds (PAC) in leaf lettuce. Z Lebensm Unters Forsch 183(3):182–185.

106. Muller JP, Steinegger A, and Schlatter C. (1993). Contribution of aluminum from packaging materials and cooking utensils to the daily aluminum intake. Z Lebens Unters Forsch 197(4):332–341.

107. Gilvydis DM, Walters SM, Spivak ES et al. (1986). Residues of captan and folpet in strawberries and grapes. J Assoc Off Anal Chem 69(5):803–806.

108. *Ibid.*

109. *Ibid.*

110. *Ibid.*

111. Frank R, Braun HE, and Ripley BD. (1990). Residues of insecticides, and fungicides in fruit produced in Ontario, Canada, 1986–1988. Food Addit Contam 7(5):637–648.

112. *Ibid.*

113. Liukkonen-Lilja H and Piepponen S. (1992). Leaching of aluminium from aluminium dishes and packages. Food Addit Contam 9(3):213–223.

114. Jelinek CF. (1982). Levels of lead in the United States food supply. J Assoc Off Anal Chem 65(4):942–946.

115. Liukkonen-Lilja H and Piepponen S, *op. cit. (see reference 113).*

116. *Ibid.*

117. Houben GF, Abma PM, van den Berg H et al. (1992). Effects of the colour additive caramel color III on the immune system: a study with human volunteers. Food Chem Toxicol 30(9):749–757.

118. Lancaster FE and Lawrence JF. (1992). Determination of total non-sulphonated aromatic amines in soft drinks and hard candies. Food Addit Contam 9(2):171–182.

119. *Ibid.*

120. Duggan JM, Dickeson JE, Tyan PF et al. (1992). Aluminium beverage cans as a dietary source of aluminium. Med J Aust 156(9):604–605.

121. *Ibid.*

122. Muller JP, Steinegger A, and Schlatter C, *op. cit. (see reference 106).*

123. Eberhartinger S, Steiner I, Washuttl J et al. (1990). The migration of acetaldehyde from polyethylene terephthalate bottles for fresh beverages containing carbonic acid. Z Lebensm Unters Forsch 191(4–5):286–289.

124. Page BD and Lacroix GM, *op. cit. (see reference 92).*

125. Castle L, Offen CP, Baxter MJ et al. (1997). Migration studies from paper and board food packaging materials. Food Addit Contam 14(1):35–44.

126. Page BD and Lacroix GM, *op. cit. (see reference 92).*

127. Juskevich JC and Guyer CG. (1990). Bovine growth hormone: human food safety evaluation. Sci 249:875–884.

128. Chopra S. (1998). Gaps analysis: report by RBST Internal Review Team, Health Protection Branch, Ottawa Canada.

129. Muller JP, Steinegger A, and Schlatter C, *op. cit. (see reference 106).*

130. Sharman M, Read WA, Castle L et al. (1994). Levels of di-(2-ethylhexyl)phthalate and total phthalate esters in milk, cream, butter and cheese. Food Addit Contam 11(3):375–385.

131. *Ibid.*

132. Liukkonen-Lilja H and Piepponen S, *op. cit. (see reference 113).*

133. Lau OW, Wong SK, and Leung KS. (1994). Naphthalene contamination of sterilized milk drinks contained in low-density polyethylene bottles. Part 1. Analyst 119(5):1037–1042.

134. Sharman M, Read WA, Castle L, *op. cit. (see reference 130).*

135. *Ibid.*

136. Waliszeweski SM, Pardio VT, Waliszewski KN et al. (1996). Levels of organochlorine pesticides in Mexican butter. J Assoc Off Anal Chem Internatl 79(3):784–786.

137. *Ibid.*

138. Page BD and Lacroix GM. (1992). Studies into the transfer and migration of phthalate esters from aluminium foil-paper laminates to butter and margarine. Food Addit Contam 9(3):197–212.

139. *Ibid.*

140. *Ibid.*

141. Kahunyo JM, Froslie A, and Maitai CK. (1988). Organochlorine pesticide residues in chicken eggs: a survey. J Toxicol Environ Health 24(4):543–550.

142. Sharman M, Read WA, Castle L, *op. cit. (see reference 130).*

143. *Ibid.*

144. Castle L, Nichol J, and Gilbert J, *op. cit. (see reference 91).*

145. Page BD and Lacroix GM, *op. cit. (see reference 92).*

146. Epstein SS. (1990). The chemical jungle: today's beef industry. Int J Health Serv 20(2):277–280.

147. Ferguson TH, Needham GH, and Wagner JF. (1988). Compudose: implant system for growth promotion and feed efficiency in cattle. J Controlled Release 8:45–54.

148. Kesler DJ and Favero RJ. (1997). Needleless implant delivery of gonadotropin releasing hormone enhances the calving rate of beef cows synchronized with norgestomet and estradiol valerate. Drug Dev Ind Pharm 23(6):607–610.

149. Moran C, Prendiville DJ, Quirke JF et al. (1990). Effects of oestridiol, zeranol or trenbolone acetate implants on puberty, reproduction and infertility in heifers.
J Reprod Fertil 892:527–536.

150. Kesler DJ and Favero RJ, *op. cit. (see reference 148).*

151. Gopinath R and Kitts WD. (1984). Plasma thyroid hormone concentrations in growing beef steers implanted with estrogenic anabolic growth promotants. Growth 48(4):515–526.

152. Moran C, Prendiville DJ, Quirke JF et al, *op. cit. (see reference 149).*

153. Gibbons SN, Kaneene JB, and Lloyd JW. (1996). Patterns of chemical residues detected in US beef carcasses between 1991 and 1993. J Am Vet Med Assoc 209(3):589–593.

154. Vazquez-Moreno L, Bermudez A, Langure A et al. (1990). Antibiotic residues and drug resistant bacteria in beef and chicken tissues. J Food Sci 55(3):632–634, 657.

155. Lorber M, Cleverly D, Schaum J et al. (1994). Development and validation of an air-to-beef food chain model for dioxin-like compounds. Sci Total Environ 156(1):389–65.

156. Ferrario J, Byrne C, McDaniel D et al. (1996). Determination of 2,3,7,8-chlorine-substituted dibenzo-p-dioxins and -furans at the part per trillion level in United States beef fat using high-resolution gas chromatography/high-resolution mass spectrometry. Anal Chem 68(4):647–652.

157. Brown EA, Biddle K, and Spaulding JE. (1986). Residue levels of hexochlorobenzene in meat and poultry in the food supply of the USA. IARC Sci Publ 77:99–108.

158. Neidert E, Saschenbrecker PW, and Patterson JR. (1984). Detection and occurrence of pentachlorophenol residues in chicken liver and fat. J Environ Sci Health 19(7):579–592.

159. Castle L, Mayo A, and Gilbert J. (1990). Migration of epoxidised soya bean oil into foods rom retail packaging materials and from plasticised PVC film used in the home. Food Addit Contam 7(1):29–36.

160. *Ibid.*

161. *Ibid.*

162. *Ibid.*

163. Garbarino JR, Hayes HC, Roth DA et al. (1995). Contaminants in the Mississippi River. US Geological Survey Circular 1133, Reston, Virginia.

164. Hileman B. (1988). The Great Lakes cleanup effort. Chem Engin News 66:22–39.

165. Cook PM, Glass GE and Tucker JH. (1974). Asbestiform amphibole minerals: detection and measurement of high concentrations in municipal water supplies. Sci 185:853–855.

166. Madati PJ and Kormondy EJ. (1989). Introduction. In: Kormondy EJ. (Ed.). International handbook of pollution control, Greenwood Press, Westport, Connecticut, pp.1–17.

167. Williams DJ. (1992). Great Lakes water quality: a case study. In: Dunnette DA and O'Brien RJ. (Eds.). The science of global change. The impact of human activities on the environment. American Chemical Society, Washington, D.C., pp.297–323.

168. *Ibid.*

169. Meier JR. (1988). Genotoxic activity of organic chemicals in drinking water. Mutat Res 196:211–246.

170. Millette JR, Clark PJ, Stober J et al. (1983). Asbestos in water supplies of the United States. Environ Health Perspect 53:45–48.

171. Environmental Working Group (1997). Weedkillers by the Glass Study. Environmental Working Group, Washington, D.C. (Website location: http://www.ewg.org).

172. *Ibid.*

173. *Ibid.*

174. *Ibid.*

175. *Ibid.*

176. *Ibid.*

177. *Ibid.*

178. Engel RR and Smith AH. (1994). Arsenic in drinking water and mortality from vascular disease: an ecologic analysis in 30 counties in the United States. Arch Environ Health 49(5):418–427.

179. Smith AH, Hopenhayn-Rch C, Bates MN et al. (1992). Cancer risks from arsenic in drinking water. Environ Health Perspect 97:259–267.

180. Muller JP, Steinegger A, and Schlatter C, *op. cit (see reference 106).*

181. Liukkonen-Lilja H and Piepponen S, *op. cit. (see reference 113).*

182. Washington State Department of Agriculture. (1991). Washington State Agricultural Chemicals Pilot Study. Pesticides in Groundwater. Report No. 2. Washington State Department of Agriculture, Olympia, Washington.

183. *Ibid.*

184. Washington State Department of Agriculture. (1991). Washington State Agricultural Chemicals Pilot Study. Pesticides in Groundwater. Report No. 3. Washington State Department of Agriculture, Olympia, Washington.

185. *Ibid.*

186. Washington State Department of Agriculture, *op. cit (see reference 182).*

187. Galal-Gorchev H. (1993). Dietry intake, levels in food and estimated intake of lead, cadmium, and mercury. Food Addit Contam 10(1):115–128.

188. Yess NJ. (1993). U.S. Food and Drug Administration survey of methyl mercury in canned tuna. J Assoc Off Anal Chem Internatl 76(1):36–38.

189. Wang L, Su DZ, and Wang YF. (1994). Studies on the aluminium content in Chinese foods and the maximum permitted levels of aluminium in wheat flour products. Biomed Environ Sci 7(1):91–99.

190. Menichini E, Bocca A, Merli F et al. (1991). Polycyclic aromatic hydrocarbons in olive oils on the Italian market. Food Addit Contam 8(3):363–369.

191. Lickly TD, Breder CV, and Rainey ML. (1995). A model for estimating the daily dietary intake of a substance from food-contact articles: styrene from polystyrene food-contact polymers. Regul Toxicol Pharmacol 21(3):406–417.

192. Galal-Gorchev H, *op. cit. (see reference 187).*

193. Kreis IA, Wijga A, and van Wijnen JH. (1992). Assessment of the lifetime accumulated cadmium intake from food in Kempenland. Sci Total Environ 127(3):281–292.

194. Tsuda T, Inoue T, Kojima M, et al. (1995). Market basket and duplicate portion estimation of dietary intakes of cadmium, mercury, arsenic, copper, manganese, and zinc by Japanese adults. J Assoc Off Anal Chem Internatl 78(6):1363–1368.

195. *Ibid.*

196. Benfenati E, Natangelo M, Davoli E et al. (1991). Migration of vinyl chloride into PVC-bottled drinking-water assessed by gas chromatography-mass spectrometry. Food Chem Toxicol 29(2):131–134.

197. Loftus NJ, Woollen BH, Steel GT et al. (1994). An assessment of the dietary uptake of di-2-(ethylhexyl) adipate (DEHA) in a limited population study. Food Chem Toxicol 32(1):1–5.

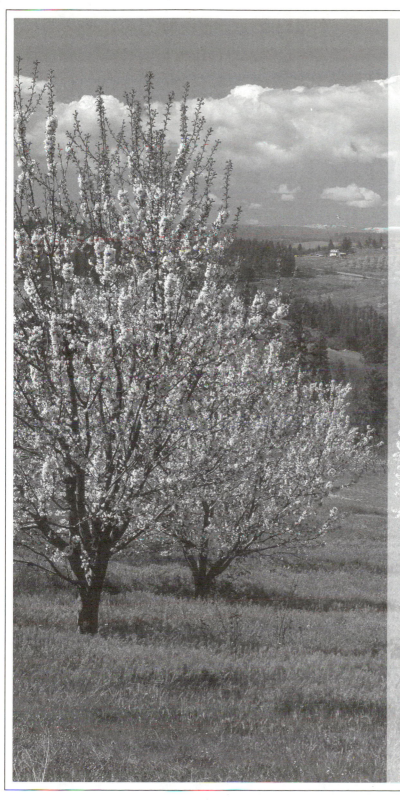

The Impact of Food Toxins on the Body

CONTENTS

Chapter 5: **The Impact of Food Toxins on the Body**

The Impact of Food Toxins on the Body

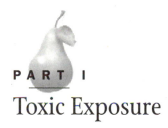

PART I

Toxic Exposure

In this chapter we will review two aspects of food toxins in relationship to the body and health. Part I looks quantitatively at the prevalence of toxins in body tissues and fluids, and also reviews the recent history of toxic surveillance by public health organizations. Part II examines the impact of food toxins on human physiology and metabolism, and identifies specific molecular mechanisms through which toxins damage health.

Governmental Surveillance

During the past three decades, surveillance of toxic exposure in the U.S. population has been a routine governmental practice. Since 1970, for example, the U.S. Environmental Protection Agency (EPA) has conducted the National Human Adipose Tissue Survey (NHATS) to determine the prevalence of fat-soluble toxins in the fat cells of U.S. citizens.[1] The 1986 version of this survey, for example, analyzed 671 adipose tissue specimens to determine the prevalence of 111 toxic compounds.[2]

Within the U.S. Department of Health and Human Services (HHS), several agencies have also conducted long-term surveillance of toxic exposure. (Before its renaming in 1980, HHS existed as the Department of Health, Education and Welfare). Under HHS jurisdiction and headquartered in Atlanta, Georgia are the Centers for Disease Control (CDC). This group of 11 public health-related organizations includes the National Center for Environmental Health (NCEH). NCEH, through its division of Environmental Health Laboratory Sciences, has been monitoring national exposure to toxins since the mid 1970s. In its current capacity, the lab conducts analyses of over 200 toxicants found in the general U.S. population, including 10 metals, 144 dioxins and furans, 20 PCBs, 42 pesticides, 32 VOCs, 19 PAHs, and tobacco smoke.

Also housed falling under HHS jurisdiction is the National Center for Health Statistics (NCHS). As of 1999, NCHS has completed three national health and nutrition surveys that contain information about food toxins. Beginning with the first National Health and Nutrition Examination Survey (NHANESI, 1971-1975) and ending with the third National Health and Nutrition Examination Survey (NHANESIII, 1988-1994), NCHS together with NCEH and its laboratory have analyzed levels of lead, cadmium, and other toxins in the U.S. population. In the NHANESII (1976-1980) survey data, for example, 99.5% of all blood sera analyzed showed presence of DDE in concentrations greater than or equal to 1 ppb.[3]

In some instances the prevalence of toxins in U.S. adults has been so high that reference ranges have been set for allowable levels. The CDC, for example, through its Environmental Health Laboratory Sciences division, has set up reference ranges for several dozen pesticide analytes in urine.[4]

Toxins can be detected in a wide range of body tissue types and fluids. Although blood and urine samples have provided the bulk of analyses to date, adipose cells, breath, bone, saliva, hair, stool, and immune cell (antibody) response have also been used to assess toxic exposure. Urinary trimetallic anhydrides, for example, have often been measured to assess exposure to benzene derivatives.

Tissue and Body Fluid Estimates

Table 5-1 summarizes recent studies on toxic exposure in the general U.S. population and in other populations worldwide. Because these studies have not attempted to identify sources of toxic exposure, they cannot speak directly to food as a source of toxins. However, the contribution of diet to toxic burdens in the range of hundreds part per billion or greater is highly

Table 5-1. *The presence of toxins in blood, urine, bone, fat cells and breath*

Tissue/Fluid	Sample Size	Toxin	% of subjects[†] mean amt. detected	Place	Year
Serum	5,994	p,p'–DDE[a]	99.5%/1–378 ppb	U.S.	1989[5]
Serum	5,994	p,p'–DDT[b]	35.7%/>1ppb	U.S.	1989[6]
Serum	5,994	β–BHC[c]	17.2%	U.S.	1989[7]
Serum	989	TCDD[d]	12.2ppt	U.S.	1997[8]
Whole blood	1,000	p-DCB[e]	98%/2.1 mcg/L	U.S.	1995[9]
Whole blood	299	Lead	11.4 mcg/L	U.S.	1996[10]
Whole blood	70	Lead	6.7 mcg/dl	U.S.	1997[11]
Whole blood	56	Mercury	18.2 ng/L	Japan	1994[12]
Whole blood	278	Cadmium	0.21–0.26 mcg/L	Malaysia	1994[13]
Adipose	1,681	PBBs[f]	97%	U.S.	1982[14]
Adipose	40	p,p'-DDE[a]	100%/60.98 ppm	Mexico	1997[15]
Adipose	40	p,p'-DDD[g]	100%/950 ppb	Mexico	1997[16]
Adipose	40	p,p'-DDT[b]	100%/31 ppm	Mexico	1997[17]
Adipose	40	Total DDT	100%/104.48 ppm	Mexico	1997[18]
Fetal adipose	34	PCBs[h]	700 ppb	Germany	1996[19]
Fetal adipose	34	HCH[i]	140 ppb	Germany	1996[20]
Fetal adipose	34	DDT[b]	700 ppb	Germany	1996[21]
Fetal adipose	34	Heptachlor	30 ppb	Germany	1996[22]
Breath	350	11 VOCs[k]	100%	U.S.	1986[23]
Urine	1,000	2,5-DCP[l]	98%	U.S.	1995[24]
Urine	1,000	1-naphthol	86%	U.S.	1995[25]
Urine	1,000	3,5,6-TCP[m]	82%	U.S.	1995[26]
Urine	1,000	2-naphthol	81%	U.S.	1995[27]
Urine	1,000	2,4-DCP[n]	64%	U.S.	1995[28]
Urine	1,000	PCP[o]	64%	U.S.	1995[29]
Urine	1,000	4-nitrophenol	41%	U.S.	1995[30]
Urine	1,000	2,5-DCP[l]	98%/200 mcg/L	U.S.	1995[31]
Urine	130	Mercury	2.33 mcg/L	Japan	1994[32]
Bone (patella)	70	Lead	29.1 ppm	U.S.	1997[33]
Bone (tibia)	70	Lead	17.5 ppm	U.S.	1997[34]

† percentage of subjects in the total sample testing positive for the presence of the toxin
[a] 2,2-bis(p-chlorophenyl)-1,1-dichloroethylene
[b] 1,1,1-trichloro-2,2-bis(p-chlorophenyl)ethane
[c] beta-benzene hexachloride
[d] 2,3,7,8-tetrachlorodibenzo-p-dioxin
[e] p-dichlorobenzene
[f] polybrominated biphenyls
[g] 1,1-dichloro-2,2-bis(p-chlorophenyl)ethane
[h] polychlorinated biphenyls
[i] hexachlorohexane
[k] volatile organic compounds, including chloroform
[l] 2,5-dichlorophenol
[m] 3,5,6-trichlorophenol
[n] 2,4-dichlorophenol
[o] pentachlorophenol

likely, particularly in locations where use and disposal of toxins has caused controversy and where persistence in the ecosystem and biomagnification through the food chain have been documented.

PART II

Methodological Issues in Food Toxicity Research

Food Versus Non-Food Toxins

Two factors make it difficult for researchers to assess the impact of food toxins on the body. The first complicating factor is the rarity of human exposure to toxins that derive exclusively from food and from no other source. On any given day, most individuals are confronted with both food and non-food toxins. Our bodies could become exposed to lead, for example, following dietary intake of poppy seeds or a glass of tap water. But during the same day, lead arsenate in the outdoor or indoor air we breathe could also be a source of exposure. Dietary intake of cabbage or sweet potato could expose our bodies to the pesticide heptachlor, but so could contact with air, since this pesticide could be absorbed transdermally (across the skin).

Functional Level of Toxic Impact

A second complicating factor in research on food toxins involves level of analysis. The degree to which food toxins can be observed to impact body function depends in large part on the level of body function that researchers choose to observe. Our bodies are simultaneously functioning at an infinite number of levels, including cellular, organ-specific, whole body, psychological/emotional, etc. We can reach different conclusions about food toxins and their impact on the body depending upon the level of function we choose to assess. For example, if we look at a morphological level and assess the formation of microscopic lesions in the brain, we can find studies showing the non-damaging effects of a food additive like aspartame (NutraSweet™ on brain function.[35] However, if we look at an intracellular, molecular level, we can find changes in NMDA-receptor activity in the brain's hypothalamic neurons following administration of this same molecule (aspartame).[36] (NMDA receptors, or *N*-methyl-D-aspartate receptors, are part of the excitatory neurotransmitter system in which the amino acids aspartic acid and glutamic acid serve as neurotransmitters. NDMA receptors are one of three receptor types found in the excitatory system, and provide binding sites on the neurons for glutamic and aspartic acid.)

Even within one single level of analysis it can be difficult to determine toxic effects. In chronic fatigue syndrome, for example, at least 25% of patients have altered cellular processes in which mitochondrial function is compromised.[37] Exposure to chlorinated hydrocarbons (like DDE and hexachlorobenzene) has been associated with these changes in mitochondrial function.[38] Chronic fatigue researchers who assess muscle or nerve cell activity might easily ascertain these changes in mitochondrial function, since both muscle and nerve cells have strong aerobic activity and high concentrations of mitochondria. But if the same researchers examine red blood cell activity instead of muscle or nerve cell activity, no mitochondrial alterations will be detected since red blood cells have no mitochondria and produce energy only through anaerobic means.

Organ-Specific Mechanisms of Toxicity

The fact that food is only one source of potential toxic exposure for humans has not been a real-life problem for researchers, since researchers have simply not tried to differentiate between the impact of food versus non-food toxins. The need for that differentiation remains ahead for future researchers who want to isolate the effect of food toxins from environmental toxins in general. The complications imposed on food toxicity research by physiological level of analysis, however, have created problems for researchers. Most textbooks of toxicology have handled the level of analysis problem by simply listing, in random, non-integrated order, all known mechanisms through which toxins cause bodily damage. These mechanisms have included processes like enzyme inhibition, enzyme overactivation, and membrane damage. In addition, textbooks have tried to provide a more integrated look at toxic action by making their discussion of toxins organ-specific. This organ-specific approach has produced categories of analysis like pulmonary toxicity, renal toxicity, cardiac toxicity, neurotoxicity, endocrine/reproductive toxicity, hepatotoxicity, and immunotoxicity. (Cadmium, for example, holds a special place in the study of renal toxicity, since this heavy metal can accumulate in the renal cortex, and produce, as an early subclinical

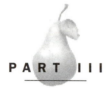

Cytosine

Thymine

Adenine

Guanine

Figure 5-1
Nitrogenous bases

manifestation of its toxicity, increased urinary excretion of plasma proteins including (2-microglobulin and retinal-binding protein.)[39]

The second half of this chapter takes a slightly different approach to the analysis of "toxic action." This latter half is organized around three concepts that can be used to understand all body processes (even if toxic action is not present). The three types of processes that will be used as organizing principles are 1) informational processes, 2) structural processes, and 3) energetic processes. It is within these three conceptual categories that the impact of food toxins on the body will be assessed. (A summary of concepts and molecular mechanisms used to assess impact of food-related toxins is presented in *Table 5-5*, on page 231 of this chapter).

PART III

Toxic Disruption of Informational Processes

Information and Genetics

Nowhere are body processes more closely identified with "information" than in the area of genetics. Ever since the Austrian monk Gregor Mendel published the results of his work with garden peas in 1866, the idea of genes as information stored in cells has shaped the evolution of human genetics. Much of our genetic language reflects this focus on information. We describe genes as carrying the information that cells need to live and divide. We often describe DNA (deoxyribonucleic acid) as "containing" genetic information. When DNA sequences are copied into strands of RNA, we say that information is being "transcribed." When messenger RNA (mRNA) sequences are converted into amino acid sequences, we say that information is being "translated." The processes of transcription and translation are also referred to as "information transfer" processes.

Genotoxicity

Interference with transmission of genetic information is commonly described as genotoxicity. Chemicals that actively damage DNA (typically in short-term gene mutation tests) are often referred to as "genotoxic agents." Damage to DNA can occur in a variety of ways. Chemically, DNA is composed of three types of molecules: bases, sugars, and phosphates. Bases are nitrogen-containing rings (*Figure 5-1*). Bases combine with sugars to form nucleosides, or with sugars and phosphates to form nucleotides. Nucleotides, in turn, join together in a helical configuration to form two basic types of nucleic acids, namely, DNA (deoxyribosenucleic acid and RNA (ribonucleic acid) (*Figure 5-2*). A gene is defined as any sequence of nucleotides to which a specific function can be assigned. There are about 100,000 genes within the nucleus of a human cell and about three billion nucleotide bases.

Strand Breaks, Cross-Linking, and Sister Chromatid Exchanges

The complexity of DNA means that damage to its structure can occur in a variety of ways. Types of DNA damage include changes in base pairs, insertion and deletion of base pairs, insertion and deletion of nucleotide pairs, and crosslinking of DNA strands.

Pentachlorophenol. An increasing number of food-related toxins appear capable of producing genotoxic effects. The pesticide pentachlorophenol (PCP), for example, found in chicken liver and chicken fat in a 1984 study,[40] has been shown to induce DNA fragmentation in the liver cells of mice.[41] These genotoxic effects appear to occur after PCP is metabolized inside of cells to tetrachlorohydroquinone (TCHQ).

Benzoyl Peroxide. Benzoyl peroxide, a GRAS-listed food additive commonly used to bleach flour and whey powder, has been shown to induce single strand breaks and cross-linking of envelopes in the DNA of human bronchial epithelial cells.[42] The genotoxicity of benzoyl peroxide should not be surprising, since the ability of this substance to act as a free radical initiator was the reason for its initial selection as a flour-bleaching agent. Several hours after benzoyl peroxide has been added to milled flour, it generates enough free radicals to initiate oxidation of flour carotenoids and in this manner destroy the coloration of the flour.

Sodium Bisulfite. Sodium bisulfite, the widely-used and GRAS-listed preservative that is added to prevent discoloration of food, has also been shown to have genotoxic effects in human lymphocytes. Increased number of sister chromatid exchanges (SCEs) and other chromosomal aberations have been shown to increase with exposure to sodium bisulfite in a dose-dependent manner.[43] Although wines, grapes, and cherries are particularly well-known examples of sulfited foods, the range of commonly-sulfited products extends from jams and jellies, syrups and molasses, to canned clams, shredded coconut, instant teas, pre-cut potatoes, and flavored gelatin.

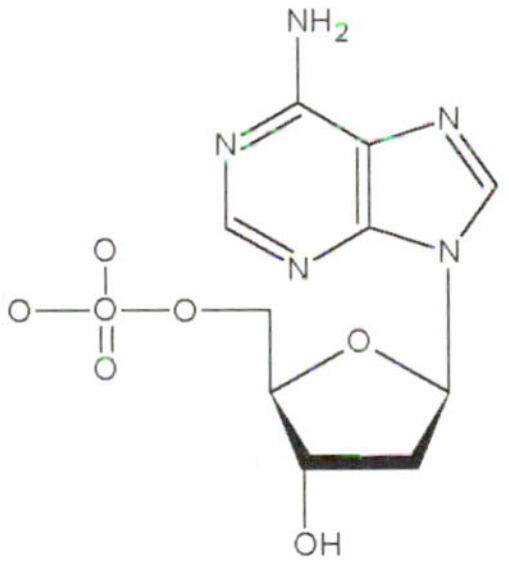

Adenine-containing nucleotide unit of DNA

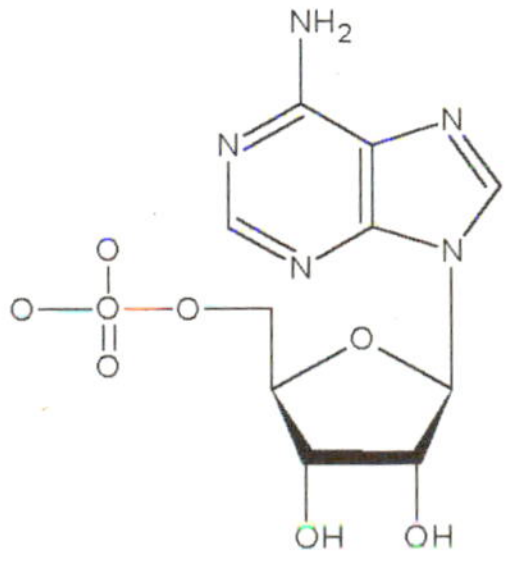

Adenine-containing nucleotide unit of RNA

Figure 5-2
DNA and RNA

Heavy Metals. Also classifiable as genotoxic are the heavy metal food contaminants cadmium, mercury, and lead. Cadmium has been show to induce DNA deletions in the yeast *Saccharomyces cerevisiae*,[44] and DNA-single strand breaks in the hepatocytes of rats.[45] Fragmentation of nuclear DNA has been observed in human T cells following exposure to methyl mercuric chloride,[46] and DNA damage has also been shown to occur, most likely as a secondary consequence of lipid peroxidation, in animal models following exposure to lead.[47]

Toxic Disruption of Transcription Factor Activity

The copying of DNA sequences onto strands of RNA (described earlier and most commonly referred to as transcription) provides another framework in which food-related substances can exert genotoxic effects. The process of transcription is partially guided by the activity of small protein molecules called transcription factors. These small protein molecules serve as modifiers of gene expression by binding to specific locations on the cell's DNA that lie adjacent to specific genes. These nearby regions are called promoter regions. By binding onto promoter regions, transcription factors can stimulate or repress the expression of specific genes. Transcription factors include proteins like p53 and AP-1, but the best-researched transcription factor is the protein NF-kappa B (nuclear factor kappa B).

NF-Kappa B Induction by Heavy Metals. NF-kappa B is part of a large family of transcription factors that have far-ranging effects on immune function, cell growth, tissue development, and aging. Control of cytokines, for example, the key intercellular messaging molecules of the immune system, has been closely tied to NF-kappa B activity.[48] With respect to aging, the binding of NF-kappa B to promoter regions on DNA in the nuclei of temporal lobe brain cells has been found to parallel induction of the COX-1 (cyclo-oxygenase 1) gene.[49] Damage to brain cells by increased activity of this COX-1 enzyme will be discussed later in this chapter (page 210, under "Cyclo-oxygenase [COX] and Lipoxygenase [LPX]").

The heavy metal lead has been shown to induce NF-kappa B activity in human lymphocytes, and to be a key component in the ability of lead to induce immunotoxicity.[50] Also identified as NF-kappa B inducers are the pesticides paraquat[51] and triphenylin.[52]

Toxic Promotion of Polyploidy

Polyploidy (also reviewed in Chapter 4, page 145, under "Consumption-Related Health Risks") refers to the circumstance in which three or more sets of chromosomes are contained in a single human cell. (Human cells are normally diploid and contain two sets of chromosomes). For other organisms that are monoploid (and contain only one set of chromosomes in their cells), the existence of two or more sets of chromosomes would be also be classified as polyploidy. Although many types of plants are commonly polypolid in their genetic makeup, polyploidy is much less common in animals and is often associated with aging or disease.

Pesticides and Packaging. Increases in polyploidy have been experimentally produced through exposure to food-related toxins. These toxins have included dieldrin,[53] the widely-used pesticide frequently found on carrots, corn, cucumbers, potatoes, and sweet potatoes, and the packaging plasticizer DEHP (di-[2-ethylhexyl]phthalate), have both been determined to increase tetraploidy in the liver cells of rats.[54]

In addition to the impact of toxins on the cell's informational library of genetic material, two other types of informational interference have also been shown to occur within the cell. One type of interference involves the blocked transfer of information across cell membranes. (The process of sending information across the membranes of cells is commonly referred to as *signal transduction*.) A second type of informational interference is related to the natural, programmed lifespan of the cell. All cells appear to have a naturally-programmed, pre-planned lifecycle in which cell death is brought about in an orderly, timed, and orchestrated way. This informational programming of cell death has been termed *apoptosis*. The presence of toxins within cells has been shown capable of altering this informational process. In the following two sections, we will look more closely at the informational processes of cell signaling and apoptosis, and review the evidence for toxic disruption of both processes.

Information and Cell Signaling

In addition to the clear informational language used to describe DNA-related events in genetics is the rapidly-increasing use of terms like "signaling," "signal sequences," "signal recognition," "signal transduction," and "intercellular communication" in molecular and cell biology. The preceding list of "cybernetic" terms revolves around the concept of information. From this informational perspective, cells are viewed as being able to act in consort with one another and remain coordinated in their activity only so long as information is continually passing back and forth between them and across their multiple membranes. According to information theory, it is this constant communication process that provides each cell with essential feedback from the body as a whole, and from the environment in which that body responds and acts.

Hormones and Intercellular Communication

The language of signaling and communication is not altogether new, of course. Hormones have long been regarded as vehicles for intercellular communication. The plant hormones known collectively as auxins were investigated at least as far back as Charles Darwin in 1880. Isolation and identification of human hormones dates back into the early 1900s, with purification of the key blood sugar-regulating hormone, insulin, occurring in 1922. In some respects, present-day work in cell signaling is an extension of hormonal-type thinking.

Receptor Binding

In many respects, our 1998 model for cell signaling is much like the 50-year-old model that we have been using to understand hormonal activity. This model involves a signaling molecule (like a hormone) that can travel at a distance through the body; a receptor site on the membrane of a cell where that molecule can bind and come to rest; and a series of protein and protein enzyme-related events that follow purposively after the binding of the hormone to the receptor.

When hormones bind to receptors on or in target cells, they produce a conformational change in the receptors. These conformational changes are recognized by other macromolecules in the cell. (Sometimes hormones bind to receptors that are not only proteins, but also enzymes. In this case, the hormones are not described as binding to receptors but rather as "allosterically modifying the enzymes." (In other words, when there is direct modification of a target enzyme by a hormone, with nothing coming in between the hormone and activation or deactivation of the enzyme, the word "receptor" is not ▶

The Signal Transduction Model

Springing forth from a hormonal messaging model (see "Hormones and Intercellular Communication" above) has been an entire field of bioscience that is focused on the passage of information across cell membranes. "Signal transduction" is the term used in this new field to describe the conveying of chemical information between cells and across cell membranes. (A simplified diagram of the signal transduction process is presented in *Figure 5-3*, on page 190). When chemical information is passed across a membrane, the signal transduction is referred to as *transmembrane* signal transduction. In this case, the primary goal of the process is to translate extracellular information into an intracellular response. Different types of extracellular signals can arrive at the plasma membrane of a cell. These types of signals include serum growth factors, hormones, and drugs or toxins. When a serum growth factor arrives at a cell membrane, for example,

BACK-TO-BASIC CONCEPTS: Hormones and Intercellular Communication

CONTINUED

used to describe the interaction.) When hormones do not bind directly to enzymes, however, but to separate, non-enzyme proteins, the process of hormonal action is described as receptor-mediated, and the separate binding protein that relays activity of the hormone is described as a "receptor."
It is also possible for a third protein, not an enzyme or a receptor, to come into play during the process of hormonal messaging. In this case, the third protein is referred to as an "acceptor protein". The hormone binds initially to this third, acceptor protein. The acceptor protein proceeds to interact with the receptor protein, and the receptor protein in turn interacts with the enzyme.

Receptor Location

Receptors can be located in the cell membrane or within the cell. If located on the cell membrane, receptors, once activated, typically respond by generating a diffusable chemical signal inside the cell. This signal is called a second messenger. Five second messengers have been the object of extensive research. These messengers include nucleotide derivatives cyclic AMP (adenosine monophosphate), cyclic GMP (guanosine monophosphate), inositol triphosphate, diacylglycerol, and calcium. Receptors for steroid hormones are located inside of cells. Once activated, these receptors can bind directly to DNA. If the binding sites are located in the promoter regions of genes, the process of steroid hormone binding to receptors can activate gene transcription. In this way, steroid hormones can act as initiators of gene activity. *Figure 5-3* illustrates basic structural components of the cell signaling process. ■

it can bind to a membrane receptor and become part of a signal transduction pathway referred to a mitogen-activated pathway. When a hormone binds to a plasma membrane receptor, it can become part of a hormone-activated transduction pathway. When a drug or toxin binds, it can become part of a stress-activated pathway. Each of these pathways has a slightly different way of altering cellular activity.

Using basic principles in cellular and molecular biology, elaborate models have been developed to account for the complexity of information delivery across cell membranes. One particularly important model involves the activity of the G-protein family.

G-Protein-Coupled Reactions (GPCRs)

G-proteins are a family of proteins that traverse the full width of the cell membrane and are associated with receptor sites that allow for modulation

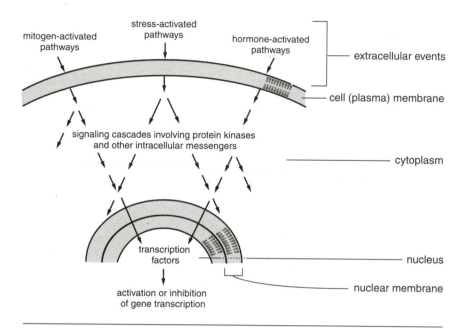

Figure 5-3
Signal transduction

of G-protein activity. Thanks to G-protein-related receptor sites, a wide variety of substances can trigger events within cells. G-protein-linked receptor sites provide binding locations for photons, hormones, prostaglandins, and peptides.

Also connected with G-proteins are effector molecules located on the inner side of the cell membrane like the enzymes adenylate cyclase, cGMP phosphodiesterase, and phospholipase C, as well as ion channels like potassium or calcium channels that provide electrochemical channels through the membrane. Through these effector molecules, activated G proteins trigger changes in signaling pathways by increasing or decreasing amounts of high-energy molecules like cAMP (cyclic adenosine monophosphate) and by opening or closing energy-regulating ion channels.[55] A schematic diagram of these events is presented in *Figure 5-4* opposite.

Adenylate Cyclase and Protein Kinases

The function of effector molecules and their exact role in signal transduction is illustrated by the example of adenylate cyclase. Adenylate cyclase is an enzyme that is stationed on the inner side of the cell membrane, where it converts ATP (adenosine triphosphate) into the second messenger cAMP (cyclic adenosine monophosphate). As a second messenger, cAMP's main

STEP I: Unoccupied membrane receptor

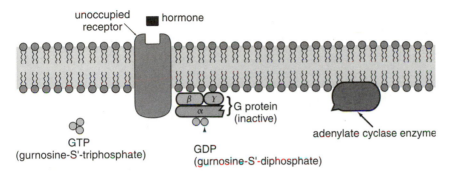

STEP 2: Receptor binding and activation of adeylate cyclase through G-protein

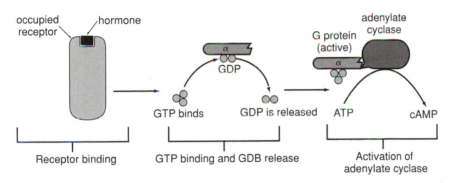

STEP 3: Activation of protein kinase

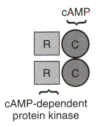

STEP 4: Downstream protein phosphorylation

Figure 5-4
G-protein coupled reactions

function is to stimulate a protein kinase enzyme. This protein kinase enzyme, in turn, carries out phosphorylation of a hydroxyl group on a serine or threonine amino acid residue of an intracellular protein.

Enzymes can be activated or inactivated by phosphorylation, and the sensitivity of enzymes to other effector molecules can be increased or decreased by the phosphorylation process. Because enzyme phosphorylation has been shown to play such a key role in the signaling process, protein kinases are commonly regarded as having a unique regulatory presence in the signaling process. Uncontrolled signaling from protein kinases has been linked to the development of inflammation, psoriasis, atherosclerosis, and cancer.[56]

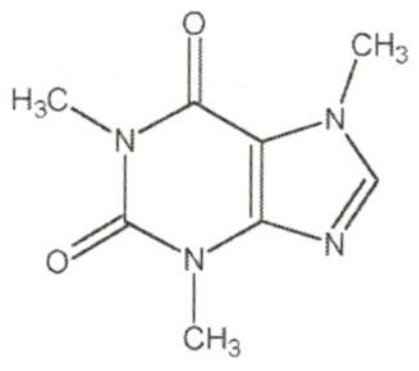

cAMP Phosphodiesterase

Since protein kinase enzymes are typically activated in the presence of a second messenger like cAMP, researchers interested in cell signaling have also investigated substances that alter the presence of cAMP and other second messengers. One mechanism for reducing the presence of cAMP is to enzymatically hydrolyze it. cAMP phosphodesterase is the name of an enzyme that slowly hydrolyzes (siphons off) cAMP following its synthesis by adenylate cyclase. Substances that inhibit cAMP phosphodiesterase can therefore mimic the action of hormones and other substances that use cAMP as a second messenger.

Phosphodiesterase Inhibition by Methylxanthines. One group of substances that are known to inhibit cAMP phosphodiesterase are the methylxanthines. Methylxanthines include caffeine (1,3,7-trimethylxanthine), theophylline (1,3-dimethylxanthine), and theobromine (3,7-dimethylxanthine). The ability of methylxanthines to alter cAMP activity means that foods containing high levels of methylxanthines, including coffee beans, black tea leaves, kola nuts, and cacao seeds should be considered as foods that affect cell signaling and signal transduction processes. *Figure 5-5* illustrates the structure of some methylxanthine molecules.

Growth Factors in Signal Transduction

Growth factors are small proteins (with molecular weights ranging from 6,000 to 13,000 daltons, and containing 50 to 100 amino acids). Unlike hormones, which typically have a specific organ as their site of synthesis, growth factors are synthesized by a variety of cells in a variety of locations. Despite their widespread synthesis, however, growth factors stimulate proliferation of very specific cells.

Growth factors include epidermal growth factor (EGF), tumor growth factor (TGF), insulinlike growth factor I (IGF-I), insulinlike growth factor II

caffeine

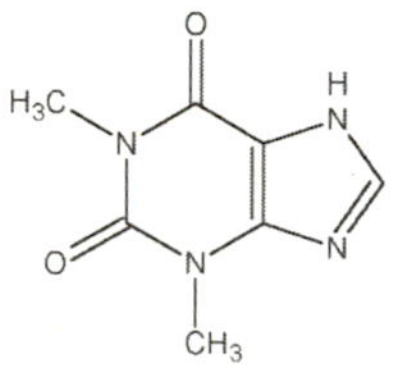

theophylline

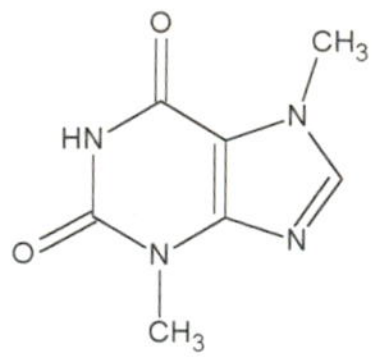

theobromine

Figure 5-5
Methylxanthines

Differences Between Hormonal and Signal Transduction Concepts

Although signal transduction models are clearly outgrowths of earlier hormonal models, present-day work in cell signaling is not merely an extension of hormonal-type thinking. Historically, the field of endocrinology has tended to focus on the idea of "action at a distance" and "hormonal "targets."

Hormones have been described as vehicles for getting cells that lie at a great distance from the site of hormone synthesis to do things that they would not ordinary do. Central to the idea of hormonal activity has been the notion of "target cells" and "target organs". These target cells have their own signals overridden by incoming hormonal signals. From this conventional perspective, the hormonal signal and the cell's response are highly determined events, with neither the hormone nor the cell having much uncertainty about the outcome. The outcome is predetermined, with no possibility for a wider variety of events to occur.

The information-based model of cell signaling, by contrast, relies strongly on the ideas of uncertainty, non-determinism, and possibility in its analysis of signal-response relationships.[57] The at-large, incoming signal is not seen as "overriding" some localized set of events. Instead, localized sets of events are envisioned as synergistically transforming in attunement with momentary and transitory whole-body and environmental processes. Intracellular processes are envisioned as cooperating with, and varying in accommodation with, events at the whole-body and environmental level. ■

(IGF-II), fibroblast growth factor (FGF), platelet-derived growth factor (PDGF), nerve growth factor (NGF), erythropoietin, macrophage colony stimulating factor (M-CSF), granulocyte colony stimulating factor (G-CSF), granulocyte-macrophage colony stimulating factor (GM-CSF), interleukin-3 (IL-3), and interleukin-2 (IL-2).

The genes for most of the growth factors and their receptors have been cloned. The intracellular domain of many of the receptors for growth factors involves tyrosine kinase activity. Normal cells cannot typically reproduce without the stimulation provided by growth factors. In the absence of growth factor presence, cell cycles become arrested. Tumor cells do not require growth factor stimulation to continue their cell cycles.

Understanding of growth factors has helped researchers evolve a more complex model of signal transduction. Because growth factors can induce different responses using the same signaling pathways in identical cells, researchers have postulated a network-type signaling process (called parallel distributed processing, or PDP) in which interconnected layers of elements combine to accomplish transfer of extracellular information across the membrane and into the interior of the cell.[58]

Toxic Disruption of Cell Signaling

Protein Kinase Disrupters

An increasing number of studies on toxic disruption of cell signaling have focused on overactivation of protein kinases, and a wide variety of food-related toxins have been shown to upregulate these enzymes. Numerous pesticides, including chlorpyrifos, endrin, fenthion, and the herbicidal by-product dioxin (TCDD, or 2,3,7,8-tetrachlorodibenzo-*p*-dioxin) have all been shown to increase protein kinase activity in the brain and liver cells of rats.[59] Heavy metals like cadmium, when introduced in the form of cadmium chloride, have been shown to produce similar effects.[60] Solvents used in food processing, including benzene and toluene,[61] have been shown to activate protein kinase C in the platelet cells of rabbits. Plasticizers found in food packaging, including DEHP (diethylhexylphthalate), have been shown activate protein kinsase C in rats[62], and in the keratinocytes of mice, a metabolic derivative (BHTOOH, or butylated hydroxytoluene hydroperoxide) of the commonly-used antioxidant preservative BHT (butylated hydroxy toluene) has been observed to activate protein kinase activity.[63]

Adenylate Cyclase Disrupters

Food-related toxins can also alter signaling processes through activation of the enzyme adenylate cyclase. The insecticide chlorpyrifos, for example, whose residues have been found on tomatoes, cucumbers, corn, and oranges, has been shown to inhibit adenylate cyclase in nerve cells and to cause neurotoxicity through this mechanism.[64]

Toxins can also disrupt cell signaling processes by directly damaging the structure of cell membranes. This mechanism of toxic impact will be reviewed on page 198, under "Direct Damage Caused By Oxidative Stress."

Information and the Apoptosis Model

Unlike the process of necrosis in which cells die as a result of unanticipated physical or biochemical injury, apoptosis refers to a process of cell death in which a pre-programmed sequence of events dismantles the cell. While the apoptosis model of cell death has yet to be fully elucidated in molecular medicine, it has clearly emerged as an information-oriented model. The enzymatic and non-enzymatic events associated with apoptosis are events that provide the cell with information about the timing of its life cycle.

Laboratory Detection of Apoptosis

Apoptosis can be detected in laboratory tests through measurement of molecular-level events. For example, early in the process of apoptosis, the plasma membrane component phosphatidylserine becomes exposed as a result of disrupted membrane asymmetry, and the protein Annexin V binds to the exposed phosphatidylserine sites. Annexin V presence can thus be used as an early marker for apoptosis.

Later on in the apoptosis sequence, endonuclease and protease enzymes, including serine protease and cysteine protease, become activated and trigger cell surface changes that attract phagocytic cells from the immune system over to the apoptotically-dismantling cell for the purpose of engulfing it and protecting the body from unwanted consequences. Changes brought about by activation of endonucleases and proteases can also be measured in the lab and are used as biomarkers of apoptosis. Other methods of apoptosis detection include measurement of DNA laddering, PARP (poly [ADP-ribose] polymerase) cleaving, and MTT (3-4,5-dimethylthiazol-2-yl-2,5-diphenyltetrazolium bromide) reduction.

Whole-Body Perspectives on Apoptosis

Researchers have speculated that the ratio of apoptotic (programmatically dying) cells to mitotic (programmatically dividing) cells and resting cells in the body may be involved in the etiology of chronic disease states. For example, elevated apoptotic cell populations have been observed in patients with chronic fatigue.[65]

Excessive induction of apoptosis, while generally considered to be an undesirable event in the maintenance of healthy tissue, has also been viewed as a desirable event in the treatment of cancerous tissue. Defects in apoptosis have frequently been found in cancer cells. These defects have generally been assumed to make the process of apoptosis unavailable as an aid in removal of cancerous cells from the body. For this reason, many researchers have attempted to find substances that are capable of inducing apoptosis for use as anti-cancer treatment agents.

Toxic Disruption of Apoptosis

General Inducers

Toxins shown capable of inducing apoptosis include PCBs, which induce apoptosis in the spleen cells of mice;[66] methyl mercuric chloride and ethyl mercuric chloride, which activate apoptosis in human T-cells;[67] cadmium chloride, which induces it in human kidney cells;[68] arsenic (as might be contained, for example, in residues from arsenical pesticides;[69] and benzene, which has been observed to induce apoptosis in the sperm cells of rats and guinea pigs.[70] Research involving subjects with Parkinson's disease has also suggested that defects in mitochondrial function, particularly in Complex I of electron transport chain processing, may be a precursor to increased apoptosis.[71] This suggestion raises the possibility that food-related toxins which can damage mitochondrial structures or disrupt mitochondrial metabolism can also contribute to induction of apoptosis in mitochondrially-compromised cells.

AHR-Binding Agents

Among the food-related toxins shown capable of inducing apoptosis are a group of substances that share a specific mechanism of action involving a specialized group of receptors found on cell membranes. Receptors in this group are called *aryl hydrocarbon receptors* (AHRs).[72] (AHRs are currently named for the environmentally-derived hydrocarbons that bind to them because naturally-occurring substances designed by the body to bind with AHRs have yet to be identified). Exactly how AHR-binding promotes changes in cell cycles is not known, but AHRs have been shown to serve as gene regulatory proteins and to alter gene expression.[73] Polycyclic aromatic hydrocabons, dioxins, and halogenated biphenyls all appear to induce apoptosis through AHR-mediated events.

P A R T   I V

Toxic Damage to Tissues and Cell Structures

All structures in the body are susceptible to physical and chemical damage. Exposure to food-related toxins can cause structural damage to tissues and cells through a variety of molecular mechanisms. In this section we address the most common mechanism of structural damage, namely, excessive oxidative stress and production of free radicals.

Oxidative Chemistry and Physiology

Most cells within the body require a continual flow of oxygen to remain healthy, and many organ systems and metabolic processes within the body are at least partially focused on delivery of oxygen to cells. Oxygen transport is complicated by the fact that oxygen is poorly dissolvable in water (so much so that only about .003% of the blood plasma can be saturated with oxygen).

Oxygen transport is not only complex, but also risky. Atmospheric (or "molecular") oxygen, symbolized as O_2, is itself a free radical. (Free radicals are defined as molecules with at least one unpaired electron in their atomic structure.) To understand the risk that accompanies all oxygen metabolism, it is necessary to look further into the issue of unpaired electrons and free radicals.

Free Radicals

Within their atomic structure, all elements, including oxygen, have unique combinations of protons, neutrons, and electrons. The atomic structure of elements, and the function of their components, are reviewed in Chapter 3 (page 112, under "Elements"). Most molecules in the body have orbital regions that are occupied by a pair of electrons with opposite spin. "Spin" refers to the rotation of an electron around an axis, much like the earth rotates around an axis that passes through the north and south poles. The spin of an electron provides it with the properties of a magnet. Like magnets, electrons can "attract" each other when their spins move in opposite directions (clockwise versus counterclockwise). Oppositional spin allows electrons to share the same orbital with a moderate degree of stability by virtue of this magnetic attraction.

Free radical molecules with unpaired electrons do not enjoy this electromagnetic stability. In order to gain more stability, unpaired electrons in their outermost shells react readily to pair up with opposite-spin electrons in other molecules. The reactivity of free radicals can also lead to a series of chain reactions in which the net result is a propagation of more free radicals.

Molecular Oxygen

Molecular oxygen (*Figure 5-6*) contains two unpaired electrons and is technically classified as a free radical. However, because the two unpaired electrons in molecular oxygen have a parallel (versus opposite) spin, the molecule is not as reactive as might be expected of a free radical.

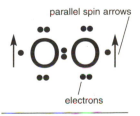

Figure 5-6
Molecular oxygen

Radical and Non-Radical Forms of Oxygen

Through a variety of enzymatic and non-enzymatic processes, molecular oxygen can be transformed into other radical and non-radical states. In most of these states, oxygen is highly reactive with other molecules, even if it lacks an unpaired electron and is classified as a non-radical. A list of radical and non-radical forms of oxygen is presented in *Table 5-2*.

Oxygen Metabolism

Within the body, the fate of molecular oxygen (O_2) is to be ultimately converted into water (H_2O). In route to that destination, oxygen can be converted into several unusually reactive forms. These forms include superoxide anion radical ($O_2^{-\bullet}$) and hydroxyl radical ($OH^\bullet$). Xanthine oxidase (XO), superoxide dismutase (SOD), catalase (CAT), and glutathione peroxidase (GPO) are unique enzymes in their ability to help regulate these conversion processes. Also critical in this regulation are enzymatic cofactors (like copper, zinc, and manganese for SOD and selenium for GPO), as well as intracellular concentrations of free iron that can stimulate conversion of hydrogen peroxide to hydroxyl radical through the Fenton reaction. A summary diagram of these events is presented in *Figure 5-7*, on page 200.

Direct Damage Caused By Oxidative Stress

In one sense, the complexity and risk associated with oxygen metabolism means that the body is constantly under "oxidative stress." In this context, "oxidative stress" simply means the inescapable presence of free radicals that accompanies oxygen metabolism. Without this "oxidative stress," many essential life-support functions in the body could not take place. These functions include inflammatory response to infection or trauma, elimination of fat-soluble toxins from the body, and production of energy within the mitochondria of cells.

Table 5-2. Radical and non-radical forms of oxygen

Oxygen radicals		Oxygen non-radicals	
$O_2^{-\bullet}$	Superoxide anion radical	$^1O_2$	Singlet Oxygen
$HO^\bullet$	Hydroxyl radical	H_2O_2	Hydrogen peroxide
$ROO^\bullet$	Peroxyl radical	$ROOH$	Organic/fatty acid hydroperoxides
$HO_2^\bullet$	Hydroperoxyl radical	O_3	Ozone

The term "oxidative stress" can also be defined, however, as a situation in which there is excessive risk associated with oxygen metabolism. This excessive risk occurs whenever oxygen metabolism is insufficiently supported within the body. The lack of support can involve lack of enzymatic activity, lack of enzymatic cofactors, imbalanced production of free radicals, excessive presence of free iron, lack of "antioxidant" nutrients, etc. For the remainder of this chapter, we will adopt this second definition of oxidative stress, namely, excessive risk associated with unsupported oxygen metabolism.

Air Pollution and Oxidative Stress

Air pollution has long been associated with excessive presence of oxygen free radicals. In atmospheric chemistry, processes in which free radicals are formed through interaction of molecules with light are referred to as primary photochemical reactions. In these reactions, a photon of light is absorbed by an airborne molecule, creating, photoelectrically, an unpaired electron state. Two key photochemical reactions include 1) the conversion of nitrogen dioxide into nitric oxide (a nitrogen free radical), and 2) the multi-step conversion of ozone into hydroxyl radical (an oxygen free radical) (*Figure 5-8*, on the following page.). Emission of agricultural and industrial pollutants into the atmosphere has repeatedly been show to induce primary photochemical reactions and to result in environmental problems like photochemical smog. As described above, these smogs depend heavily on excessive formation of free radicals.

Common Air Pollutants

Toxins contributing to these air pollution problems include aldehydes (e.g., formaldehyde) and ketones (e.g., acetone or methyl ethyl ketone) derived from solvents like benzene and toluene; by-products of fossil fuel combustion (e.g., sulfur and nitric oxides); and by-products of herbicide production (e.g., dioxin). All of these toxins have also been shown to exist in the U.S. food supply. The issue of photochemical smog and primary photochemical reactions has been thoroughly reviewed by Hippeli and Elstner.[74]

Oxidative Stress in the Body

Like excessive production of free radicals in the earth's atmosphere, excessive production of free radicals in the body has been shown to have a long list of unwanted consequences. Most of these consequences involve damage to tissue structure. In this section of the chapter, we review the kinds of structural damage that have been associated with overproduction of free radicals and oxidative stress.

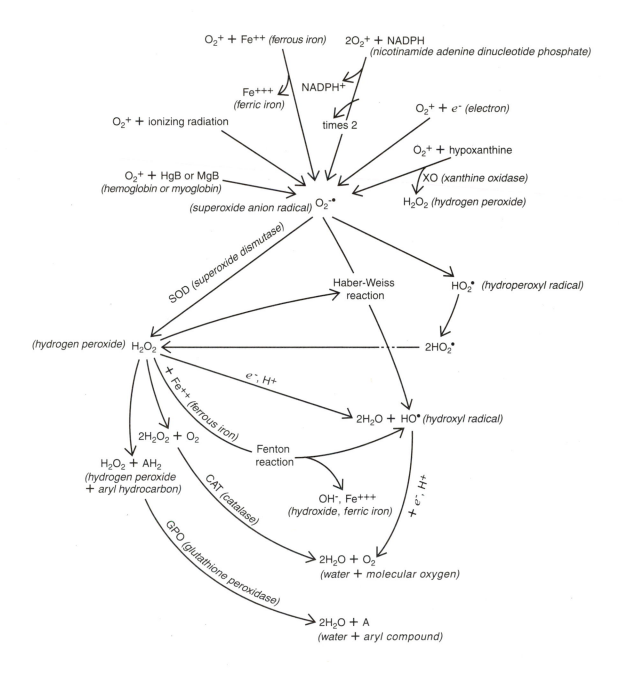

Figure 5-7
Oxygen metabolism

Damage to Plasma Membranes

Because of their high unsaturated fatty acid content, plasma membranes (the outermost membranes of cells that enclose all of their fluids and contents) are unusually susceptible to oxidative stress. Many researchers view oxidative damage to plasma membrane fats as a gateway event in the ability of oxygen to further disrupt cellular function.[75] Oxidative damage to lipids in the plasma membrane is often initiated by a hydroxyl free radical and its ability to convert a plasma lipid into a lipid carbon-centered radical. (Molecular oxygen itself can react with membrane lipids to form lipid carbon-centered radicals, as well as perhydroxy radicals.) Hydroxyl radicals are able to accomplish this feat by removing a hydrogen atom from a methylene group in the lipid's hydrocarbon chain (*Figure 5-9*, on the following page). The presence of double bonds in unsaturated fatty acids

Photolysis of nitrogen dioxide

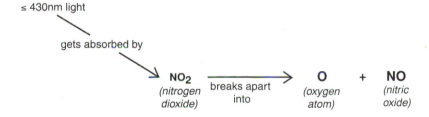

≤ 430nm light

gets absorbed by

NO_2
(nitrogen dioxide) — breaks apart into → O
(oxygen atom) + NO
(nitric oxide)

Oxidation of atomic hydrogen to a hydroperoxyl radical

H + O_2 + M ⟶ $HOO^{\bullet}$ + M
(hydrogen atom) (molecular oxygen) (molecule, usually nitrogen or oxygen) (hydroperoxyl radical) (molecule, usually nitrogen or oxygen)

Oxidation of nitric oxide to nitrogen dioxide and reduction of hydroxyl radical by hydroperoxyl radical

$HOO^{\bullet}$ + NO ⟶ $HO^{\bullet}$ + NO_2
(hydroperoxyl radical) (nitric oxide) (hydroxyl radical) (nitrogen dioxide)

Figure 5-8
Photochemical production of free radicals

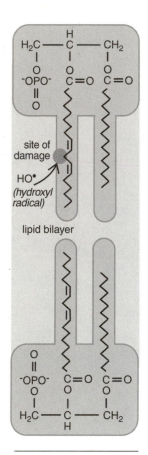

Figure 5-9
Lipid membrane damage by hydroxyl radical

makes this process easier, since double bonds weaken carbon-hydrogen bonds in carbons that lie next to the site of double-bonding. Hydroxyl radicals are the most active of all oxygen radicals. The rates at which hydroxyl radicals can react with surrounding structures approaches the speed of diffusion, although they must be in extremely close proximity (within a few angstroms) of those structures.[76]

Peroxidation of Membrane Lipids. The interaction of hydroxyl radicals (as well as other free radicals, including peroxyl radicals and alkoxyl radicals) with membrane lipids can also trigger an ongoing series of free radical reactions. For example, interaction of lipid carbon-centered radicals with molecular oxygen can generate lipid peroxyl radicals. These lipid peroxyl radicals can go on to interact with other lipid and fat components in the membrane. This chain-like series of reactions eventually ends with the formation of hydroperoxides and cyclic peroxides. Collectively, these molecules are referred to as *lipid peroxides*, and their process of formation as *lipid peroxidation*. Numerous laboratory tests have been developed to measure the presence of lipid peroxides. The chemistry of lipid peroxidation and the lab tests available for its detection have been comprehensively reviewed by Gutteridge,[77] Esterbauer[78] and Benzie.[79]

Lipid peroxidation has been shown to be a common mode of action for numerous food-related toxins. These toxins include organochlorine insecticides like endosulfan,[80] herbicides like paraquat[81] and herbicide production by-products like TCDD,[82] as well as solvents like trichloroethylene,[83] metals like aluminum,[84] heavy metals like cadmium[85] or lead,[86] and particulates like asbestos.[87] Most of the above-cited research studies on lipid peroxidation has utilized the TBARS (thiobarbituric acid reactive substances) test to measure free radical damage to membranes. TBARS results have typically been reported in nanamoles of thiobarbituric acid reactive substances per gram of protein. Increases of 25-30% in TBARS levels have been common following toxic exposure.

Damage to Mitochondrial Membranes

Approximately 90% of all oxygen taken into the body ultimately finds its way into mitochondria.[88] Mitochondria are highly specialized, energy-rejuvenating components of cells. Embryologically, in their initial stages of development, all cells in the body contain mitochondria. An adult body, with approximately 30 trillion cells, contains approximately 100 quadrillion mitochondria. Mitochondria are uniquely structured to provide for oxidation (breakdown) of fats, and for recycling of the body's most critical energy storage molecule, ATP (adenosine triphosphate).

Because 90% of the body's oxygen is delivered to the mitochondria, these organelles continually face a heightened risk of oxidative stress. Approximately 4% of all oxygen in mitochondria has been estimated to undergo incomplete reduction and to routinely form oxygen radicals including superoxide radical ($O2^{-\bullet}$) and hydroxyl radical ($OH^{\bullet}$).[89] The constant formation of these oxygen radicals in close proximity to the unsaturated lipid-containing membranes of the mitochondria makes them uniquely susceptible to oxidative damage.

Because oxidative damage to the mitochondrial membranes disrupts energy-driven processes throughout the body, structural damage to mitochondrial membranes can also be regarded as disruption of the body's energetic processes. In keeping with this second way of classifying oxidative damage to mitochondrial membranes, we will review the consequences of these events beginning on page 230, under "Toxic Disruption of Mitochondrial Function"

Other Types of Direct Damage Caused by Oxidative Stress

Induction of Apoptosis. Although induction of apoptosis is reviewed earlier in this chapter, it is worth repeating the research conclusion that oxidative stress is a major mechanism for inducing apoptosis. The close connection between unsupported oxygen metabolism and increased programming of cell death makes intuitive sense. Whole-body health would clearly be benefited by sensitivity to immanent danger on the part of every cell, and by cell responses that eliminated that danger, even if these responses brought cell death. The connection between oxidative stress and apoptosis also makes sense within the context of research. Previously-cited studies with chronic fatigue syndrome (CFS) patients, for example, have moved equally in two directions. In one direction has been the confirmation of apoptosis as a relevant consideration in understanding CFS. Compared to the number of cells undergoing mitosis or simply resting, cells undergoing apoptosis are unexpectedly common in CFS. In another direction, and equally compelling, has been confirmation of mitochondrial disruption as a key component of CFS. A similar research overlap has occurred in the study of Parkinson's disease, where increased mitochondrial defects, particularly in Complex I of electron transport chain processing, have been observed alongside of observations involving increased apoptosis among nerve cells.

Adrenochrome Production. A final type of oxidative damage worthy of mention within this section is unwanted oxidation of catecholamine neurotransmitters in the nervous system. Neurotransmitters (NTs) are molecules used to

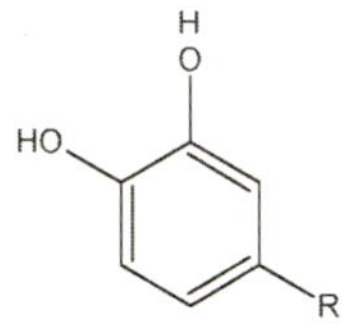

Figure 5-10
Catechol

carry messages from one nerve cell to the next. The majority of neurotransmitters are protein-related and are sometimes as simple as a single amino acid. The catecholamine neurotransmitters are a special category of NTs and include epinephrine (adrenalin), norepinephrine (noradrenalin), dopa, and dopamine. Catecholamines are named for their two common chemical characteristics: a catechol nucleus, consisting of a twice-hydroxylated benzene ring (*Figure 5-10*) and a single amine group (NH_2). This second chemical feature qualifies catecholamines as monoamines. Nerve cells and adrenal cells are the only cell types that produce catecholamines.

For the past forty years, pioneers in orthomolecular medicine, including Abram Hoffer, M.D., Ph.D., have used high-dose vitamin and mineral support of catecholamine metabolism in keeping with a metabolic theory of schizophrenia that included excessive oxidation of catecholamine neurotransmitters. Adrenolutin, for example, one catecholamine oxidation product, has been proposed as an appropriate plasma marker for overall catecholamine oxidation.[90] Adrenochrome, another oxidized form of adrenalin (epinephrine), appears to be produced in the presence of reactive oxygen molecules and may itself function as a radical.[91]

Oxidative Stress and Chronic Disease

Thus far in the chapter we have reviewed a variety of ways in which oxidative stress can cause direct damage to tissues and cells. Mechanisms have included direct damage to cellular membranes and membrane lipids, including plasma, mitochondrial, and nuclear membranes; induction of apoptosis, and adrenochrome production. (Subsequently in the chapter, we review two additional ways in which oxidative stress can cause cell damage: through excessive inflammatory response and through imbalanced cellular detoxication). In light of these multiple mechanisms, it is not surprising that oxidative stress has been linked with a wide variety of chronic diseases. This list includes adult respiratory distress syndrome (ARDS),[92] general aging,[93] amyotrophic lateral sclerosis (ALS),[94] cataract,[95] numerous cancers,[96] gastric ulcer,[97] inflammatory bowel disease,[98] myocardial infarct,[99] and Parkinson's disease.[100] Because dietary deficiencies and imbalances are widely-regarded as contributing factors to virtually all health-compromising conditions, the connection of these diseases with diet is not surprising. What also needs to be taken into account, however, is the ability of food-related toxins to set into motion mechanisms of injury, and in so doing, to create or exacerbate nutrient deficiency and contribute to disruption of health.

Toxin-Related Aspects of Excessive Inflammation

"Inflammation" is a term used to describe one of the body's fundamental, naturally-occurring responses to injury. Injuries to the body that evoke inflammation include chemical injuries (like toxic exposure), physical injuries (like trauma or burns), and microbial injuries (like exposure to a virus). Inflammation is usually thought of as a response to injury, i.e., the start of a healing process that would not be occurring unless damage to the body had already been caused by some external (or internal) agent.

This basic understanding of inflammation has been extended in the recent immunology literature. Researchers have begun to recognize that inflammation cannot be damage-reducing and healing unless is it also well-timed and well-regulated. When inflammation lacks proper timing and regulation, it can become damage-creating and disease-producing.

Overview of the Inflammatory Response

Regardless of the triggering event, inflammation involves three inter-connected changes in body function. First, blood flow to the injured area is increased to allow for increased delivery of cells and nutrients to the area. Second, capillary walls in the area become more permeable to allow for the passage of larger molecules like specialized immune cells out of the blood and into the area. Third, the specialized immune cells, having gained access to the injured area, respond to the injury through a variety of molec-ular events.

While our bodies constantly rely on inflammation as a means of responding to physical and chemical injury, there are circumstances under which inflammation can occur inappropriately. This inappropriateness may involve activation of an immune response in the absence of real injury, overactivation and exaggeration of a response in the presence of a real injury, or chronic response that is overly prolonged in spite of a recov-ery from real injury. Many inappropriate immune responses can be classi-fied as hypersensitivities and immunologists generally recognize four basic types of hypersensitivity response. (The four types are simply referred to as Type I, Type II, Type III, and Type IV hypersensitivity reactions). In this section, we look in detail at Type I responses since they have been most closely linked with toxic exposure.

Type 1 Hypersensitivity

Function and Tissue Distribution of Mast Cells

The central event in Type I responses involves a process called *mast cell degranulation*. Mast cells are a type of white blood cell, and more specifically, a subdivision of white blood cells called *granulocytes*. Three primary types of granulocytes are found in human blood: neutrophils, basophils, and eosinophils. Mast cells are most closely related to basophils, but are found in tissue rather than blood. Despite this difference in anatomical location, many researchers believe that mast cells and basophils are actually one and the same type of cell.

Mast cells are found in two types of tissue: 1) mucosal tissue that lines body cavities like the respiratory tract, intestinal tract, urinary and reproductive tracts; and 2) connective tissue that is found throughout the body, but is particularly abundant in bone, skin, and in the areas around blood vessel walls. Mucosal mast cells (MMCs) and connective tissue mast cells (CTMCs) are both subject to the process of degranulation.

Mast Cell Degranulation (MCD)

Fc Receptors. Mast cell degranulation (MCD) begins with two triggering events that occur on the membrane of the mast cell. First, a pair of antibodies, usually immunoglobulin E (IgE) antibodies, binds to a pair of specialized receptors found on the membrane of the mast cell. These receptors are called *Fc receptors*. Second, this pair of receptor-bound IgE antibodies must then be linked together by a third molecule. (This linking together of the bound Fc receptors is called *receptor crosslinking*). A variety of molecules can accomplish this crosslinking. Once the Fc receptors have been crosslinked, degranulation is triggered in the mast cell.

Cross-Linking by Dietary Lectins and Antigens. Antigenic proteins found in food (for example, the alpha-gliadins found in wheat) are one example of an Fc-crosslinking molecule. The ability of food antigens like alpha-gliadins to trigger mast cell degranulation is the basis of most food allergies involving an immediate reaction to food. Strawberry-induced urticaria (hives) is probably the best-known example of such a reaction. Specialized glycoproteins found in all virtually all foods, called lectins, can also crosslink Fc receptors and trigger degranulation. The ability of food lectins to perform crosslinking has served as the basis for dietary recommendations based on lectin classification of foods. Diets using the Lewis antigen blood typing system are an example of this approach.

Other Food-Related MCD Triggers. Food-related toxins have also been shown to trigger mast cell degranulation. These toxins include the pesticides malathion[101] and diquat,[102] the heavy metal lead,[103] and the solvent toluene.[104] It should be noted that these studies of food-related toxins have determined increased mast cell degranulation following toxic exposure in animals and human subjects but have not ascertained the specific mechanisms linking toxins with increased degranulation. None of the above-mentioned toxins would be likely to serve as a direct crosslink between Fc receptors.

Basic Consequences of Mast Cell Degranulation

Release of Inflammatory Mediators. The crosslinking of Fc receptors on the membrane of the mast cell triggers two parallel processes inside the cell. (A schematic diagram of these processes is presented in *Figure 5-11*). The first of these processes is degranulation. During this process, a set of granules that have been previously stored inside the cell are released into the surrounding extracellular space. The released granules contain a variety of injury response-related substances, including histamine for dilating blood

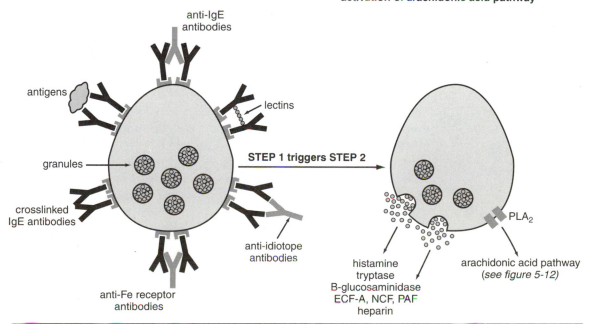

STEP 1:
Fc receptor-mediated triggering of degranulation

STEP 2:
Release of granules and
activation of arachidonic acid pathway

anti-IgE antibodies

antigens

lectins

granules

STEP 1 triggers STEP 2

crosslinked IgE antibodies

PLA_2

anti-idiotope antibodies

histamine
tryptase
B-glucosaminidase
ECF-A, NCF, PAF
heparin

arachidonic acid pathway
(*see figure 5-12*)

anti-Fe receptor antibodies

Figure 5-11
Mast cell degranulation

vessels and increasing capillary permeability; heparin for preventing coagulation; proteolytic enzymes for activating inflammation-based proteins; and chemotactic factors for helping mobilize and direct immune cells toward appropriate targets.

Activation of the Arachidonic Acid (AA) Pathway. The second process set into motion by crosslinking is activation of the arachidonic acid (AA) pathway. Activation of this pathway is accomplished through activation of its initial enzyme, phospholipase A2. Because the arachidonic acid pathway has great potential for increasing oxidative stress and because food-related toxins have also directly linked to its activity, we will now review this pathway in more detail.

Oxidative Aspects of the Arachidonic Acid Pathway

Metabolic Overview. The arachidonic acid pathway (*Figure 5-12*) is named for its chemical starting point, namely, arachidonic acid (AA) (*Figure 5-13*). This 20-carbon, omega 6 fatty acid is contained in the plasma membranes of most cells. Because AA is typically attached to the second carbon in plasma membrane phospholipids, the activation of the enzyme phospholipase A2 is typically regarded as the first step in the arachidonic acid pathway since it unfastens AA from the membrane and makes it available for metabolism.

A common purpose of the arachidonic acid pathway is to convert AA into a family of substances collectively referred to as *eicosanoids*. This conversion requires activity of several oxidative enzymes, including cyclooxygenase and lipoxygenase (reviewed subsequently in this section). The role of these oxidative enzymes in the synthesis of eicosanoid molecules provides a key link between excessive inflammation and oxidative stress.

Like AA, all eicosanoids are twenty-carbon molecules. Unlike AA, however, they are not simply found in straight-chain form, but typically contain a 5-carbon ring and at times, other ring-like configurations. Also, unlike AA, eicosanoids can be classified as hormones since they exhibit a wide range of regulatory activities including control of inflammation, blood pressure, diuresis, smooth muscle contraction, gastric secretion, nerve conduction, and platelet aggregation. Unlike most hormones, however, which are typically synthesized by specific glands and subsequently travel through the blood and exert similar effects on multiple target sites, eicosanoids are synthesized by a variety of cell types found throughout the body, including epithelial cells, platelets, and leukocytes, but have effects which are limited to the tissue in which they are synthesized. Major categories of eicosanoids include prostaglandins and prostacyclins (PGs), leukotrienes (LTs), and thromboxanes (TXs).

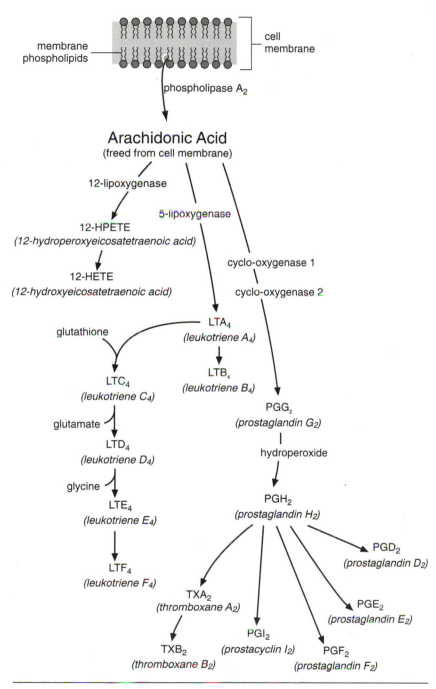

Figure 5-12
Arachidonic acid pathway

Figure 5-13
Arachidonic acid

Eicosanoid Production. Four types of eicosanoids are commonly referred to in the research literature as "pro-inflammatory." These four types include the series 2 prostaglandins (PGD_2, PGE_2, PGF_2, PGG_2, PGH_2); the series 2 thromboxanes (TXA_2, TXB_2); and the series 4 (LTA_4, LTB_4, LTC_4, LTD_4, LTE_4, LTF_4) and series 5 leukotrienes (LTA_5, LTB_5, LTC_5, LTD_5, LTE_5, LTF_5). In order for cells to produce these pro-inflammatory hormones, activity of two key enzyme families is required. For production of series 2 prostaglandins and thromboxanes, AA must be enzymatically processed by cyclo-oxygenase 1 (COX-1) or cyclo-oxygenase 2 (COX-2). For production of series 4 or series 5 leukotrienes, AA must be enzymatically processed by 5-lipoxygenase (5-LPX).

Cyclo-oxygenase (COX) and Lipoxygenase (LPX). Altered cyclo-oxygenase and/or lipoxygenase activity has been associated with a wide variety of chronic diseases. These diseases include inflammatory bowel conditions like Crohn's or ulcerative colitis, in which upregulation of COX-2 occurs in apical epithelial cells;[105] gastric ulcer;[106] inflammatory joint disease, in which gene expression for COX-1 and COX-2 is increased in sinovial fluid cells;[107] Alzheimer's disease, in which cells of the superior temporal lobe neocortex see increased transcription of the COX-2 gene;[108] asthma;[109] atherosclerosis, in which oxidation of LDL (low-density lipoprotein) in the bloodstream by monocytes appears to lipoxygenase dependent;[110] and diabetes.[111]

In the context of immune function, excessive inhibition of COX and LPX enzymes can be as disruptive to health as overactivation, since some immune cells (for example, phagocytes) use activation of COX and LPX enzymes as a mechanism for generating oxygen radicals that can damage the cell walls of pathogenic bacteria. Here food-related toxins may play an important immune-compromising role since several toxins have been shown to inhibit COX and/or LPX activity. These food-related toxins include the carbamate insecticides (including carbaryl, found predominantly on fruits, including bananas, grapes, grapefruit, oranges, peaches, and watermelon);[112] dioxin (TCDD);[113] the widely-used antioxidant preservative BHT (butylated hydroxytoluene);[114] and the packaging plasticizer mono-ethylhexyl phthalate (MEHP).[115]

Toxin-Related Aspects of Imbalanced Detoxication

Beginning with Part IV of this chapter (page 196) we reviewed basic connections between imbalanced oxidative metabolism and damage to the body at a cellular level. We looked at direct forms of oxidative damage, including damage to plasma membranes, membrane lipids, mitochondrial membranes, and catecholamine neurotransmitters. We also reviewed the ability of oxidative stress to trigger cell cycle damage in the form of increased apoptosis.

Next, we turned our attention to a less direct form of oxidative damage, namely, damage caused by overactivation of oxidative enzymes during excessive inflammation. In this section, we focused on the ability of food-related toxins to trigger overactivation of the arachidonic acid pathway, overproduction of pro-inflammatory eicosanoid mediators, and exacerbation of oxidative stress.

Now we will review a second indirect form of oxidative damage that is parallel to the damage caused by excessive inflammation. This second form of indirect damage is related to the body's metabolic processes that are commonly referred to as processes of detoxication.

Overview of Cellular Detoxication

Basic Function of Detoxication

Detoxication is the technical term for describing cellular deactivation of toxins. (The terms "detoxification" and "detoxication" are often used interchangeably, although many researchers use the term "detoxication" to refer to natural dismantling of foreign substances that takes place routinely in the cells of healthy persons, and the term "detoxification" to refer to clinical situations in which patients have been exposed to unnaturally high toxic loads and must undergo treatment to regain their health).

Tissue Distribution of Detoxicating Enzymes

Detoxication occurs in a wide variety of human cell types and organ systems. Cytochrome P450 enzyme systems, a hallmark of cellular detoxication, have been identified in the epithelial linings of the body's key "entry portals" including the respiratory tract, digestive tract, and urinary tract. The systems have also been identified in primary immune-related organs, including the skin and liver; in specialized immune cells, including macrophages, monocytes and lymphocytes; in reproductive-related organs like the placenta; in endocrine organs like the adrenals; and in the brain.[116] Although widespread availability of detoxication clearly reflects localized capability for dismantling of toxins, many of the toxic substances introduced into the body (especially through the GI tract) are sent to the liver for deactivation.

Metabolic Phases in Detoxication

The detoxication process consists of two distinct phases. These phases are typically referred to as Phase I and Phase II. The separation of detoxication into phases is related to a specific characteristic of the toxins, namely, the degree to which they dissolve in water. Toxins that are completely water-soluble can typically by-pass the entire cellular detoxication process and be directly eliminated from the body either through the urine (renal excretion) or stool (biliary excretion). In contrast, toxins that are highly water-insoluble must always pass through both phases of cellular detoxication, and in fact may be stored for years inside fat cells or in the fatty portions of any cell membrane before ultimately becoming mobilized and undergoing detoxication.

The chemistry of food-related toxins reviewed in Chapter 3 largely determines their relationship to detoxication. As discussed in that chapter, many food-related toxins are derived from saturated hydrocarbons and contain few electrically charged regions. These toxins have little affinity for interaction and for this reason are highly persistent in the environment. As a group, these food-related toxins are described as hydrophobic (water-avoiding), lipophilic (fat-loving), and non-polar (lacking permanent, net negative or net positive electrochemical sites which would allow them to interact with polarized molecules like those constituting water). The hydrophobic, lipophilic, non-polar nature of these toxins prevents them from passing directly out of the body through the urine or stool and requires instead that they be uptaken into cells and sent through both phases of detoxication. The two-phase detoxication process is designed to convert non-polar, water-insoluble molecules that have little means to leave the body into polar, water-soluble versions that can gain access to the blood and urine and thus be eliminated from the body.

Toxin-Related Aspects of Phase I Metabolism

Functional Overview of Phase I

Phase I of the detoxication process is designed to take molecules that are non-polar and lipophilic (fat-loving) and create in them more polar, electrochemically-charged regions. This task is carried out by oxidoreductase enzymes. Oxidoreductases are one of six basic families of enzymes, and their function is to transfer electrons between molecules. The oxidoreductase family of enzymes includes oxidases, dehydrogenases, hydroperoxidases, and oxygenases, and reductases. The specialized network of oxidoreductase enzymes used in Phase I of detoxication is specifically referred to as the cytochrome P450 enzyme system. Because of its critical relationship to toxicity and oxidative stress, we will look more closely at the its function and components.

The Cytochrome P450 System

Many enzymes belonging to the oxidoreductase family contain iron atoms to assist with electron transfer from one molecule to another. Iron atoms facilitate electron transfer by readily switching between ferrous (Fe^{++}) and ferric (Fe^{+++}) states. The most common form of iron in human metabolism is heme iron, and proteins containing this form of iron are called heme proteins. Many of these heme proteins function as enzymes.

Cytochromes constitute one family of iron-containing enzymes, and all cytochromes contain iron in its heme form. (These heme proteins were originally named according to patterns of light absorption observed in laboratory tests, and these patterns are still represented by italicized lower case letters and numerical subscripts, e.g., cytochrome a_1, cytochrome b, cytochrome c_1, etc.) Cytochromes are typically found anchored to the membranes of the endoplasmic reticulum or to the mitochondrial membranes within cells.

The cytochrome P450 enzyme system both conforms and differs from the cytochrome rules described above. Like the cytochromes previously described, the P450 system contains specific cytochrome enzymes (P450s) that have been named for their light absorption patterns (maximum absorption of a 450-nanometer wavelength when carbon monoxide-bound). They also have transfer of electrons as their primary enzymatic function. Unlike the specific examples of cytochromes cited above, however, the P450 system includes enzymes that are not themselves cytochromes. The non-cytochrome members of the P450 system include other heme enzymes like peroxidases and catalases, as well as non-heme enzymes containing iron-sulfur clusters (like the enzyme xanthine oxidase), and flavoprotein enzymes (like microsomal flavin-containing monooxygenase). The cytochrome and non-cytochrome members of the cytochrome P450 system work together in Phase I detoxication to transfer electrons to and from fat-soluble toxins.

P450 Gene Families

Cytochrome P450 protein enzymes have been divided up according to the gene families from which their proteins are expressed. Over 200 genes expressing P450 proteins have been identified and grouped into 36 gene families.[117] Although twelve of these gene families have been shown to exist in humans,[118] the majority of Phase I detoxication appears to be accomplished by three families of P450 enzymes. These enzyme families are CYP1, CYP2, and CYP3. (The names of the cytochrome P450 families refer once again back to genes. For cytochrome enzymes to be included in a specific CYP family, their proteins must show at least 40% homology[119]).

Following the CYP1, CYP2, and CYP3 designations of P450 enzyme families, subfamilies of P450 enzymes are designated by capital letters (ranging from "A" to "H"). Subfamily members of the CYP1 family, for example, include CYP1A, CYP1B, CYP1C, etc. Specific enzymes within subfamilies are indicated by an additional arabic numeral, ranging from 1 to 23. The CYP1A subfamily, for example, contains the specific cytochrome P450 enzymes CYP1A1, CYP1A2, CYP1A3, etc.

P450 Substrate

Cytochrome P450 enzymes are responsible for conducting Phase I detoxication not only on food-related toxins, but on virtually all molecules that require conversion into more water-soluble forms in order to be eliminated from the body. Like food-related toxins, most prescription and over-the-counter medications require processing by the P450 system. In addition, most fat-soluble regulatory molecules produced inside the body require P450 Phase I processing. These fat-soluble regulatory molecules include steroid hormones like estrogens, neurotransmitters like serotonin or epinephrine, fatty acid derivatives like prostaglandins, and emulsification agents like bile acids.

The capabilities of a specific enzyme subfamily, or a specific subfamily enzyme may become overloaded if demands for Phase I processing from multiple sources become too great. For example, Phase I detoxication of the anti-inflammatory drug acetaminophen (Tylenol™ requires activity of the enzyme CYP1A2[120]. But if events triggering the inflammation included exposure to the solvent toluene,[121] or the herbicidal by-product dioxin,[122] (both of which also require the activity of CYP1A2 for Phase I processing), CYP1A2 capabilities might be exceeded. Adding routine intake of caffeine to the clinical picture would further compromise CYP1A2 function, since caffeine also requires Phase 1 processing by this member of the P450 family.[123]

Toxic Induction of P450 Enzymes

"Induction" of the cytochrome P450 system refers to the ability of a substance to stimulate activity of the P450 enzymes, or to trigger expression of CYP genes that serve as the templates for constructing P450 enzymes. A long list of food-related toxins has been shown to induce the P450 system. (*Table 5-3*). This list includes solvents like benzene used in pesticide formulation,[124] grain fumigants like EDB,[125] synthetic flavorings like methyl isobutyl ketone,[126] and coal tar dye colorings containing polycyclic aromatic hydrocarbons.[127] Food pesticides and fungicides have also been shown to inhibit cytochrome P450 enzymes. These inhibitors include the fungicides captan,[128] thiram[129] and zineb[130], and the pesticides parathion[131] and diethyldithiocarbamate.[132]

Phase I Overactivity and Underactivity

Inappropriate induction or inhibition of the P450 system can be equally problematic for human health. Excessive inhibition of P450 activity can leave numerous fat-based substances active in the body for prolonged periods of time, and can produce steroid hormone imbalances, imbalances in eicosanoid hormones, and other metabolic disruptions. But excessive induction of the P450 system is generally regarded by researchers as the more dangerous of the possibilities, for two reasons. These reasons involve potential initiation of radical activity, and depletion of nutrient reserves.

The first threat posed by excessive induction of the P450 system is creation of molecules that are actually more dangerous to the body than the initial toxins being detoxicated. By taking non-polar, infrequently reactive molecules and using electron transfer to create electrically charged, reactive regions, the P450 system prepares toxins to become more water soluble, but also, by necessity, renders them more electrochemically reactive. Molecules transformed by the P450 system may exist temporarily as radical species

*Table 5-3. **Induction of cytochrome P450 enzymes by food-related toxins***

Toxin	Relationship to food	CYP classification (if known)
Acetone[133]	Pesticide solvent	
Arsenic[134]	Arsenical pesticides	CYP1A1
Benzene[135]	Solvent	CYP2E1
Bromobenzene[136]	Fumigant precursor	
Carbon tetrachloride[137]	Former fumigant	CYP2E1
Ethylene dibromide[138]	Fumigant	
Ethylene dichloride[139]	Fumigant	
Hexane[140]	Solvent	
Kepone[141]	Pesticide	
Methoxychlor[142]	Insecticide	CYP3A4
Methyl isobutyl ketone[143]	Synthetic flavoring	
Methylene chloride[144]	Decaffeinator	
Polychlorinated Biphenyls[145]	Pesticide preparations, Air, soil and water contaminants	CYP1A, CYP2B
Polycyclicaromatic hydrocarbons[146]	Soil contaminants	CYP1A1
Styrene[147]	packaging migrant	CYP2E1
Toluene[148]	Solvent	CYP2E1, 1A1, 2B1, 2B2, 3A1
Vinyl chloride[149]	Packaging migrant	CYP2E1
Xylene[150]	Solvent	

containing an unpaired electron following the process of electron transfer.

What normally prevents cellular damage in the wake of this heightened reactivity is initiation of Phase II. During this second phase of detoxication a new chemical group is attached to the reactive region created during Phase I. Once this new chemical group has been attached the detoxicated molecule is typically returned to a less reactive state and becomes sufficiently water-soluble for urinary excretion.

In addition to the threat of unwanted reactivity, excessive induction of the P450 system also poses a second threat to the body's metabolic balances. This threat involves depletion of specific detoxication-related nutrients. To understand the nature of this second threat, a more detailed review of Phase II detoxication processes is required.

Toxin-Related Aspects of Phase II Metabolism

Functional Overview of Phase II

Like its Phase I counterpart, Phase II detoxication also operates with a full complement of enzymes from one of six basic enzyme families. In Phase I, that enzyme family was the oxidoreductase family. In Phase II, it is the transferase family. Transferase enzymes are proteins that help transfer small chemical groups between molecules, and they are typically named after the type of group which gets transferred. Sulfotransferases, for example, transfer sulfur-containing groups; methyltranferases transfer methyl groups; acetyltransferases transfer acetyl groups. The transfer reactions that occur during Phase II detoxication are also typically referred to as conjugation reactions, in reference to the joining together of Phase I-activated toxins and Phase II-provided chemical groups.

*Table 5-4. **Phase II conjugation reactions***

Category	Group transferred	Enzymes involved
Sulfur conjugation	Inorganic sulfur	ATP sulfurase, sulfotransferases
Glutathione	Glutathione	*S* transferases
Methylation	Methyl group	Methyltransferases
Glucuronidation	Glucuronic acid	Glucuronosyltransferases, UDP-glucuronosyltransferases
Acetylation	Acetyl group	Acetyltransferases
Acylation	Glycine Glutamine Taurine	Acyltransferases

Phase II Conjugation Reactions

Researchers generally recognize five basic types of conjugation reactions as the backbone of Phase II detoxication (*Table 5-4*). These five basic types of conjugation include 1) sulfation (also called sulfonation), in which an inorganic form of sulfur, or the sulfur-containing tripeptide glutathione gets transferred; 2) methylation, in which a methyl group is transferred; 3) glucuronidation (also called gluconation), in which a form of the molecule glucuronic acid is transferred; 4) acetylation, in which an acetyl group is transferred; and 5) acylation, in which one of three amino acids (glycine, glutamine, or taurine) is transferred. When Phase II acylation involves the amino acid glycine, the transfer process is specifically referred to as glycation. An even greater level of specification that is particularly important during Phase II is the transfer of glycine to a molecule of benzene. (*Figure 5-14*). This transfer produces a new molecule called hippuric acid. Because glycation of benzene is a common Phase II conjugation reaction, hippurate formation is often listed as a basic category of Phase II conjugation along with sulfation, methylation, etc.

Unique Aspects of Phase II Sulfur Metabolism

Sulfotransferases. Also worthy of mention in relationship to basic aspects of Phase II are several unique aspects of transfers involving sulfur. First is the complexity of the sulfotransferase (ST) system. The sulfotransferase gene family has been determined to have five major isoforms (forms similar in function but having different substrate affinities, maximum activity, or regulatory properties), to be highly polymorphic (occurring in several forms within a population), and to exist in a wide variety of tissue including brain, liver, small intestine, endometrium, and scalp.[151] The sulfotransferase gene family is typically regarded as having two major divisions.

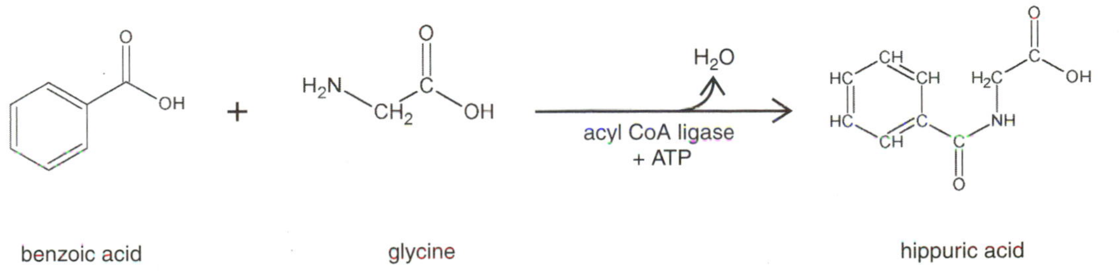

benzoic acid   glycine   hippuric acid

Figure 5-14
Glycination of benzoic acid

The PST (phenol sulfotransferase) division acts on all phenolic substances, including thyroid hormones, neurotransmitters, and many commonly-used drugs like acetaminophen (Tylenol™). PST enzymes also act on numerous food-related toxins including the carbamate herbicide chlorpropham;[152] the organochlorine herbicide and pesticide pentachlorophenol;[153] and the food texturizing agents ethylene glycol, diethylene glycol, and propylene glycol.[154]

The HST (hydroxysteroid sulfotransferase) division acts on a wide variety of steroid compounds in the body, including the hormones cortisol, estrone, beta-estradiol, and testosterone; digestive agents like bile salts; and cell membrane constituents like cholesterol. Many of the substances acted upon by the HST division of the ST gene family are endogenous (naturally produced inside the body) rather than exogenous (environmentally derived). A schematic diagram of the entire sulfotransferase gene family is depicted in *Figure 5-15.*

Another unique aspect of the ST system is its ability to further activate Phase I metabolites, allowing them to participate in new types of reactions. For example, the activity of ST enzymes is required to keep estrogen hormones circulating in the blood since over 90% of all estrogens circulate in a sulfated form.[155] (A similar situation exists for catecholamine neurotransmitters like dopamine, epinephrine, and norepinephrine). In addition, the actual synthesis of steroid hormones like estrogen may often require a

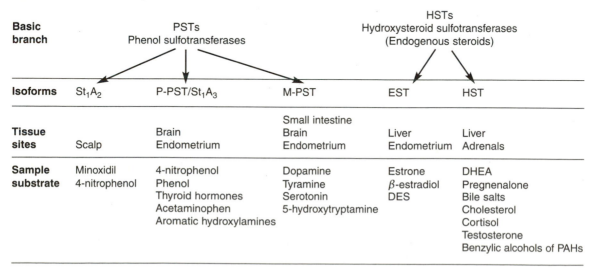

Basic branch	PSTs Phenol sulfotransferases			HSTs Hydroxysteroid sulfotransferases (Endogenous steroids)	
Isoforms	St_1A_2	P-PST/St_1A_3	M-PST	EST	HST
Tissue sites	Scalp	Brain Endometrium	Small intestine Brain Endometrium	Liver Endometrium	Liver Adrenals
Sample substrate	Minoxidil 4-nitrophenol	4-nitrophenol Phenol Thyroid hormones Acetaminophen Aromatic hydroxylamines	Dopamine Tyramine Serotonin 5-hydroxytryptamine	Estrone β-estradiol DES	DHEA Pregnenalone Bile salts Cholesterol Cortisol Testosterone Benzylic alcohols of PAHs

Figure 5-15
The sulphotransferase gene family

sulfation step. Synthesis of estrogen *in utero*, for example, requires sulfation of DHEA in the fetal adrenal glands before placental synthesis of estrogen from DHEA becomes possible.[156]

Glutathione Conjugation. Usually included within the category of Phase II sulfur conjugations are enzyme transfers involving the tripeptide glutathione. Glutathione is generally regarded as the most important non-protein thiol (sulfhydryl-containing molecule) in humans. The term "thiol" is derived from the Greek word for sulfur (*theion*), and its "-ol" ending refers to the chemical observation that sulfhydryl groups, which contain one sulfur and one hydrogen atom (-SH), act like analogs of alcohol groups which contain one oxygen and one hydrogen (-OH). In chemistry, thiols are also referred to as mercaptans.

Although it is composed of amino acids, glutathione (GSH) is classified as a tripeptide instead of a protein because of its short, three amino acid length. Glycine, glutamic acid, and cysteine are the three amino acids from which GSH is synthesized. Synthesis occurs in a wide variety of cells, and requires proper function of two enzymes, gamma-glutamylcysteine synthase and glutathione synthase. Enzymatic combination of the three amino acids results in the production of gamma-glutamylcysteinylglycine (GSH).

GSH conjugation during Phase II detoxication requires activity of glutathione *S*-transferases, or GSTs. The enzymology of GSTs has recently been reviewed by Ketterer and Christodoulides, and numerous food-related toxins have been identified as candidates for GST detoxication.[157] Food-related toxins requiring GSH conjugation include the anti-microbial agent (and by-product of ethylene glycol production) ethylene oxide;[158] the solvent and decaffeinator methylene chloride,[159] the fumigant methyl bromide;[160] the U.S. prohibited but internationally still-used fungicide and fumigant, ethylene dibromide (EDB);[161] the widely-used food packaging materials styrene and polystyrene;[162,163] and the pesticides methyl parathion[164] and chlorvinphos.[165]

Clinical Research on Sulfur Supplementation. The uniqueness of sulfur conjugations in Phase II detoxication has prompted researchers to investigate the use of sulfur-containing supplements in treatment of toxicity-related conditions. Dimethyl sulfoxide (DMSO), for example, has been used in treatment of toxicity-related conditions like ulcerative colitis;[166] N-acetyl cysteine (NAC) has been shown to protect against pulmonary damage caused by inhalation of the toxin perfluoroisobutene in rats;[167] methionine (MET) supplementation has been used to help offset enzyme induction following exposure to polychlorinated biphenyls in rats;[168] and taurine (TAU) supplementation has been shown to protect the rat liver against toxic damage by the hepatocarcinogen 2-acetylaminofluorene.[169] Because many of these sulfur-containing compounds have antioxidant and metal-chelating ability in addition to their role as GST conjugates, their therapeutic benefit may be primarily related to maintenance of an adequate, functional supply of sulfur-containing compounds in cells which would subsequently assure regeneration of GSH for Phase II detoxication.

Unique Aspects of Phase II Methyl Metabolism

COMT Enzymes. Also worthy of special mention in a review of Phase II detoxication is the process of methylation enacted by methyltransferase (MT) enzymes. Two key families of MT enzymes have been found in a wide variety of human tissue. The first MT family, referred to as catechol-O-methyltransferase (COMT) family, has been determined to operate in cells of the brain, liver, kidney, intestine, skin, blood vessel walls, salivary glands, pituitary gland, and peripheral nerves. In addition, COMT enzymes are found in all red blood cells and fat cells. COMT activity appears required for intracellular synthesis of both vitamin K and coenzyme Q (ubiquinone).[170] Although most studies of detoxication have focused on problems related to underactivity of COMT enzymes, overactivity has also received interest. For example, COMT inhibitors have recently been under investigation as pharmcologic agents of potential use in Parkinson's disease.[171]

HIOMT Enzymes. The second MT family has been designated as the HIOMT (hydroxyindole-O-methyltransferase) family. HIOMT enzymes have been located in the red blood cells, pineal cells, retinal cells, cells within the cerebellum of the brain, and in specialized intestinal cells called APUD (amino precursor uptake and/or decarboxylation) cells.[172]

MT activity has been shown to be essential for Phase II detoxication of numerous food-related toxins. These toxins include arsenic and arsenic-based pesticides;[173] the previously used fumigant carbon tetrachloride;[174] and the heavy metals lead and mercury.[175]

SAM Cycle Interactions. Two aspects of methyl metabolism complicate our understanding of MTs in their role as protectors against toxicity. First is the unique nutrient cycle required to maintain an adequate supply of methyl groups in the body. Methyl metabolism, also called one-carbon metabolism, involves creation and transfer of one carbon, three hydrogen methyl groups (-CH$_3$ groups). Numerous vitamins, vitamin derivatives, amino acids, and amino acid derivatives participate in a methyl-supplying cycle referred to as the *S*-adenosylmethionine (SAM) cycle (*Figure 5-16*, on the following page). Key nutrients in the SAM cycle include vitamins B-6, B-12, folate and choline, as well as the amino acids glycine and serine. The trimethylated, glycine-derived hydroxide salt *betaine* and the dimethylated serine-derived alcohol *dimethylaminoethanol* are also key metabolites in this cycle. Disruption of the SAM cycle disrupts the supply of methyl groups needed for Phase II methyltransferase activity. For this reason, underactivity of MT enzymes may not be a primary factor in disrupted detoxication, but a secondary factor that naturally results from imbalances and/or

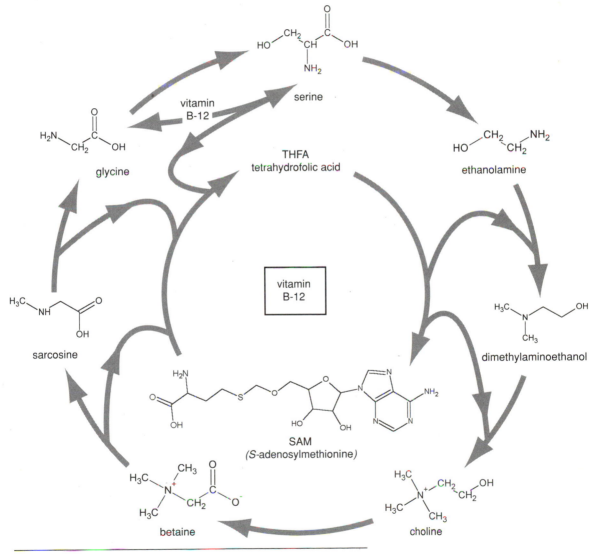

Figure 5-16
S-adenosylmethionine (SAM) cycle

deficiencies in the SAM cycle. In keeping with this distinction, many clinicians have approached underactivity of MT enzymes through direct oral supplementation of SAM cycle metabolites (including SAM) when treating exposure to methylation-requiring toxins like lead.[176]

Methyl Regulation of Gene Expression. A second complicating factor in Phase II methylation activity is the role of MT enzymes in regulating gene expression. Methylation along gene promoter regions in the DNA strands found inside the cell nucleus has long been identified as a key mechanism in gene regulation. In general, methylation has been determined to act as a mechanism that inhibits gene transcription,[177] and hypomethylation of genes has been identified as a contributing factor to diseases like Alzheimer's (in which it is the amyloid precursor protein gene that has been determined to be hypomethylated).[178] Gene-related methyltranferase functions are likely to play at least as great a role as Phase II-related methyltransferase functions in the connection between methylation-requiring toxins and disease.

An alternative way of understanding the above complexities of methyl metabolism is to consider all enzymatic and non-enzymatic methyl-related functions as part of an interconnected pattern in which compromise at any one juncture shifts the entire pattern and causes disruption. Support for this holistic view has been offered by research findings that have linked multiple forms of methyl deficiency with toxin-related chronic disease. Interpreted in this holistic way as a broad category of metabolic compromise, "undermethylation" has been linked to schizophrenia,[179] Alzheimer's disease,[180] Parkinson's disease and general aging,[181] depression,[182] and numerous cancers.[183]

Phase II Overactivity and Underactivity

Considered as a whole, Phase II detoxication reactions can be regarded as requiring a vast array of food-derived nutrients. Looking only at the above discussions of sulfur and methyl metabolism, for example, we would be able to compile a list of at least eighteen nutrients directly involved in Phase II detoxication. These nutrients would include as direct substrates in metabolic pathways the amino acids cysteine, glycine, glutamine, serine, taurine and the tripeptide glutathione; and the vitamins B-6, B-12, folate, and choline. Required enzymatic cofactors would include the minerals phosphorus and selenium and vitamins B-2, B-3 and C , all required for GSH cycling; the mineral molybdenum, required as a cofactor in operation of the enzyme sulfite oxidase; and in maintenance of the SAM cycle, the additional nutrients magnesium and pantothenic acid. If we extended this list by adding to it micronutrients *indirectly* involved in methylation and sulfation by virtue of their roles in amino acid or vitamin synthesis, it would be difficult to name *any* conventionally-recognized vitamin or mineral that did not play an important role in Phase II conjugation.

The importance of nutrient sufficiency in Phase II detoxication has important implications for the establishment of nutrient requirements. Because of its potential drain on nutrient stores, toxicity must be considered as a risk factor for dietary insufficiency. Just as nutritionists have always recognized dietary insufficiency as a risk factor for chronic disease, toxicity may need to be recognized as risk factor for dietary insufficiency. It is not difficult to imagine a situation in which dietary intake would be sufficient to avoid disease risk under toxin-free circumstances, yet insufficient to avoid this same disease risk under circumstances of high toxicity. Because the same nutrient pool serves toxicity-related and toxicity-unrelated needs, circumstances of high toxicity may tip the scales of nutrient availability from adequacy to inadequacy in an individual.

The importance of nutrient sufficiency in Phase II detoxication also means that dietary recommendations at a public health level may need to account for toxic exposure on a population basis. Desirable daily nutrient intake in a given population may be significantly impacted by degree of toxic exposure, and circumstances of routine exposure might require upward revision of baseline dietary recommendations.

Toxin Classification and Phase II Conversions

All toxins have potential access to Phase II detoxicating enzymes, and this access is best understood with respect to the chemical classification of each toxin. Phenols, for example, have direct access to methylating, sulfating, and glutathione-conjugating enzymes. Aromatic thiols, on the other hand, must be converted into ketones, and then into secondary alcohols, before they can become sulfated or glucuronidated. A summary of these relationships is presented in *Figure 5-17*, on the following page.

Imbalanced Detoxication in the GI Tract

All lipophilic toxins pass through cellular detoxication, including numerous toxins that are completely unrelated to diet. When placed against this background of toxins unrelated to food and diet, food-related toxins can be seen as sharing certain basic characteristics. For example, unlike inhaled contaminants or contaminants absorbed transdermally (across the skin), food toxins always arrive first at the GI (gastrointestinal) tract. Because the GI is the first organ system to be presented with all food toxins, it is also the organ most likely to have altered function following exposure to them. In addition, because GI-absorbed food toxins are sent directly through the portal circulation to the liver, the liver is another organ system particularly affected by food toxins.

GI Sensitivity to Toxic Overload

Within the above context, we would expect to see particularly problematic consequences following compromised detoxication of food-related toxins in both the GI tract and the liver. These expectations appear to have been met in the research literature. In the stomach of the rat, for example, Phase II detoxication activities have been determined to be quite low. The rat stomach has been determined to have less than 6% of the glutathione-*S*-transferases found in the rat small intestine[184] and only one third of the glucuronosyl transferases.[185] Sulfotransferase activity has also been determined to be low.[186] Naturally-depressed Phase II activity in the stomach may help explain why exposure to certain food-related toxins raises the risk

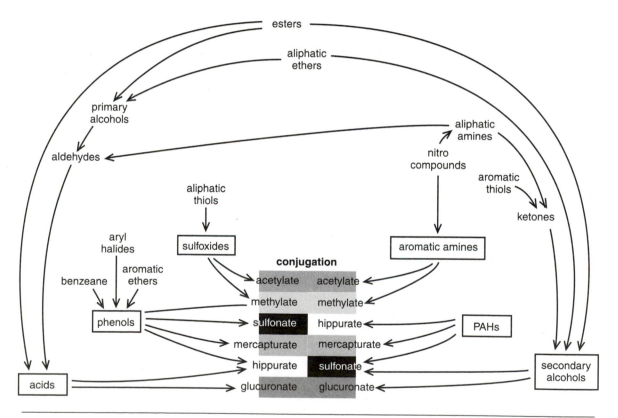

Figure 5-17
Phase II access by chemical group

Mechanisms of Toxic Action in a Cancer Model

The Initiation-Promotion Model

Beginning in the early 1990s, many investigators in the area of cancer research began to embrace a two-stage model of cancer formation. In the first stage, called initiation, a series of metabolic changes was observed to take place and to result in damage to DNA in the cell nucleus. "Initiation" therefore means "initiation of damage to the genetic information contained in DNA". If the cell can repair this damage prior to replication (reproducing itself through the process of mitosis), the cell does not become cancerous. If, however, the cell goes on to replicate (reproduce itself) before this DNA damage is repaired, the cell moves on toward the possibility of becoming fully cancerous and is described as having passed into the second stage of the cancer process, namely, promotion.

When a cell has passed into the promotion stage, the damage to its DNA that occurred during initiation is viewed as irreversible. However, the second stage cell is still described as "pre-neoplastic" (not fully cancerous) because a certain degree of normal growth control can still be maintained within the cell despite irreversible DNA damage. With the addition of a promoting agent, however, a pre-neoplastic cell can be transformed into fully cancerous (neoplastic) cells. Such a cell no longer possesses its normal growth control.

Toxin-Related Aspects of Carcinogenesis

During the initiation as well as the promotional stage of carcinogenesis, the cell is undergoing changes in its informational, structural, and energy-based processes. Structural changes include alteration in its cytoskeleton and inner membranes, and along with these alterations, disrupted membrane fluidity. Informational changes include decreased apoptosis, decreased growth factor input into the cell's mitotic processes, and altered cyclic nucleotide levels no longer appropriate for supporting cell signaling. Disruptions in energy processes include inappropriate ion fluxes, imbalanced protein secretion, inappropriate gap junction activity, and inappropriate transport energetics across several sub-cellular membranes. Once the cell has become fully neoplastic, changes in all of these areas have run their full course, and the cell can no longer act in consort with surrounding tissue.

This molecular-level description of carcinogenesis leads to a simple, unmistakable conclusion: exposure to food-related toxins can contribute to carcinogenesis, since food-related toxins have been shown to affect all of the informational processes that get disrupted during carcinogenesis. When mercury, cadmium, PCBs, benzene, and arsenical pesticides disrupt apoptosis, they are also adding to the risk of carcinogenicity, since disruptions in apoptosis are a hallmark of that process. When pesticides like chlorpyrifos or endrin, or heavy metals like cadmium, or solvents like benzene and toluene, or plasticizers like DEHP (diethyl-hexylphthalate) disrupt protein kinase activity, these disruptions contribute to the risk of carcinogenecity, because disruptions in protein kinases are characteristic of carcinogenesis. ■

of cancer more dramatically here than in other locations. In studies of humans involving fetal stomach cells, for example, benzo(a)pyrene and some N-nitrosamines in the stomach have been shown to be activated in that location by Phase I enzymes and to bind directly to DNA in stomach cells rather than undergoing Phase II detoxication.[187] A similar situation has been observed in rats with respect to esophageal cells.[188]

Imbalances in the Small Intestine. The small intestine (SI) has been shown to have higher Phase I activity than any other GI locale,[189] and SI tissue has been shown to readily activate food-related toxins like aromatic amines[190] and benzo(a)pyrene.[191] At the same time, however, only 3% of GI tumors occur here. This apparent contradiction may be at least partially explained by the high level of Phase II activity in the small intestine.[192] Glucuronosyl transferase activity, for example, has been show to be 300%-600% greater here than in any other area of the GI.[193] Glutathione-S-transferase activity has been found to be 20–30 times greater.[194] Sulfotransferase activity has also shown to be higher in this GI location.[195] Ability to sulfate toxins like *p*-nitrophenol appears to be better in the small intestine than in the colon.[196]

Imbalances in the Large Intestine. In the large intestine (LI), major Phase II enzymes (for example, glutathione-s-transferase and UDP-glucuronosyl-transferase) appear to be lower in concentration than in the SI. Simultaneously, there appears to be greater activity of beta-glucuronidase,[197] an enzyme that can convert non-toxic glucuronides into toxic metabolites. Relatively low Phase II activity, high beta-glucuronidase activity, and reduced isoenzyme variety in the Phase I area may leave the colon more susceptible to cancer.

Bacteria in the large intestine also play a key role in detoxication and in further activation of toxins. Bioactivating enzymes in LI bacteria include nitroreductases that reduce nitroaromatics; azo reductases that reduce water-soluble food colorings like Methyl Orange, Methyl Yellow and Congo Red; glycosidases that activate compounds containing glycosidic linkages; and, as previously mentioned, beta-glucuronidase. LI bacteria also contain enzymes that can bioactivate bile acids arriving through the stool. These enzymes include 7-alpha-hydroxysteroid dehydrogenase that converts the bile acid cholic acid into deoxycholic acid and the bile acid chenodeoxy-cholic acid into lithocholic acid. Both of these conversions have been repeatedly linked to the development of colorectal cancer,[198] particularly in beef-consuming individuals whose bile acid secretion and fecal microflora show distinct patterns.[199] An outstanding review of detoxication-GI relationships compiling most of the references cited above has been published by Chadwick, George and Claxton (1992).[200]

PART V

Toxic Disruption of Energetic Processes

Overview of Mitochondrial Function

Embryologically, in their initial stages of development, all cells in the body contain specialized energy-rejuvenating components called mitochondria. (An adult body, with approximately 30 trillion cells, contains approximately 100 quadrillion mitochondria.) Mitochondria are uniquely structured to provide for oxidation (breakdown) of fats, and for recycling of the body's most critical energy storage molecule, ATP (adenosine triphosphate). This high-phosphate, aerobically-produced molecule is a critical presence in virtually all cells (except red blood cells) and fueling a wide spectrum of cellular events. These events include active and bulk transport of molecules across membranes, breakdown and synthesis of macronutrients, muscle contraction, operation of transmembrane sodium-potassium pumps, phagocytosis, pinocytosis, and receptor-mediated endocytosis.

Tissue Distribution of Mitochondria

Cardiocytes

The recycling of ATP by mitochondria is an aerobic (oxygen-driven) event, and tissues that have particularly active oxygen metabolism also have particularly large numbers of mitochondria. Cardiac muscle, for example, one of the few tissues in the body that is continuously aerobic, is parti-cularly dependent upon mitochondria and their function. Mitochon-dria occupy 40% of the cytoplasmic space within myocardial cells, and 80% of the energy used by cardiocytes comes from oxidation of fat inside the mitochondria.

Hepatocytes

As a tissue type, liver cells (hepatocytes) are also aerobically active. The high-level aerobic activity of liver cells is related to their oxidase enzyme system for detoxifying toxic substances. (This system, called the cytochrome P450 system, is reviewed earlier in this chapter, page 213, under "The Cytochrome P450 System"). A liver cell may contain as many as 1500-2500 mitochondria.

ATP Recycling

Membrane Transport

A complex set of events must take place in order for mitochondria to recycle ATP. (*Figure 5-18* illustrates the basic features of mitochondrial metabolism). Entry into mitochondria is complicated by the presence of an inner and outer membrane. In particular, the inner membrane is particularly

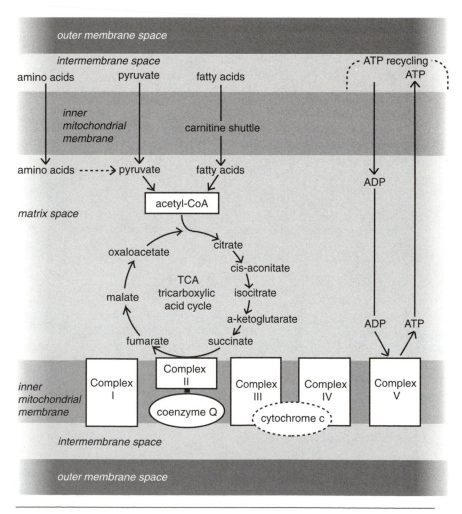

Figure 5-18
Mitochondrial metabolism

impermeable to many substances. Among all amino acids in the body, for example, only the branched chain amino acids (BCAAs, including leucine, isoleucine, and valine) are allowed to cross the inner membrane. The most common molecules to pass into the mitochondria are fatty acids, and even here, a complex transport system involving the activity of an amino acid-like substance, carnitine, is required.

Krebs Cycle Activity

Inside of the mitochondria, a two-step process is used to recycle the high-phosphate energy carrier, ATP. First, macronutrient molecules, including amino acids and fatty acids that have crossed the outer and inner mitochondria membranes must be metabolically transformed to gain entrance into the tricarboxylic acid (TCA) cycle (also called the "Krebs cycle," in honor of its 1953 Nobel-Prize winning discoverer, Hans Krebs). Upon entering the cycle, these molecules have some of their electrons (in the form of hydrogen atoms) systematically stripped off. Once these hydrogens have been stripped off, they are immediately added to vitamin B-2 (flavin adenine dinucleotide, or FAD) and B-3 (nicotinamide adenine dinucleotide, or NAD) metabolites to form FADH and NADH. The formation of these metabolites completes step one of the ATP recycling process, and it is in the form of FADH and NADH that electrons are transported over to step two in mitochondrial processing.

Electron Transport Chain Activity

During step two of the ATP recycling process, FADH- and NADH-based electrons are fed into complex system of enzymes referred to as the electron transport chain (ETC). This enzyme system is actually composed of five

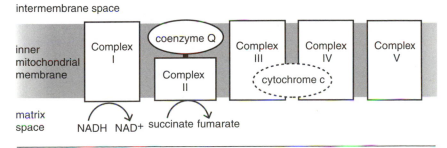

Figure 5-19
The electron transport chain

separate enzyme complexes, known as Complex I, II, III, IV and V. (*Figure 5-19* illustrates the basic structure of a mitochondrial electron transport chain). Although the activities associated with ETC enzymes actually occur within the matrix space of the mitochondrion, the enzymes themselves are imbedded in the inner mitochondrial membrane and help explain its unusually high protein content. Along a single inner membrane there may be as many as 17,000 ETCs.

Re-Phosphorylation of ADP

In order for FADH- and NADH-based electrons to be transported along the electron transport chain, the FADH and NADH hydrogen atoms must be split apart into their constituent parts (one electron and one proton). While hydrogen-derived electrons are transported along the ETC, hydrogen-derived protons are simultaneously pumped out of the matrix space through channels in the inner membrane. In this way a special voltage gradient is created across the inner mitochondrial membrane. This voltage gradient provides the right circumstance for a third phosphate group to be added to the molecule ADP (adenosine diphosphate), thus converting it into the preferred energy transport molecule, ATP (adenosine triphosphate).

Toxic Disruption of Mitochondrial Function

Food-related toxins have been shown to disrupt mitochondrial function through a variety of different mechanisms. Since many disruptive mechanisms are specific to the mitochondrial membrane, we will begin with a review of the ways in which membrane function can be compromised.

Altered Membrane Permeability

Altered permeability of the inner mitochondrial membrane (IMM) is a common consequence of toxic exposure. Altered permeability in this context typically means excessive permeability and inability of the IMM to homeodynamically regulate entry or removal of molecules. The entire research area of altered mitochondrial permeability has recently been reviewed by Reed.[201] The pesticide chlordecone (Kepone™),[202] the packaging plasticizers DEHP (di[2-ethylhexyl]phthalate) and MEHP (mono[2-ethylhexyl]phthalate),[203] and the heavy metal mercury[204] have all been shown to increase the permeability of the IMM and disrupt mitochondria function through this mechanism. Heavy metals like mercury appear to alter mitochondrial membrane function by disrupting calcium homeostasis and thereby depolarizing the membrane. Alongside of this calcium disruption and membrane polarization, mercury-containing compounds appear to deplete the mitochondria's supply of reduced glutathione and thereby place their IMMs at high risk of peroxidation.[205] The insecticide toxaphene has also been shown to disrupt calcium transport in the mitochondrion through inhibition of enzyme adenosine triphosphatase.[206]

Uncoupling

Another common consequence of food-related toxic exposure is referred to as mitochondrial uncoupling. The term "uncoupling" refers to a disengagement of two processes that are normally closely linked in mitochondrial metabolism. The first process, described earlier in this section, involves oxidation of macronutrients through activity of the Krebs cycle and electron transport chain. The second process involves a "recharging" of ATP through phosphorylation of ADP using electrochemical energy generated during the first process. When "coupled," these two processes are collectively referred to as *oxidative phosphorylation*. However, several food-related toxins have been shown to "uncouple" oxidative phosphorylation. When oxidative phosphorylation is uncoupled, completion of step one (the oxidative step involving the Krebs cycle and ETC activity) does not lead to step two (the "phosphorylation" step involving regeneration of ATP). By uncoupling these two steps, food-related toxins can severely compromise the body's energy metabolism by reducing its key source of aerobic energy, ATP.

The packaging plasticizers DEHP (di[2 ethylhexyl]phthalate) and MEHP (mono[2-ethylhexyl]phthalate) have both been shown to uncouple oxidative phosphorylation,[207] as have all of the following food-related toxins: polychlorinated biphenyls;[208] the food packaging material styrene;[209] the solvents toluene[210] and trichloroethane;[211] the pre-harvest defoliant, general herbicide, and dioxin-producing organochlorine, pentachlorophenol;[212] the fungicide 2,4,6-trichlorophenol;[213] the pesticides 2,6-dinitrophenol,[214] DDT and DDE;[215] and the widely used food preservatives BHA and BHT.[216]

Mitochondrial Disruption and Chronic Disease

Disruption of mitochondrial function by food-related toxins might represent a critical link between diet and chronic disease since compromise of mitochondrial function has been associated with several conditions that affect large cross-sections of the U.S. population. In the view of some researchers, aging itself may be viewed as having a direct relationship with oxidative stress and mitochondrial disruption since mutations in mitochondrial DNA appear to occur with increasing frequency in older individuals in association with oxidative stress.[217, 218] Oxidatively-induced mitochondrial damage has been associated with the occurrence of both Parkinson's disease and Alzheimer's disease. Excellent research reviews in this area have been published by Beal[219] and Jenner.[220]

PART VI

Toxic Impact: Summary of Concepts

The second half of this chapter uses three organizing concepts to assess the impact of food-related toxins on health. The concepts are 1) information, 2) structure, and 3) energy. Information is used as an organizing concept in order to make sense of research findings that link food toxins to genetic damage. This concept is also used to understand the ability of food toxins to change messaging across cell membranes and to alter the timing of cell death.

The concept of structure is used to understand the real-life targets of toxin-generated oxidative stress. The structures of plasma membranes, nuclear membranes, and mitochondrial membranes are viewed as structures highly susceptible to damage under conditions of oxidative stress, and food toxins are viewed as substances highly capable of creating these conditions.

The concept of energy is used primarily to understand the impact of food toxins on mitochondrial function. Like bent metal contacts in a battery charger that should press up against the ends of a battery but do not, food toxins are viewed as preventing the body's "battery charger" (the mitochondrion) from recharging the "battery" (ATP) the concept of energy is also used to help explain the ability of food toxins to interrupt messaging across cell membranes insofar as this messaging is energy-driven.

A summary of the above concepts together with examples of molecular mechanisms is presented in *Table 5-5*.

*Table 5-5. **Summary of concepts for assessing toxic impact***

Informational

Genotoxicity	Altered cell signaling	Altered cell cycles
Strand breaks	Altered signal transduction	Induction of apoptosis
Cross-linking	Adenylate cyclase disruption	Inhibition of apoptosis
Sister chromatid exchanges	Altered growth factors	Altered transcription factors
Popyploidy		

Structural/Oxidative

Membrane damage	Excessive inflammation	Imbalanced detoxification
Plasma membranes	Excessive mast cell degranulation	Excessive P450 induction
Mitochondrial membranes	Excessive activation of arachidonic acid pathways	Excessive P450 inhibition
Nuclear membranes	Excessive COX and LPX activity	Insufficient Phase II conjugation
Membrane lipids	Imbalanced eicosanoid production	GI bacterial imbalance

Energetic

Disrupted signaling	Mitochondrial energetics disruption
Disrupted ion flux	Altered membrane permeability
Second messenger imbalances	Uncoupling
Disrupted membrane transport	Disrupted electron transport
Disrupted gap junction activity	Krebs cycle imbalances

1. Murphy R and Harvey C. (1985). Residues and metabolites of selected persistent halogenated hydrocarbons in blood from a general population survey. Environ Health Perspect 60:115–120.

2. Lordo RA, Dinh KT, and Schwemberger JG. (1996). Semivolatile organic compounds in adipose tissue: estimated averages for the US population and selected subpopulations. Am J Publ Heal 86(9):1253–1259.

3. Stehr-Green PA. (19889). Demographic and seasonal influences on human serum pesticide residue levels. J Toxicol Environ Heal 27(4):405–421.

4. Hill RH, Head SL, Baker S et al. (1995). Pesticide residues in urine of adults living in the United States: reference range concentrations. Environ Res 71(2):99–108.

5. Stehr-Green PA, *op. cit. (see reference 3)*.

6. *ibid*.

7. *Ibid*.

8. Henriksen GL, Ketchum NS, Michalek JE et al. (1997). Serum dioxin and diabetes mellitus in veterans of Operation Ranch Hand. Epidem 8(3):252–258.

9. Hill RH Jr, Ashley DL, Head Sl et al. (1995). *P*-dichlorobenzene exposure among 1,000 adults in the United States. Arch Environ Health 50(4):277–280.

10. Hammand TA, Sexton M, and Langenberg P. (1996). Relationship between blood lead and dietary iron intake in preschool children. Ann Epidemiol 6(1):30–33.

11. Kim R, Landrigan C, Mossmann P et al. (1997). Age and secular trends in bone lead levels in middle-aged and elderly men: three-year longitudinal follow-up in the Normative Aging Study. Am J Epidemiol 146(7):586–591.

12. Yamamura Y, Yoshinaga Y, Arai F et al. (1994). Background levels of total mercury concentrations in blood and urine. Sangyo Igaku 36(2):66–69.

13. Chia SE, Chan OY, Sam CT et al. (1994). Blood cadmium levels in nonoccupationally exposed adult subjects in Singapore. Sci Total Environ 145(1–2):119–123.

14. Wolff MS, Anderson HA, and Selikoff IJ. (1982). Human tissue burdens of halogenated aromatic chemicals in Michigan. JAMA 247(15):2112–2116.

15. Rivero-Rodriguez L, Borja-Aburto VH, Santos-Burgoa C et al. (1997). Exposure assessment for workers applying DDT to control malaria in Veracruz, Mexico. Environ Health Perspect 105(1):98–101.

16. *Ibid*.

17. *Ibid*.

18. *Ibid*.

19. Bosse U, Bannert N, Niessen KH et al. (1996). Chlorinated carbohydrate content of fetal and pediatric organs and tissues. Zentralbl Hyg Umweltmed 198(4):331–339.

20. *Ibid*.

21. *Ibid*.

22. *Ibid*.

23. Wallace L, Pellizzari E, Hartwell T et al. (1986). Concentrations of 20 volatile organic compounds in the air and drinking water of 350 residents of New Jersey compared with concentrations in their exhaled breath. J Occup Med 28(8):603–608.

24. Hill RH Jr, Head SL, Baker S et al. (1995). Pesticide residues in urine of adults living in the United States: reference range concentrations. Environ Res 71(2):99–108.

25. *Ibid*.

26. *Ibid*.

27. *Ibid*.

28. *Ibid*.

29. *Ibid*.

30. *Ibid*.

31. Hill RH Jr, Ashley DL, Head Sl et al, *op. cit. (see reference 9)*.

32. Yamamura Y, Yoshinaga Y, Arai F et al, *op. cit. (see reference 12)*.

33. Kim R, Landrigan C, Mossmann P et al, *op. cit. (see reference 11).*

34. *Ibid.*

35. Reynolds WA, Butler V, and Lemkey-Johnston N. (1976). Hypothalamic-morphology following ingestion of aspartame or MSG in the neonatal rodent and primate: a preliminary report. J Toxicol Environ Health 2:471–480.

36. Olney JW. (1980). Excitatory neurotoxins as food additives: an evaluation of risk. Neurotoxicol 2:163–192.

37. Barnes RJ, Taylor DJ, Kemp GJ et al. (1993). Skeletal muscle bioenergetics in the chronic fatigue syndrome. J Neurol Neurosurg Psychiatr 56:679–683.

38. Dunstan RH, Donohoe M, Taylor W et al. (1995). A preliminary investigation of chlorinated hydrocarbons and chronic fatigue syndrome. Med J Austral 163:294–297.

39. Bernard A and Lauwerys R. (1986). Effects of cadmium exposure in man. In: Foulkes EC. (Ed). Cadmium toxicology. A handbook of experimental pharmacology. Springer-Verlag, New York, pp.136–177.

40. Neidert E, Saschenbrecker PW and Patterson JR. (1984). Detection and occurrence of pentachlorophenol residues in chicken liver and fat. J Environ Sci Health 19(7):579–592.

41. Wang YJ, Ho YS, Chu SW et al. (1997). Induction of glutathione depletion, p53 protein accumulation and cellular transformation by tetrachlorohydroquinone, a toxic metabolite of pentachlorophenol. Chem Biol Interact 105(1):1–16.

42. Saladino AJ, Willey JC, Lechner JF et al. (1985). Effects of formaldehyde, acetaldehyde, benzoyl peroxide, and hydrogen peroxide on cultured normal human bronchial epithelial cells. Canc Res 45(6):2522–2526.

43. Meng Z and Zhang L. (1992). Cytogenetic damage induced in human lymphocytes by sodium bisulfite. Mutat Res 298(2):63–69.

44. Brennan RJ and Schiestl RH. (1996). Cadmium is an inducer of oxidative stress in yeast. Mutat Res 356(2):171–178.

45. Bagchi D, Vuchetich PJ, Bagchi M et al. (1997). Induction of oxidative stress by chronic administration of sodium dichromate (chromium VI) and cadmium chloride (cadmium II) to rats. Free Rad Biol Med 22(3):471–478.

46. Shenker BJ, Datar S, Mansfield K et al. (1997). Induction of apoptosis in human T-cells by organomercuric compounds: a flow cytometric analysis. Toxicol Appl Pharmacol 143(2):397–406.

47. Skoczynska A. (1997). Lipid peroxidation as a toxic mode of action for lead and cadmium. Med Pr 48(2):197–203.

48. Beauparlant P and Hiscott J. (1996). Biological land biochemical inhibitors of the NF-kappa B/Rel proteins and cytokine synthesis. Cytokine Growth Factor Rev 7(2):175–190.

49. Lukiw WJ and Bazan NG. (1998). Strong nuclear factor-kappa-B-DNA binding parallels cyclooxygenase-2 gene transcription in aging and in sporadic Alzheimer's disease superior temporal lobe neocortex. J Neurosci Res 53(5):583–592.

50. Pyatt DW, Zheng JH, Stillman WS et al. (1996). Inorganic lead activates NF-kappa B in primary human CD4+ T lymphocytes. Biochem Biophys Res Commun 227(2):380–385.

51. Vogt M, Bauer MK, Ferrari D et al. (1998). Oxidative stress and hypoxia/reoxygenation trigger CD95 (APO-1/Fas) ligand expression in microglial cells. FEBS Lett 429(1):67–72.

52. Marinovich M, Viviani B, Corsini E et al. (1996). NF-kappa B activation by triphenyl triggers apoptosis in HL-60 cells. Exp Cell Res 226(1):98–104.

53. Van Ravenzwaay B and Kunz W. (1988). Quantitative aspects of accelerated nuclear polyploidization and tumour formation in dieldrin-treated CF-1 mouse liver. Br J Canc 58(1):52–56.

54. Ahmed RS, Price SC, Grasso P et al. (1990). Hepatic nuclear and cytoplasmic effects following intermittent feeding of rats with di(2-ethylhexyl)phthalate. Food Chem Toxicol 28(6):427–434.

55. Bourne HR, Sanders DA, and McCormick F. (1990). The GTPase superfamily: a conserved switch for diverse cell functions. Nature 348(6297):125–132.

56. Levitzki A and Gazit A. (1995). Tyrosine kinase inhibition: an approach to drug development. Sci 267(24 March):1782–1788.

57. Campbell J. (1982). Grammatical man. Touchstone, New York, pp.28–31.

58. Schamel WWA and Dick TP. (1996). Signal transduction: specificity of growth factors explained by parallel distributed processing. Med Hypoth 47:249–255.

59. Bagchi D, Bagchi M, Tang L et al. (1997). Comparative in vitro and in vivo protein kinase C activation by selected pesticides and transition metal salts. Toxicol Lett 91(1):31–37.

60. *Ibid*.

61. Roghani M, Da Silva C, Guvelli D et al. (1987). Benzene and toluene activate protein kinase C. Carcinogen 8(8):1105–1107.

62. Bojes HK and Thurman RG. (1994). Peroxisomal proliferators inhibit acyl CoA synthetase and stimulate protein kinase C in vivo. Toxicol Appl Pharmacol 126(2):233–239.

63. Guyton KZ, Gorospe M, Kensler TW et al. (1996). Mitogen-activated protein kinase (MAPK) activation by butylated hydroxytoluene hydroperoxide: implications for cellular survival and tumor promotion. Canc Res 56(15):3480–3485.

64. Huff RA, Corcoran JJ, Anderson JK et al. (1993). Chlorpyrifos oxon binds to neuronal muscarinic receptors and inhibits adenylate cyclase in a receptor-independent manner. Neurotoxicol 14(4):553.

65. Vodjani A, Ghoneum M, Choppa PC et al. (1997). Elevated apoptotic cell population in patients with chronic fatigue syndrome: the pivotal role of protein kinase RNA. J Int Med 242:465–478.

66. Yoo BS, Jung KH, Hana SB et al. (1997). Apoptosis-mediated immunotoxicity of polychlorinated biphenyls (PCBs) in murine splenocytes. Toxicol Lett 91(2):83–89.

67. Shenker BJ, Datar S, Mansfield K et al. (1997). Induction of apoptosis in human T-cells by organomercuric compounds: a flow cytometric analysis. Toxicol Appl Pharmacol 143(2):397–406.

68. Hamada T, Sasaguri T, Tanimoto A et al. (1996). Apoptosis of human kidney 293 cells is promoted by polymerized cadmium-metallothionein. Biochem Biophys Res Commun 219(3):829–834.

69. Kitamura K, Yoshida H, Ohno R et al. (1997). Toxic effects of arsenic (As3+) and other metal ions on acute promyelocytic leukemia cells. Int J Hematol 65(2):179–185.

70. Ku WW, Wine RN, Chae BY et al. (1995). Spermatocyte toxicity of 2-methoxyethanol (ME) in rats and guinea pigs: evidence for the induction of apoptosis. Toxicol Appl Pharmacol 134:100.

71. Swerdlow RH, Parks JK, Miller SW et al. (1996). Origin and functional consequences of the complex I defect in Parkinson's disease. Ann Neurol 40(4):663–671.

72. Zaher H, Fernandez-Salguero PM, Letterio et al. (1998). The involvement of aryl hyddrocarbon receptor in the activation of transforming growth factor-beta and apoptosis. Mol Pharmacol 54(2):313–321.

73. Gasiewicz TA. (1997). Dioxins and the Ah receptor: probes to uncover processes in neuroendocrine development. Neurotox 18(2):393–413.

74. Hippeli S and Elstner EF. (1991). Oxygen radicals and air pollution. In: Sies H. (Ed). Oxidative stress: oxidants and antioxidants. Academic Press, New York, Chapter 1, pp. 3–55.

75. Niki E, Yamamota Y, Komuro E et al. (1991). Membrane damage due to lipid oxidation. Am J Clin Nutr 53:201S–205S.

76. Beal MF. (1995). Aging, energy, and oxidative stress in neurodegenerative diseases. Ann Neurol 38:357–366.

77. Gutterdge JMC. (1995). Lipid peroxidation and antioxidants as biomarkers of tissue damage. Clin Chem 41(12):1819–1828.

78. Esterbauer H. (1996). Estimation of peroxidative damage: a review. Pathol Biol (Paris) 44(1):25–28.

79. Benzie IF. (1996). Lipid peroxidation: a review of causes, consequences, measurement, and dietary influences. Int J Food Sci Nutr 47(3):233–261.

80. Hincal F, G'urbay A, and Giray B. (1995). Induction of lipid peroxidation and alteration of glutathione redox status by endosulfan. Biol Trace Elem Res 47(1–3):321–326.

81. Takenaka T and Goto F. (1994). Alteration of lipid peroxidation and the activity of peroxide metabolism enzymes in the liver, kidney and lung following the administration of paraquat in mice. Masui 43(1):34–40.

82. Alsharif NZ, GrandJean CJ, Murray WJ et al. (1990). 2,3,7,8-tetrachorodibenzo-p-dioxin (TCDD)-induced decrease in the fluidity of rat liver membranes. Xenobiotica 20(9):979–988.

83. Cluet JL, Boisset M, and Boudene C. (1986). Effect of pretreatment with cimetidine or phenobarbitol on lipoperoxidation in carbon tetrachloride- and trichloroethylene-dosed rats. Toxicol 38(1):91–102.

84. Fraga CG, Oteiza PI, Golub MS et al. (1990). Effects of aluminum on brain lipid peroxidation. Toxicol Lett 51(2):213–219.

85. Senturk UK, Oner G, and Izgut-Uysal VM. (1994). Cadmium induced lipid peroxidation in kidney function. J Basic Clin Physiol Pharmacol 5(3–4):305–313.

86. Skoczynska A, *op. cit. (see reference 47)*.

87. Iguchi H, KoJo S, and Ikeda M. (1993). Lipid peroxidation and disintegration of the cell membrane structure in cultures of rat lung fibroblasts treated with asbestos. J Appl Toxicol 13(4):269–275.

88. Cadenas E. (1989). Biochemistry of oxygen toxicity. Ann Rev Biochem 58:79–110.

89. *Ibid*.

90. Dhalla KS, Ganguly PK, Rupp H et al. (1989). Measurement of adrenolutin as an oxidation product of catecholamines in plasma. Mol Cell Biochem 87(1):85–92.

91. Matthews SB, Henderson AH, and Campbell AK. (1985). The adrenochrome pathway: the major route for adrenalin catabolism by polymorphonuclear leucocytes. J Mol Cell Cardiol 17(4):339–348.

92. Cross CE, van der Vliet A, O'Neill CA et al. (1994). Reactive oxygen species and the lung. Lancet 344:930–933.

93. Ames BN, Shigenaga MK, and Hagen TM. (1993). Oxidants, antioxidants, and the degenerative diseases of aging. Proc Natl Acad Sci USA 90:7915–7922.

94. Rabizadeh S, Gralla EB, Borchelt DR et al. (1995). Mutations associated with amyotrophic lateral sclerosis convert superoxide dismutase from an antiapoptotic gene to a proapoptotic gene: studies in yeast and neural cells. Proc Natl Acad Sci USA 92(70:3024–3028.

95. Knekt P, Heliovaara M, Riassanen A et al. (1992). Serum antioxidant vitamins and risk of cataract. Br Med J 305:1392–1394.

96. Cerutti PA. (1994). Oxy-radicals and cancer. Lancet 344:862–863.

97. Das D, Bandyopadhyay D, Bhattacharjee M et al. (1997). Hydroxyl radical is the major causative factor in stress-induced gastric ulceration. Free Rad Biol Med 23(1):8–18.

98. Buffinton GD and Doe WF. (1995). Depleted mucosal antioxidant defences in inflammatory bowel disease. Free Rad Biol Med 19(6):911–918.

99. Singh RB, Niaz MA, Agarwal P et al. (1995). Effect of antioxidant-rich foods on plasma ascorbic acid, cardiac enzyme, and lipid peroxide levels in patients hospitalized with acute myocardial infarction. JADA 95:775–780.

100. Logroscino G, Marder K, Cote L et al. (1996). Dietary lipids and antioxidants in Parkinson's disease: a population-based, case-control study. Ann Neurol 39(1):89–94.

101. Rodgers K and Xiong S. (1997). Effect of administration of malathion for 90 days on macrophage function and mast cell degranulation. Toxicol Lett 93(1):73–82.

102. Anton P, Theodorou V, Fioramonti J et al. (1998). Low-level exposure to diquat induces a neurally mediated intestinal hypersecretion in rats: involvement of nitric oxide and mast cells. Toxicol Appl Pharmacol 152(1):77–82.

103. Laschi-Loquerie A, Descotes J, Tachon P et al. (1984). Influence of lead acetate on hypersensitivity. J Immunopharmacol 6(1–2):87–93.

104. Huang J, Wang X-P, Chen B-M et al. (1991). Immunological effects of toluene diisocyanate exposure on painters. Arch Environ Contamin Toxicol 21(4):607–611.

105. Singer II, Kawka DW, Schloemann S et al. (1998). Cyclooxygenase 2 is induced in colonic epithelial cells in inflammatory bowel disease. Gastroenterol 115(2):297–306.

106. Shigeta J, Takahashi S, and Okabe S. (1998). Role of cyclooxygenase-2 in the healing of gastric ulcers in rats. J Pharmacol Exp Ther 286(3):1383–1390.

107. Iniguez MA, Pablos JL, Carreira PE et al. (1998). Detection of COX-1 and COX-2 isoforms in synovial fluid cells from inflammatory joint diseases. Br J Rheumatol 37(7):773–778.

108. Lukiw WJ and Bazan NG, *op. cit. (see reference 49)*.

109. Sousa A, Pfister R, Christie PE et al. (1997). Enhanced expression of cyclooxygenase isozyme 2 (COX-2) in asthmatic airways and its cellular distribution in aspirin-sensitive asthma. Thorax 52(11):940-945.

110. McNally AK, Chisolm GM 3rd, Morel DW et al. (1990). Activated human monocytes oxidize low-density lipoprotein by a lipoxygenase-dependent pathway. J Immunol 145(1):254-259.

111. Asano M and Okuda Y. (1997). Abnormal arachidonate metabolites in diabetes mellitus. Nippon Rinsho 55(Suppl):705–710.

112. Krug HF, Hamm U, and Berndt J. (1988). Mechanism of inhibition of cyclo-oxygenase in human blood platelets by carbamate insecticides. Biochem J 250(1):103–110.

113. Lawrence BP and Kerkvliet NI. (1998). Role of altered arachidonic acid metabolism in 2,3,7,8-tetrachlorodibenzo-p-dioxin-induced immune suppression in C57Bl/6 mice. Toxicol Sci 42(1):13–22.

114. Metz SA. (1987). Lipoxygenase inhibitors reduce insulin secretoin without impairing calcium mobilization. Endocrinol 120(6):2534–2546.

115. Ledwith BJ, Pauley CJ, Wagner LK et al. (1997). Induction of cyclooxygenase-2 expression by peroxisome proliferators and non-tetradecanoylphorbol 12,13-myristate-type tumor promoters in immortalized mouse liver cells. J Biol Chem 272(6):3707–3714.

116. Wislocki PG, Miva GT, and Lu AYH. (1980). Reactions catalyzed by the cytochrome P450 system. In: Jakoby WB (Ed). Enzymatic basis of detoxication. Vol. 1. Academic Press, New York.

117. Halpert JR, Guengerich FP, Bend JR et al. (1994). Contemporary issues in toxicology. Selective inhibitors of cytochromes P450. Toxicol Appl Pharmacol 125:163–175.

118. Nelson DR, Kamataki T, Waxman DJ et al. (1993). The P450 superfamily: update on new sequences, gene mapping, accession numbers, early trivial names of enzymes, and nomenclature. DNA Cell Biol 12:1–51.

119. Earl-Salotti GL and Charland SL. (1994). The effect of parenteral nutrition on hepatic cytochrome P-450. JPEN 18:458–465.

120. Raucy JL, Lasker JM, Liever CS et al. (1989). Acetaminophen activation by human liver cytochromes P450IIE1 and P450IA2. Arch Biochem Biophys 271:270–283.

121. Nakajima T and Wang RS. (1994). Induction of cytochrome P450 by toluene. Int J Biochem 26(12):1333–1340.

122. Olson JR. (1994). Hepatic uptake and metabolism of 2,3,7,8-tetrachlorodibenzo-*p*-dioxin and 2,3,7,8-tetrachlorodibenzofuran. Fund Appl Toxicol 22:631-640.

123. Butler MA, Iwasaki M, Guengerich FP et al. (1989). Human cytochrome P-450PA (P450IA2), the phenacetin o-deethylase, is primarily responsible for the hepatic 3-demethylation of caffeine and N-oxidation of carcinogenic arylamines. Proc Nat Acad Sci USA 86:7696–7700.

124. Keyon EM, Kraichely RE, Hudson KT et al. (1996). Differences in rates of benzene metabolism correlate with observed genotoxicity. Toxicol Appl Pharmacol 136(1):49–56.

125. Guengerich FP. (1994). Metabolism and genotoxicity of dihaloalkanes. Adv Pharmacol 27:211–236.

126. Vezina M, Kobusch AB, du Souich P et al. (1990). Potentiation of chloroform-induced hepatotoxicity by methyl isobutyl ketone and two metabolites. Can J Physiol Pharmacol 68(8):1055–1061.

127. Levin W et al. (1982). Oxidative metabolism of polycyclic aromatic hydrocarbons to ultimate carcinogens. Drug Metab Rev 13:555–580.

128. Dalvi RR and Mutinga ML. (1990). Comparative studies of the effects of liver and liver microsomal drug-metabolizing enzyme system by the fungicides captan, captafol, and folpet in rats. Pharmacol Toxicol 66:231–233.

129. Shukla Y, Baqar SM, and Mehrotra NK. (1996). Carcinogenic and co-carcinogenic studies of thiram on mouse skin. Food Chem Toxicol 34:283–289.

130. Borin C, Periquet A, and Mitjavila S. (1985). Studies on the mechanism of nabam- and zineb-induced inhibition of the hepatic microsomal monooxygenases of the male rat. Toxicol Appl Pharmacol 81:460–468.

131. Butler AM and Murray M. (1993). Inhibition and inactivation of constitutive cytochromes P-450 in the rat liver by parathion. Mol Pharmacol 43:902–908.

132. Stott I, Murthy A, Robinson A et al. (1997). Low-dose diethyldithiocarbamate attenuates the hepatotoxicity of 1,3-dichloro-2-propanol and selectively inhibits CYP2E1 activity in the rat. Hum Exper Toxicol 16(5):262–266.

133. Casazza JP, Felver ME, and Veech RL. (1984). The metabolism of acetone in the rat. J Biol Chem 259:231–236.

134. Albores A, Sinal CJ, Cherian MG et al. (1995). Selective increase of rat lung cytochrome P450 1A1 dependent monooxygenase activity after acute sodium arsenite administration. Can J Physiol Pharmacol 73(1):153–158.

135. Keyon EM, Kraichely RE, Hudson KT et al, *op. cit (see reference 124).*

136. Zheng J and Hanzlik RP. (1992). Bromo(monohydroxyl)phenyl mercapturic acids: a new class of mercapturic acids from bromobenzene-treated rats. Drug Metabol Dispos 20:688-694.

137. Guengerich FP and Shimada T. (1992). Human cytochrome P450 enzymes and chemical carcinogenesis. Chapter 2. In: Jeffrey EH. (Ed). Human drug metabolism from molecular biology to man. CRC Press, Boca Raton, pp.5–12.

138. Guengerich FP, *op. cit. (see reference 125).*

139. Cheever KL, Cholkis JM, el-Hawari AM et al. (1990). Ethylene dichloride: the influence of disulfiram or ethanol on oncogenicity, metabolism and DNA covalent binding in rats. Fund Appl Toxicol 14(2):243–261.

140. Lapadula DM. (1991). Induction of cytochrome P450 isozymes by simultaneous inhalation exposure of hens to *n*-hexane and methyl iso-butyl ketone (MiBK). Biochem Pharmacol 41(6–7):877–883.

141. Kocarek TA. (1991). Selective induction of cytochrome P450e by kepone (chlordecone) in primary cultures of adult rat hepatocytes. Mol Pharmacol 40(2):203–210.

142. Stresser DM and Kupfer D. (1997). Catalytic characteristics of CYP3A4: requirement for a phenolic function in ortho hydroxylation of estradiol and mono-O-demethylated methoxychlor. Biochem 36(8):2203–2210.

143. Vezina M, Kobusch AB, du Souich P et al, *op. cit. (see reference 126).*

144. Hogan GK, Smith RG, and Cornish HH. (1976). Studies on the microsomal conversion of dichloromethane to carbon monoxide. Toxicol Appl Pharmacol 37:112–119.

145. Madra S and Smith AG. (1992). Induction of cytochrome P450 activities by polychlorinated biphenyls in isolated mouse hepatocytes. Influence of Ah-phenotype and iron. Biochem Pharmacol 44(3):455–464.

146. Ross PH, van Afferden M, Strotkamp D et al. (1996). Liver microsomal levels of cytochrome P450IA1 as a biomarker for exposure and bioavailability of soil-bound polycyclic aromatic hydrocarbons. Arch Environ Contam Toxicol 30(1):107–113.

147. Guengerich FP and Shimada T, *op. cit. (see reference 137)*.

148. Nakajima T and Wang RS. (1994). Induction of cytochrome P450 by toluene. Int J Biochem 26(12):133301340.

149. Guengerich FP and Shimada T, *op. cit. (see reference 137)*.

150. Ungv·ry G. (1990). The effect of xylene exposure on the liver. Acta Morphol Hungar 38:245–258.

151. Coughtrie MWH. (1996). Sulphation catalysed by the human cytosolic sulphotransferases—chemical defense or molecular terrorism? Hum Exper Toxocol 15:547–555.

152. Maziasz TJ, Liu J, Madhu C et al. (1991). The differential effects of hepatotoxicants on the sulfation pathway in rats. Toxicol Appl Pharmacol 110(3):365–373.

153. Boles JW and Klaassen CD. (1998). Effects of molybdate and pentachlorophenol on the sulfation of dehydroepiandrosterone. Toxicol Appl Pharmacol 151(1):105–109.

154. Sumner SCJ, Stedman DB, Clarke DO et al. (1992). Characterization of urinary metabolites from (1,2 methoxy-13C)-2-methoxyethanol in mice using 13C nuclear magnetic resonance spectroscopy. Chem Res Toxicol 5(4):553–560.

155. Hobkirk R. (1993). Steroid sulfation—current concepts. Trends Endocrinol Metab 4:69–74.

156. Barker EV, Hume R, Hallas A et al. (1994). Dehydroepiandrosterone sulfotransferase in the developing human fetus—qualitative biochemical and immunological characterization of the hepatic, renal, and adrenal enzymes. Endocrinol 134:982–989.

157. Ketterer B and Christoulides LG. (1994). Enzymolotgy of cytosolic glutathione S-transferases. Part I. In: Anders MW and Dekant W. Advances in pharmacology. Vol. 27. Conjugation-dependent carcinogenicity and toxicity of foreign compounds. Academic Press, San Diego.

158. Mori K. (1989). Testicular toxicity and alterations of glutathoine metabolism resulting from chronic inhalation of ethylene oxide in rats. Toxicol Appl Pharmacol 101:299–309.

159. Danovik DA and Bailer AJ. (1994). The impact of exercise and inter-subject variability on dose estimates for dichloromethane derived from a physiologically based pharmacokinetic model. Fundam Appl Toxicol 22:20–25.

160. Davenport CJ. (1992). Effects of methyl bromide on regional brain glutathoine, glutathione S-transferase, monoamines and amino acids in F3344 rats. Toxicol Appl Toxicol 112:120–127.

161. Guengerich FP. (1995). Conjugation of carcinogens by theta class glutathione S-transferases: mechanisms and relevance to variations in human risk. Pharmacogenetics 5:S103–107.

162. Anonymous. (1994). Styrene-7,7-oxide. IARC monographs on the evaluation of the carcinogenic risks of chemical to humans 60:321–346.

163. Hiratsuka A, Yokoi A, Iwata H et al. (1989). Glutathione conjugation of styrene 7,8-oxide enantiomers by major glutathione transferase isoenzymes isolated from rat livers. Biochem Pharmacol 38(24):4405–4414.

164. Radulovic LL, LaFerla JJ and Kulkarni AP. (1986). Human placental glutathione S-transferase-mediated metabolism of methyl parathion. Biochem Pharmacol 35(20):3473–3480.

165. Kao C-H and Sun C-N. (1991). In vitro degradation of some organophosphorus insecticides by susceptible and resistant diamondback moth. Pesticid Biochem Physiol 41(2):132–141.

166. Salim AR. (1992). Role of oxygen-derived free radical scavengers in the management of recurrent attacks of ulcerative colitis. J Lab Clin Med 119:740–747.

167. Lailey AF. (1997). Oral N-acetylcysteine protects against perfluoroisobutene toxicity in rats. Hum Exp Toxicol 16:212–216.

168. Hitomi Y and Yoshida A. (1991). Effects of supplementing methionine and threonine to a non-protein diet on the induction of enzymes by polychlorinated biphenyls in rats. Agric Biol Chem 55(1):7–12.

169. You JS and Chang KJ. (1998). Taurine protects the liver against lipid peroxidation and membrane disintegration during rat hepatocarcinogenesis. Adv Exp Med Biol 442:105–112.

170. Lee PT, Hsu AY, Ha HT et al. (1997). A C-methyltransferase involved in both ubiquinone and menaquinone biosynthesis: isolation and identification of the *Escherichia coli* ubiE gene. J Bacteriol 179(5):1748–1754.

171. Gottwald MD, Bainbridge JL, Dowling GA et al. (1997). New pharmacotherapy for Parkinson's disease. Ann Pharmacother 31(10):1205–1217.

172. Martin C. (1985). Endocrine physiology. Oxford University Press, New York, pp.854–860.

173. Hopenhayn-Rich C, Biggs ML, Kalman DA et al. (1996). Arsenic methylation patterns before and after changing from high to lower concentrations of arsenic in drinking water. Environ Health Perspect 104:1200–1207.

174. Varela-Moreiras G, Alonso-Aperte E, Rubio M et al. (1995). Carbon tetrachloride-induced hepatic injury is associated with global DNA hypomethylation and homocysteinemia: effect of S-adenosylmethionine treatment. Hepatol 22(4Pt. 1):1310–1315.

175. Aposhian HV. (1983). DMSA and DMPS—water soluble antidotes for heavy metal poisoning. Ann Rev Pharmacol Toxicol 23:193–215.

176. Paredes SR, Kozicki PA, and Batlle AM. (1985). S-adenosyl-L-methionine a counter to lead intoxication? Comp Biochem Physiol [B] 82(4):751–757.

177. Ayala FJ and Kiger JA Jr. (1984). Modern genetics. Second edition. Benjamin Cummings, Menlo Park, California, pp.515–518.

178. West RL, Lee JM and Maroun LE. (1995). Hypomethylation of the amyloid precursor gene in the brain of an Alzheimer's disease patient. J Mol Neurosci 6(2):141–146.

179. Smythies JR. (1997). Oxidative reactions and schizophrenia:a review-discussion. Schizophr Res 24(3):357–364.

180. West RL, Lee JM and Maroun LE, *op. cit. (see reference 178).*

181. Hoffman RM. (1997). Methionase: a therapeutic for diseases related to altered methionine metabolism and transmethylation: cancer, heart disease, obesity, aging, and Parkinson's disease. Hum Cell 10(1):69–80.

182. Bottiglieri T. (1996). Folate, vitamin B12, and neuropsychiatric disorders. Nutr Revs 54(12):382–390.

183. Laird PW. (1997). Oncogenic mechanisms mediated by DNA methylation. Mol Med Today May: 223–228.

184. Siegers CP, Riemann D, Thies E et al. (1988). Glutathione and GSH-dependent enzymes in the gastrointestinal mucosa of the rat. Canc Lett 40:71–76.

185. Hanninen O, Aitio A, and Hartiala K. (1968). Gastrointestinal distribution of glucuronide synthesis and the relevant enzymes in the rat. Scand J Gastroent 3:461–464.

186. Schwenk M. (1989). Glucuronidation and sulfation in the gastrointestinal tract. In: Eichelbaum FM, Forth W, Meyer U et al. (Eds). Progress in Pharmacology and Clinical Pharmacology Vol. 7/2, Intestinal Metabolism of Xenobiotics. VCH Publishers, Deerfield Beach, Florida, 155–169.

187. Autrup H, Harris CC, Wu S-M, et al. (1984). Activation of chemical carcinogens by cultured human fetal liver, esophagus, and stomach. Chem-Biol. Interact 50:15–25.

188. Autrup H. 1982. Carcinogen metabolism in human tissues and cells. Drug Metabol Revs 13:603–646.

189. Laitinen M and Watkins JB. (1986). Mucosal biotransformations. In: Rozman K and Hanninen O. (Eds). Gastrointestinal Toxicology. Elsevier, Amsterdam, 412–434.

190. Fourage M, Mercier M, and Poncelet F. (1982). Mutagenicity of 3 aromatic amines in the presence of fractions from various tissues. Toxicol Lett 11:313–320.

191. Walters JW and Combes RD. (1986). Activation of benzo(a)pyrene and aflatoxin B1 to mutagenic chemical species by microsomal preparations from rat liver and small intestine in relation to microsomal epoxide hydrolase. Mutagen 1:45–48.

192. Siegers CP, Riemann D, Thies E et al. (1988). Glutathione and GSH-dependent enzymes in the gastrointestinal mucosa of the rat. Canc Lett 40:71–76.

193. Hanninen O, Aitio A, and Hartiala K. (1968). Gastrointestinal distribution of glucuronide synthesis and the relevant enzymes in the rat. Scand J Gastroent 3:461–464.

194. Siegers CP, Riemann D, Thies E et al, *op. cit. (see reference 192).*

195. Cappiello M, Giuliani L, and Pacifici GM. (1990). Differential distribution of phenol and catechol sulphotransferases in human liver and intestinal mucosa. Pharmacol 40:69–76.

196. Chhabra RS and Fouts JR. (1976). Biochemical properties of some microsomal xenobiotic-metabolizing enzymes in rabbit small intestine. Drug Metabol Desposit 4:208–214.

197. Koster AS, Frankhuizen-Sierevogel AC, and Noordhoek J. (1985). Distribution of glucuronidation capacity (1-naphtol and morphine) along the rat intestine. Biochem Pharmacol 34:3527–3532.

198. Drasar BS and Hill MJ. (1972). Intestinal bacteria and cancer. Am J Clin Nutr 25:1399–1404.

199. Hentges DJ, Maier BR, Burton GC et al. (1977). Effect of a high-beef diet on the fecal bacterial flora of humans. Canc Res 37:568–571.

200. Chadwick RW, George SE, and Claxton LD. (1992). Role of the gastrointestinal mucosa and microflora in the bioactivation of dietary and environmental mutagens or carcinogens. Drug Metab Revs 24(4):425–492.

201. Reed DJ. (1996). Oxidative stress and mitochondrial permeability transition. Chapter 11 in: Packer L and Cadenas E. (Eds). Biothiols in health and disease. Marcel Dekker, New York, pp. 231–263.

202. Solieau SD and Moreland DE. (1983). Effects of chlordecone and its alteration products on isolated rat liver mitochondria. Toxicol Appl Pharmacol 67(1):89–99.

203. Melnick RL and Schiller CM. (1985). Effect of phthalate esters on energy coupling and succinate oxidation in rat liver mitochondria. Toxicol 34(1):13–27.

204. Lund BO, Miller DM, and Woods JS. (1993). Studies on Hg(II)-induced H2O2 formation and oxidative stress *in vivo* and *in vitro* in rat kidney mitochondria. Biochem Pharmacol 45(10):2017–2024.

205. *Ibid.*

206. Trottman CH, Prasada Rao KS, Morrow W et al. (1985). In vitro effects of toxaphene on mitochondrial calcium ATPase and calcium uptake in selected rat tissues. Life Sci 36(5):427–433.

207. Melnick RL and Schiller CM, *op. cit. (see reference 203).*

208. Ebner KV and Braselton WE Jr. (1987). Structural and chemical requirement for hydroxychlorobiphenyls to uncouple rat liver mitochondria and potentiation of uncoupling with aroclor 1254. Chem Biol Interact 63(2):139–155.

209. Mickiewicz W and Rzeczycki W. (1988). Effect of styrene and other alkyl benzene derivatives on oxidation of FAD- and NAD-linked substrates in rat liver mitochondria. Biochem Pharmacol 37(23):4439–4444.

210. *Ibid.*

211. Takano T, Miyaka Y, and Motohashi Y. (1985). An uncoupling effect of 111 trichloroethane on the mixed-function oxidase system in rat liver. J Toxicol Sci 10(3):249.

212. Narasimhan TR, Mayura K, Clement BA et al. (1992). Effects of chlorinated phenols on rat embryonic and hepatic mitochondrial oxidative phosphorylation. Environ Toxicol Chem 11(6):805–814.

213. Escher BI, Snozzi M, Habrli K et al. (1997). A new method for simultaneous quantification of uncoupling and inhibitory activity of organic pollutants in energy-transducing membranes. Environ Toxicol Chem 16(3):405–414.

214. *Ibid.*

215. Ferreira FML, Madeira VMC, and Moreno AJ. (1997). Interactions of 2,2-bis (*p*-chlorophenyl)-1,1-dichloroethylene with mitochondrial oxidative phosphorylation. Biochem Pharmacol 53(3):299–208.

216. Fusi F, Valoti M, Sgargli G et al. (1991). The interaction of antioxidants and structurally related compounds with mitochondrial oxidative phosphorylation. Meth Find Exp Clin Pharmacol 13(9):599–604.

217. Cortopassi GI and Arnheim N. (1990). Detection of a specific mitochondrial DNA deletion in the tissues of older humans. Nucleic Acids Res 18:6927–6933.

218. Munscger C, Muller-Hocker J, and Kadenback B. (1993). The point mutation of mitochondrial DNA characteristic for MERRF disease is also found in healthy people of different ages. FEBS Lett 317:27–30.

219. Beal MF. (1995). Aging, energy, and oxidative stress in neurodegenerative diseases. Ann Neurol 38:357–366.

220. Jenner P. (1994). Oxidative damage in neurodegenerative disease. Lancet 344 (Sept 17):796–798.

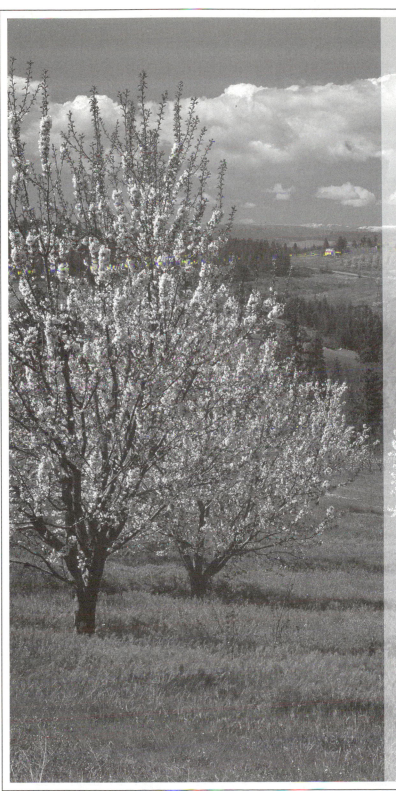

The Challenge
of Food Toxicity

CONTENTS

Chapter 6: **The Challenge of Food Toxicity**

The Challenge
of Food Toxicity

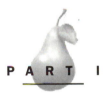

P A R T I

Taking Stock of Current Resources

This text has attempted to document the presence of non-naturally occurring toxins in the U.S. food supply and to review the molecular mechanisms through which these toxins compromise health. Although briefly mentioned at various junctures within the text, the tasks faced by clinicians in responding to food toxicity (both clinically and ecologically) have not been addressed.

Clinical Resources

Within the clinical arena, resources for dealing with the impact of food-related toxins are readily accessible to the vast majority of clinicians. Clinical ecology, environmental medicine, and industrial toxicology have all evolved as specialty areas in which clinical training is available. Clinicians working in these areas have pioneered laboratory assessment techniques and treatment protocols specifically designed to address toxic exposure. Toxicity assessment based on blood, urine, stool, hair or breath samples is offered by laboratories on a nationwide basis, and testing has evolved to include identification of toxin-specific antibodies or polymerase chain reaction (PCR)-based assay to assess disruption of gene expression. Treatment protocols for toxicity are also available on a continuing education basis by professional organizations like the American Association for Environmental Medicine (AAEM).

Policy-Related Resources

The widespread availability of clinical resources for dealing with food-related toxicity stands in stark contrast, however, to the virtual non-existence of resources available for addressing toxicity at the level of the nationalized food supply. Specific individuals, like Dr. Joan Dye Gussow (Mary Swartz Rose Professor Emeritus at Teacher's College, Columbia University, New York) and Frances Moore Lappé (co-founder of Food First: The Institute for Food and Development Policy in San Francisco) have done lifelong pioneering work in this area, and organizations like EarthSave (Santa Cruz, California), the Environmental Research Foundation (Annapolis, Maryland), and the Pesticide Action Network of North America (San Francisco, California) have worked to promote ecological awareness in relation to the food supply. Notwithstanding these efforts, however, there remains no practical framework for effecting improvement in the food supply through adoption of ecologically-based practices.

Reasons for Policy-Related Inactivity

The lack of a framework for addressing toxicity at the food supply level may be related to many different factors. For some practitioners, direct involvement in the political arena may seem unprofessional or simply unrelated to the focus of their work. For other practitioners, improvement of food supply dynamics may be a goal, but one that has no clear avenues of approach.

Lack of knowledge may also be a factor in the failure to establish a framework in which toxicity of the food supply can be addressed. In this final section of the text we will focus on three areas in which the lack of practitioner knowledge may be partly responsible for policy-related inactivity. These three areas are: 1) actual dynamics of the food supply and identification of participants in the process; 2) medical philosophies used to assess impact of food-related toxins; and 3) relationships between biogeochemical cycles and nutrition.

PART II

Dynamics of the U.S. Food Supply

Economic Aspects

Gross Revenues

Depending upon the economic indicator chosen as a point of reference, the U.S. food supply can be viewed as the one of the most successful components of the U.S. economy. In 1997, the food industry (including food producers, food and food/drug stores, and food services) brought in over $435 billion dollars in total revenues, and ranked 11th among all sectors of the economy.[1] This ranking based on total revenues placed the food sector above numerous other industrial sectors, including insurance, aerospace, and pharmaceuticals. If the beverage sector (including alcoholic beverages) had been added to the food sector, combined food and beverage sector revenues would have surpassed $500 billion and brought in more revenue than the largest industrial sector (motor vehicle and parts).[2]

Rates of Return

Other economic indicators placed the food sector on equally successful footing. When return on equity or return on assets were used as indicators, beverages ranked fourth and food seventh among all industrial sectors.[3] Food ranked in the top thirty and beverages in the top ten industrial sectors when ranked according to return on revenues.[4] Based on revenues per employee, food ranked 21st among all sectors.[5]

Total Domestic Expenditure

Services required for maintenance of the food supply, including transportation, shipping, and importing of goods also add to the magnitude of food-related expenses. The total for these expenses surpassed the $700 billion dollar level for the first time in 1997, with the domestic portion of these expenses (including agricultural and transportation costs) accounting for approximately two thirds of the total.[6] This domestic food expenditure also represented about 8.5% of a $5.19 trillion-dollar GNP (gross national product) in 1997.[7]

Like total food-related expenses, direct purchase of foods by consumers also fell into the $500 billion dollar range. In 1997, U.S. consumers spent $561 billion dollars on domestically-produced foods,[8] representing a per capita expenditure of approximately $2,250.

Political Aspects

Farming Operations

In contrast to the success of the food sector within the total U.S. economy was the lack of success among individuals and corporations inside the food sector itself. At the most basic level of participation, i.e., farming and live-stock husbandry, diminishing participation and difficulty of success were reflected in a variety of statistics. Approximately 400,000 U.S. farms stopped production between the years 1982 and 1997,[9] and among the 2 million farms that survived, income and acreage discrepancies increased. Over 61% of the surviving farms (almost 1,250,000 farms, with the term "farm" defined as any establishment from which $1,000 or more of agricultural products was sold or would normally have been sold during the year) reported gross sales of less than $20,000 in 1997. These same 1,250,000 farms operated only 16.9% of the total farmed acreage.[10] In contrast, the top 3% of all surviving farms (approximately 60,000 farms, each having a min-imum gross sales of $500,000 or more) operated an almost identical percent of acreage (16.5%).[11]

Factory Operations

Successful participation in the food sector was as difficult on the factory side as it was on the side of farming. In 1997, among several thousand total food-related companies, the gross sales of only 36 companies accounted for more than one third of all dollars spent by consumers on domestically-produced food. [12] (The top 36 revenue producers grossed $205 billion in 1997, and consumers spent $561 billion). The top ten food industry participants also brought in more revenues than the next twenty five par-ticipants combined.

Philosophical Aspects

The previously-described economic and political aspects of the food supply reveal a basic dichotomy. When looking at economic performance within the economy as a whole, the food sector appeared stable and successful.

However, when looking at the individual experience of farmers and manufacturers within the food sector, the food supply appeared less stable and less well-situated for long-term success.

This dichotomy within the food supply can also be viewed from a philosophical perspective. In this section of the text, we will look at the experience of farmers, manufacturers, and consumers from a philosophical perspective and try to make conceptual connections between economic and political aspects of the food supply.

Food as a Commodity: The Example of Beef

On a per capita basis, 192 pounds of beef were eaten by U.S. adults in 1997.[13] For each consumer eating his or her 192 pounds, this beef was likely to have been recognized as a specific type of food, and the cow from which it came as a specific kind of animal. From a philosophical perspective, consumers did not have to think about their basic concept of cows in order to purchase or consume the beef.

In contrast to this beef consumer's perspective was the perspective of beef manufacturers. Instead of viewing the cow as a specific form of animal, successful beef production in 1997 required the cow to be envisioned as a random and potentially limitless assortment of commodities. Economic success in beef manufacturing meant conceptualization of the cow's skin as a source of shoes, luggage, and wallets. The ear hair had to be viewed as art brushes. The hair on the rest of the body had to treated as upholstery, drum heads, and violin strings. The bones had to be viewed as knife handles. The hooves had to seen as sources of gelatin and photographic film, and the hide-and-hoof combination as a source of glue, plywood, and matches. Organs and glands had to be treated as suppliers of cortisone, insulin, corticotropic hormone, asphalt binders, and chemicals allowing tires to run cooler. Fats had to be regarded as the stearin found in chewing gum, candies, and soaps. With all of these products combined, the cow (1,000 pounds) found itself divided virtually in half, with 36% of its weight (358 pounds) representing random commodities, and 43% (432 pounds) representing edible beef cuts.

Beyond Efficient Use of Resources

From one vantage point, the commodity concept of food makes perfect sense. Efficient use of resources has always been a hallmark of successful civilizations, and the U.S. food industry was not the first enterprise to develop innovative uses for animal parts. Implements made from bones have been found in hundreds of cultural archives dating back thousands of years. But two features serve to separate these eternal traditions from U.S. food supply dynamics: 1) the invisibility of origins within final food products, and 2) removal of the conversion process from the public life.

Invisibility of Origins. When looking at cultural artifacts from previous civilizations, it has almost always been possible to recognize the origins of artifacts in their look, texture, shape, and imperfections. Striations and inconsistencies in the skins of animals used for canoe siding or percussion instruments have almost always been visible to the eye and have retained the capacity to remind observers of their source.

No such recognition of origins has taken place in the final appearance of U.S. food products. Within the national food supply, dismantling of food has made food origins virtually invisible. Consumers of General Foods Jell-O™ Brand Cherry Flavored Gelatin have not been able to recognize its origins in "the hides of animals prepared for slaughter"[14] (gelatin) or coal tar (artificial coloring). When chewing Wrigley's Hubba Bubba™ Original Flavor Bubble Gum, consumers have not been able to detect the presence of coal tar (used as a source of cresol required for synthesis of the antioxidant preservative BHT, and also as a source of color). Nor have they been able to recognize the sweetness of the gum as having originated in a sulfuric acid and bacterially-derived enzyme bath used to hydrolyze glycosides in corn starch and produce an extremely low-cost sweetener (corn syrup). Unlike cultural implements carved from bone which reveal their origins through color, texture, shape, and imperfections, jello and bubble gum have successfully hidden these origins from consumers.

De-Publicizing of Food Production Processes. The final appearance of food products is not the only place where origins have been hidden from consumers. Origins have also been hidden by a de-publicizing of food production processes. Ironically, at a time when consumers have been described as having increased awareness of diet and nutrition, they also appear to have been increasingly removed from the food supply process itself. For example, according to a 1997 American Dietetic Association Survey, 39% of U.S. adults said they were doing all they could to achieve a healthful diet; 51% liked to hear about new dietary research; 67% were aware of the Food Guide Pyramid; and 69% said they altered food purchases based on labels.[15] Cumulatively, these response levels suggested widespread awareness of diet-related issues.

At the same time, however, a small national survey (n=715) measuring consumer attitudes toward food and environment found that only half of all respondents described themselves as knowledgeable about foods.[16] In addition, one out of every five respondents agreed that "as long as you stick to a familiar brand, there can't be much wrong with it."[17] This self-described lack of knowledge and lack of deliberate inquiry on the part of consumers was also reflected in a small market research study involving the cosmetic appearance of oranges. In the initial phase of the study, eight out ten subjects in the study expressed an unwillingness to purchase oranges with substantial surface scarring and imperfections. During phase two, after being made aware of the inverse relationship between pesticide use and degree of scarring, subjects expressed a willingness to reconsider their position. Having been made aware of the role of pesticides in production of non-scarred and unblemished fruit, almost two thirds of the subjects expressed a willingness to purchase the substantially scarred and blemished fruit.[18]

Production processes that dismantle food have never been conducted in public view. For example, General Foods has never publicized the animal hide origin of its jello, presumably due to risk of consumer alienation from the product. Similarly, consumers of Premium Quality Maraschino Cherries (S & W Fine Foods, San Ramon, California) cannot tell that the cherries were originally golden brown, and the National Cherry Growers and Industries Foundation (Seattle, Washington) has predicted that a substantial loss in sales would result from removal of the erythrosine (Food, Dye & Coloring Red No. 3) in cherries. But the obscuring of food conversion processes from the general public has also taken place for other reasons, including business reasons related to legality and patents.

Many of the processes used to convert food into shelvable products are proprietary and patented. General Mills, for example, the $6 billion dollar multi-national based in Minneapolis, Minnesota that merged with Nestlé in 1989 owns a patent on the use of juice vesicle solids in cake mix. Ralston Purina, the St. Louis, Missouri-based company and producer of Chex™ cereals, Chicken of the Sea™ brand tuna, Wonder™ Bread, and Hostess™ snack cakes, owns a patent on the use of soy protein isolates for use in creme fillings.

Also contributing to the proprietary nature of the food supply process are alliances between food producers and other types of manufacturers who rely on patents and proprietary information. The most common of these alliances are formed with the pharmaceutical and chemical manufacturers. Representatives from Abbot, American Cyanamid, Burroughs, Merck, SmithKline Beckman, Warner-Lambert, and other pharmaceuticals sit on the boards of directors of numerous food companies, and pharmaceuticals almost universally own patents related to food production. Merck, for example, the Whitehouse Station, New York-based pharmaceutical and 46th largest corporation in the U.S. according to the 1998 Fortune 500, owns patents on components used in soft-serve yogurt, containerized yogurt, cake icings, jelly confectionary products, yeast doughs, tapioca pudding, and milk shakes.

Non-Food Orientation of Food Companies: The Example of Borden

The dismantling of food into a random collection of commodities has its parallel in the restructuring of food companies into companies with no recognizable food focus. The history of Borden, Inc. provides a classic example of this restructuring process.

In 1857, when Gail Borden created the Borden company and Eagle Brand™ Sweetened Condensed Milk, the company was focused on manufacturing of a single product readily identifiable as food. The Borden logo, "Elsie the Cow," became a widely-recognized feature of its sweetened condensed milk. The food product only contained two ingredients: whole milk and sugar.

The history of Borden, however, has reflected a continual dismantling of its food basis and restructuring of the company in a way that has made it less and less recognizable as a food sector participant. In route to its 1995 stature as a multi-billion dollar company, Borden was able to take increasing control of business components required for production of its premiere condensed milk product. For example, the importance of grains required for cattle feed offered the opportunity for creation of a grain-based pasta subdivision that began to manufacture 17 different brand-labeled pastas. (Creamette™ became the best recognized). The cattle's hooves and hides invited interest in the manufacture of glue, and Borden's soon launched it's Elmer's™ consumer adhesives subdivision (which also went on to produce Mystik™ tape). Knowledge of adhesives at the consumer level eventually led to the creation of Borden Chemicals and Plastics (BCP), formed as a limited partnership to advance product potential in the area of industrial adhesives. Over time, the BCP division developed three principle product groupings of its own: polyvinyl chloride (PVC) polymer products, methanol and methanol derivatives, and nitrogen products. Industrial adhesives, coatings, and resins (including wall coverings, siding, and vinyl films) became a primary product line. In addition, BCP also formed a subsidiary, Melamine Chemical, to expand its involvement in industrial adhesives through the production of melamine-based products.

In 1995 the Borden company went private by means of a leveraged buyout. Officials of the holding company Kohlberg, Kravis, Roberts and Company (KKR) acquired 100% of Borden stock in exchange for KKR's shares in another corporation, RJR Nabisco. By 1997, with total revenues of $5.7 billion dollars, and a net profit of $82 million, Borden chose to sell its original start-up division, dairy products, to Southern Foods and Milk Products, thus removing it from the dairy business altogether. In 1998, part of the BCP wall-covering and vinyl film business was also sold to Blackstone Partners, a corporate buyout firm.

Following its buyout by KKR in 1995, Borden's was also assigned the task of managing Corning Consumer Products, a company owned by KKR and well-known for its three main lines of consumer kitchenware products, namely, Pyrex™, Corelle™, and Corning™.

By 1997, a company that had entered the food sector with an identity based on Elsie the Cow and Eagle Brand™ Sweetened Condensed Milk no longer participated in the dairy business and produced the majority of its revenue from the sale of products unrelated to food. Like the dismantling of food into random collections of commodities, the fragmentation of corporate identities within the food sector attests to the foundation of cultural forgetfulness upon which our current food practices rest.

The multiple involvements of corporations like Borden's in manufacturing processes that impact the environment is an aspect of the U.S. food supply that has also gone unrecognized by many consumers and healthcare professionals. For example, through extensive educational promotion, direct advertisement in the *Journal of the American Dietetic Association*, and virtually universal presence at in-patient facilities nationwide, companies like Novartis have made their development of medical nutrition products familiar to most healthcare practitioners. Novartis, a multi-billion-dollar corporation created in 1996 by the merger of CIBA-Geigy and Sandoz, has played a leading role in dietetics through development of medical nutrition products including weight management formulas like Optifast™ and foodservice-focused liquid supplements like Resource™. Novartis (or its predecessor subdivisions, Sandoz and CIBA-Geigy) has also ranked in the top ten list of contributors to the American Dietetic Association's National Center for Nutrition and Dietetics (NCND) since its inception.

The involvement of Novartis in agrichemical production, however, may be have been largely unrecognized by dietitians and other healthcare professionals. Novartis currently ranks as the largest pesticide-producing company in the world, and in 1997, Novartis sold over four billion dollars' worth of pesticides and other agrichemicals on an international basis. The appearance of these agrichemicals as ppm- and ppb-residues in the food supply and their impact on human health has been a key focus of this text.

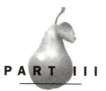

PART III

Medical Philosophies and Food-Related Toxicity

In the everyday world of patients, diseases, and nutritional practice, health-care providers have been unlikely to spend much time philosophizing about their profession. The need for practical solutions in the nutritional management of a large number of patients has typically left little time for thinking about philosophies of nutrition or medicine. Without consciously reflecting on philosophical matters, however, many practitioners have actually adopted an identifiable philosophy of health, and it is a philosophy that has worked directly against recognition of food toxicity as a relevant factor in medical care. In this section, we will look at several aspects of this widely-held medical philosophy and its impact on nutrition.

The Symptom-Diagnosis-Disease Model

The terms "symptom," "diagnosis," and "disease" have become so commonplace in medical and nutritional practice that they have ceased to sound philosophical to the vast majority of healthcare practitioners. Taking inventory of a patient's symptoms has become a routine part of medical and nutritional practice. The same can be said for making a diagnosis, or thinking about a patient in terms of his or her disease.

Definition of Terms

The term "symptom" technically refers to "any functional evidence of a disease or of a patient's condition" or "a change in a patient's condition indicative of some bodily or mental state."[19] Unlike "signs," which are also "indications" of problems or "evidence of disease" but can only be observed by trained practitioners, symptoms can typically be identified and described by the patients who experience them. Examples of commonly-reported symptoms are fatigue, fever, and pain.

Diagnosis is defined as "the art of distinguishing one disease from another"[20] and "disease" is defined as "a definite morbid process having a characteristic train of symptoms that may affect the whole body or any of its parts and whose etiology, pathology, and prognosis may be known or unknown."[21] Diseases are distinguished from one and other on the basis of symptoms, and diagnosis involves the differentiation of one symptom pattern from another.

Rheumatoid Arthritis from a Symptom-Based Perspective

The relationship between symptoms, diagnosis, and disease can be illustrated by the example of rheumatoid arthritis. The symptoms of rheumatoid arthritis often include morning stiffness of 30–60 minutes' duration in multiple joints and decreased stiffness after joint usage.[22] These symptoms (among many others) are used to help differentiate rheumatoid from osteoarthritis, since patients with osteoarthritis often have little or no exacerbated stiffness in the morning and have increased (rather than decreased) discomfort following sustained activity.[23]

Once a symptom pattern has been identified, a practitioner will often make a preliminary diagnosis which he or she then proceeds to confirm (or reject) with the help of laboratory data. In the case of rheumatoid arthritis, for example, laboratory data may include synovial fluid analysis to confirm total white blood cell and polymorphonuclear leukocyte (PMN) levels, or blood work to determine levels of rheumatoid factor or antinuclear antibody.[24] If the results of laboratory testing confirm a symptom pattern, an official diagnosis (in this case, "rheumatoid arthritis" corresponding to an ICD-9 code of 714.0) is made. As it does in this example, this diagnosis may correspond directly to the name of the patient's disease. Upon confirmation of the diagnosis, the healthcare practitioner tells the patient that he or she "has" rheumatoid arthritis. At this point, the first stage of the healthcare intervention is complete.

Philosophical Implications of the Disease Model

The above-described steps have served a practical role in the healthcare delivery system. In particular, they have provided a framework for routine contact between an extremely large number of physicians (almost 700,000 in 1994, or approximately 1 for every 383 individuals),[25] and an equally large number of patients. In 1993, for example, approximately 717.2 million visits were made to physician offices,[26] and over 30 million persons were hospitalized and received almost 40 inpatient procedures.[27] At the same time, however, these steps have also represented the creation of a medical philosophy.

The symptom-diagnosis-disease model has carried with it two far-reaching philosophical implications, and both have worked directly against recognition of food-related toxicity. The first of these implications involves the role of purpose in disease, and the second involves the appropriate context for recognizing illness.

Disconnecting Purpose From Disease

In the symptom-diagnosis-disease model described above, there is no suggestion of an underlying purpose or design at work in the manifestation of symptoms or in the development of disease. In fact, for many practitioners, the appearance of symptoms and the development of disease reflect the body's inability to continuing functioning in accordance with its natural purposes. The assignment of an ICD-9 code like 714.0 for rheumatoid arthritis means the musculoskeletal and immune systems are no longer functioning as they were designed to function.

The idea of rheumatoid arthritis as a purposeful event that reflects some grand design or cosmic intention is not a natural component of the symptom-diagnosis-disease model. In this model, the ultimate reasons for disease are not relevant to its diagnosis, and "diseases of unknown origin" constitute the single largest category of disease in the ICD-9 classification system.

Illness as a Potentially Incongruous Event

A second philosophical implication of the symptom-diagnosis-disease model has been the establishment of illness as a potentially incongruous event. By focusing attention on the appearance and disappearance of symptoms from a patient's life, the disease model has also served to focus attention on change. Symptoms themselves are defined as changes in a patient's condition, and this idea carries with it an expectation of impermanence. A symptom-less person might suddenly and unexpectedly develop symptoms, just as a person with a disease might find his or her symptoms suddenly abating.

In the symptom-diagnosis-disease model, changes in symptoms like the ones described above have become the standard for evaluating health. In the total absence of symptoms, a person can be described as healthy. Along with the appearance of a specific symptom pattern comes the declaration of disease. If symptoms disappear on a short-term basis, disease is described as having fallen into remission. If symptoms disappear over an extended and ongoing period of time, disease is described as cured.

The above perspective has permitted the event of illness to become saddled with a potentially high degree of incongruity. In the above model, health may give way to disease or disease to health abruptly and arbitrarily. Ailments, and particularly small everyday problems like the common cold, can appear to happen as if by chance. Even more dramatic, chronic conditions like heart disease, cancer, or diabetes may seem to depend on a roll of the dice" or "the luck of the draw."

Inconsistency with an Environmental Approach

The idea of illness as an incongruous event that depends on the appearance and disappearance of symptoms is an idea that is inconsistent with an environmental approach to nutrition. While a symptom-based approach to illness can capture the diversity that is characteristic of an environmental approach (there are over 10,000 diseases in the 9th edition of the International Classification of Diseases used as a basis for insurance coding in the United States),[28] it cannot situate disease within the context of wholeness and interaction that characterizes the ecosystem and the life of organisms within it. To better illustrate the incompatibility of these approaches, we will briefly revisit the condition of rheumatoid arthritis from a perspective founded upon wholeness, interaction, and congruity of health-related events.

Philosophical Alternatives to a Disease Model

Chapter 1 of this text presents a description of nutrition and ecology that treats the two fields of study as highly compatible in terms of their underlying principles and values. The concepts of wholeness, diversity, interaction, and synchronized events are described as shared aspects of nutrition and ecology, and a return of environmental standards to nutrition is described as a desirable alternative to current standards.

These same values of wholeness, diversity, interaction, and synchronized events also provide the starting point for development of alternatives to a symptom-diagnosis-disease model. In the same way that food can be viewed as something seasonal and geographically unique from an environmental perspective, so disease can be viewed as something carefully timed and uniquely situated from an environmentally-consistent perspective.

Similarly, the multiple levels of interaction (plant-microbe, animal-plant, animal-light cycle, etc.) that are required for development of food can also be viewed as prerequisite to the development of disease. If a condition like rheumatoid arthritis is approached in this way, the incongruity of morning stiffness and its inability to be treated with diet become questionable conclusions. In the following section, we will revisit the condition of rheumatoid arthritis from an environmentally-consistent perspective that emphasizes the values of wholeness, diversity, interaction, and uniqueness.

Rheumatoid Arthritis Revisited

The Role of Oxidative Stress

Movement of most body parts, including the joints, requires oxygen. Exercising cells may need 15 times as much oxygen as resting cells.29 The body is most efficient at producing energy when oxygen is available. While the presence of oxygen brings along with it an energy-related advantage, it also carries an added health risk. Reactive oxygen species (or ROS) can be excessively formed during the process of oxygen metabolism and can cause damage to cells and cell parts. Prevention of excessive ROS formation requires the activity of specific oxygen-processing enzymes and ROS-neutralizing molecules. Oxidative stress is defined as the outcome of any situation in which reactive oxygen species are not properly balanced by ROS-neutralizing molecules or by activity of specific oxygen-processing enzymes. (The topic of oxidative stress is reviewed at length in Chapter 5, page 196, under "Toxic Damage to Tissues and Cell Structures"). Research in four different areas has suggested that the origins of rheumatoid arthritis involve oxidative stress in the joints. These four areas of research include: 1) lack of motion and hypoxic-reperfusion injury, 2) inflammatory messengers and collagen instability, 3) estradiol and decreased nitric oxide production, and 4) oxidation of glycosaminoglycans.

Lack of Motion and Hypoxic-Reperfusion Injury. Articulations are places where bones come together, and in the human body, the vast majority of articulations are classified as "synovial articulations" (or synovial joints). In synovial joints, a fluid-containing cavity separates the bones from each other. Synovial cavities are also lined with synovial membranes that hold the synovial fluid in place. These membranes do not rest directly against the bones, but against cartilage, a special tissue that acts as a coating on the ends of the bones. The cartilage coating is referred to as articular cartilage, and the coated ends of the bones are called the articular surfaces of the joint.

Articular cartilage is referred to as "avascular" since it does not receive direct blood flow from the body's circulatory system. Like several other types of tissue (including lymphatic tissue, for example), the cartilage depends on movement for delivery of nutrients to its components. Motion of the ligaments (bone-to-bone connectors) and tendons (bone-to-muscle connectors) surrounding a joint facilitate delivery of nutrients to cartilage, in part by allowing nearby blood vessels to fully dilate and bring more nutrients in closer proximity to the avascular joint region. As long as pressure in the exercising blood vessels exceeds pressure in the synovial cavity, delivery of nutrients to the joint can proceed. However, when movement is absent and synovial pressure becomes greater than pressure in nearby blood vessels, the oxygen-carrying blood vessels can collapse and create a process called hypoxic-reperfusion injury.[30] This process involves one of the great ironies of oxygen metabolism. Although oxidative stress would logically be expected to peak along with peak presence of oxygen in the blood or in the tissue, production of ROS and damage to cells is usually greatest when oxygen concentrations are unusually low. This precise set of circumstances involving differential pressures in the joint and blood vessels, temporarily low concentrations of oxygen, excessive production of ROS, and damage to synovial structures has been determined to occur in the development of rheumatoid arthritis. As this condition begins to develop, damage to the synovial cavity has been shown to correlate with fluctuating oxygen pressure in the joint, overproduction of ROS, lack of oxygen-processing enzymes, and lack of free-radical scavenging molecules.[31] Each of these interactions suggests a role for oxidative stress in the origin of rheumatoid arthritis.

Inflammatory Messengers and Collagen Instability. A second type of evidence linking the origins of rheumatoid arthritis to oxidative stress involves the nature of connective tissue. Unlike most other tissues in the body, connective tissue is predominantly non-cellular and is primarily composed of an extracellular matrix (ECM). Three basic components are found in the ECM: fibers (especially collagen fibers), ground substance, and fluid. The best-studied components of the ECM are collagen fibers. Collagen fibers are constructed from protein, and when considered as a type of protein, are the most common type in the body, accounting for 30 percent of all body protein by weight. The stability of collagen protein has been shown to be highly sensitive to levels of inflammatory messenger molecules in the synovial fluid. When levels of these inflammatory messaging molecules (like interleukin-1 or tumor necrosis factor alpha) are high, collagen damage and rheumatoid arthritis risk are greatly increased.[32]

These observations provide a second type of evidence linking the origins of rheumatoid arthritis to oxidative stress.

Estradiol and Decreased Nitric Oxide Production. Abatement of symptoms in women with rheumatoid arthritis during periods of pregnancy has repeatedly sparked debate about the potential role of estrogen metabolism in the origins of the disease. Recent research in this area has also suggested a link between the origins of rheumatoid arthritis and oxidative stress. Researchers at the University of Goteborg, Sweden, have shown that administration of the most active form of estrogen, estradiol, greatly suppresses collagen damage in cell cultures, and does so by modifying oxidative metabolism. More specifically, administration of estradiol serves to decrease nitric oxide production.[33] Nitric oxide gas, like other free radical molecules, can produce tissue damage when produced in excess and in the presence of imbalanced oxygen metabolism. The determination of nitrotyrosine (a nitric oxide-related molecule) in the serum and synovial fluid of rheumatoid arthritis patients has provided further evidence of a rheumatoid arthritis-oxidative stress connection.[34]

Oxidation of Glycosaminoglycans (GAGs). A final type of evidence linking rheumatoid arthritis to oxidative stress involves the oxidation of glycosaminoglycans (GAGs). Two major families of molecules are present in the ground substance portion of connective tissue: GAGs and glycoproteins. (GAGs have also been traditionally referred to as mucopolysaccharides). GAGs are classified as linear polysaccharides because they are composed of a central, repeating disaccharide (two-sugar) unit strung out in a long chain. This disaccharide unit usually consists of a sugar-like unit called a uronic acid and a second sugar-like unit called a hexosamine. Glucuronic acid is the most common uronic acid in GAGs, and glucosamine and galactosamine are the most common hexosamines. With the exception of hya-luronic acid, all GAGs are sulfated.

In addition to the role of GAGs in determining the structure, viscosity and permeability of ground substance in connective tissue, they also play metabolic roles in the health of connective tissue and joints. Transport of ions, diffusion of nutrients, retention of water, binding of growth factors, intercellular signaling and collagen synthesis have all been shown to depend on GAG function.[35]

Hyaluronic acid (HA), which contains glucosamine and glucuronic acid, is the predominant GAG in the articular surface and also serves as a key component in synovial fluid. Although the exact connection between GAGs and oxidative stress is not clear, hyaluronic acid has been shown to undergo oxidation by ROS,[36] and oxidation of lipids in areas surrounding

GAGs has been shown to disrupt GAG metabolism.[37] These disruptions in GAG provide further evidence of a link between oxidative stress and the development of rheumatoid arthritis.

The Congruity and Purpose of Diet

Frances Zeeman, Professor of Nutrition at the University of California at Davis, and author of the widely-used textbook *Clinical Nutrition and Dietetics*, has described rheumatoid arthritis as a "chronic debilitating disease of unknown etiology" for which "there is no known cure, and treatment is not very successful." "As a result," she has written, "patients are prone, in desperation, to adopt unproved treatments, including fad diets. Among the so-called remedies suggested are…(elimination) of potatoes, tomatoes, eggplant, red or green peppers…dairy products, meat…."[38] Her description of rheumatoid arthritis as a disease of unknown origin has been echoed by Kathleen Mahan and Sylvia Escott-Stump in the ninth edition of their textbook, *Krause's Food, Nutrition and Diet Therapy*.[39]

These views of the relationship between diet and rheumatoid arthritis are inconsistent with the research evidence linking its etiology to oxidative stress. If oxidative stress is viewed as an underlying mechanism in the development of rheumatoid arthritis, then dietary practices contributing to the likelihood of oxidative stress would also be expected to contribute to increased risk of rheumatoid arthritis. Similarly, dietary practices helping to lower oxidative stress would also be expected to help prevent or reduce symptoms of rheumatoid arthritis. Both expectations appear to have been met in the research literature on rheumatoid arthritis and diet.

Dietary Antioxidants as Preventive Factors in Rheumatoid Arthritis. Studies on rheumatoid arthritis and nutrition have shown dietary antioxidants to be critical balancing factors in the prevention of molecular events involved in joint dysfunction. These events have included prevention of fibronectin fragment-mediated cartilage chondrolysis by n-acetyl-cysteine (NAC) and dimethyl sulfoxide (DMSO);[40] prevention of T cell hyporesponsiveness by restoration of glutathione and NAC levels;[41] prevention of excessive chemiluminescence in synovial fluid granulocytes by glutathione and catalase;[42] and prevention of increased inflammatory cytokine activity by NAC.[43] Status of the anti-oxidant, vitamin E, has also been shown to be inversely associated with metabolic dysfunction in rheumatoid arthritis patients.[44]

Fasting and Vegetarian Diets as Treatment Factors in Rheumatoid Arthritis. Kjeldsen-Kragh and colleagues at the Institute of Immunology and Rheumatology at the National Hospital in Oslo, Norway have carried out a long-term, prospective study on rheumatoid arthritis patients who fasted for 7–10 days, were placed on a gluten-free vegan diet for three months, and then were maintained on a lactovegetarian diet for a period of one and one-half years. A matched control group of rheumatoid arthritis patients followed their normal, meat-containing diet throughout the study period. Prior to the beginning of the study, both experimental and control subjects were meat-eating and had not significantly altered their diet in an effort to improve symptoms. Results of the study showed that for 14 out of 15 variables measured, lactovegetarian subjects had favorable outcomes in comparison with control subjects. Laboratory outcomes reaching statistical significance included total leukocyte count, presence of IgM antibodies, presence of rheumatoid factor, and complement proteins C3 and C4.[45]

The findings of Kjeldsen-Kragh and colleagues further substantiate a connection between rheumatoid arthritis and oxidative stress because vegetarian diets have long been associated with improved antioxidant intake in comparison with omnivorous diets. For example, in a 1995 study comparing subjects eating uncooked, vegan diets to matched controls eating omnivore diets, intake of beta-carotene, vitamin C, and vitamin E was significantly higher in vegan subjects.[46] Activity of the oxidative stress-reducing enzyme superoxide dismutase was also significantly higher in vegan subjects.[47] Incidence of oxidative stress-related cancers, including breast cancer,[48] colon cancer,[49] and lung cancer[50] (following adjustment for cigarette smoking practices) has also been shown to be lower in vegetarian versus meat-eating populations. In comparison with vegetarian regimens, diets high in animal products have been shown to be associated with increased formation of reactive oxygen species in the feces,[51] and inflammation-related oxidative stress triggered by excessive intake of arachidonic acid has been shown to be a characteristic of omnivore versus vegetarian diets.[52,53]

Food Toxicity and Rheumatoid Arthritis. The development of rheumatoid arthritis has been associated with exposure to a wide variety of xenbiotics,[54] and many of these toxic substances have been recognized as contaminants in the U.S. food supply. For example, increased production of reactive oxygen species through exposure to benzene and benzene derivatives, carbon tetrachloride, chloroform have been well-documented in the research literature. Environmental exposure to each of these substances has also been linked to the development of inflammatory conditions like rheumatoid arthritis.[55,56] As reviewed in Chapter 4, carbon tetrachloride and chloroform have both been identified as common contaminants in municipal tap water, and benzene derivatives have been observed to be equally common constituents of meats like beef and poultry. There has also been at least one research report suggesting that dietary toxins may have increased access to the joints of rheumatoid arthritis patients following excessive intestinal permeability in those patients.[57]

From a nutritional perspective based on wholeness, interaction, congruity and purposefulness of health and disease, the above research findings make sense. What they reflect is a conviction that the appearance and disappearance of symptoms can never be arbitrary events occurring without purpose in the life of a patient, but will always be events intricately interwoven with the patient's way of life, including diet. One of the greatest challenges of food toxicity involves acknowledgment of these inescapable interrelationships, and embrace of dietary interventions that move beyond the philosophical restrictions of a symptom-based model.

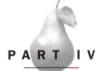

PART IV

Biogeochemical Cycles and Sustainability

A final challenge posed by the problem of food toxicity is the challenge of incorporating a biogeochemical perspective into the design and operation of the U.S. food supply. Food production and delivery in the U.S. have negatively impacted biogeochemical cycles in the global ecosystem, and over time, disruption of these cycles has increased reliance on toxic steps to maintain the existing food supply. In this section we will look more closely at the relationship between biogeochemical cycles and their food-based disruption.

In the field of biogeochemistry, researchers have tracked the flow of nutrients through the atmosphere, oceans, rivers, soil, and living organisms. As a result of their research, several well-recognized biogeochemical cycles have been established. These cycles include the hydrology cycle (involving water), the carbon and nitrogen cycles (usually referred to as "gaseous cycles" since their cycling involves a major phase in which the nutrients are atmospherically present as gases), and the sulfur and phosphorus cycles (usually referred to as "sedimentary cycles," since their cycling relies heavily upon sedimentation—the process of settling downward, becoming deposited and accumulating in soil or rock).

Basic Types of Nutrient Cycles

The Hydrology Cycle

Groundwater and Runoff

Half of all U.S. citizens depend on groundwater as their primary source of drinking water,[58] and almost 90% of all public water supply systems in the U.S. make some use of groundwater.[59] The term "groundwater" is typically defined as subsurface water that pools in fully saturated soils and rock formations. The pooling of water in these locations is part of a global water cycle typically referred to as the hydrology cycle.

The hydrology cycle rests on a delicately-balanced relationship between precipitation from the atmosphere and evaporation from the oceans and land. Both of these events average approximately 496,000 cubic kilometers per year).[60] The downhill, gravitationally-based flow of above-ground water is called *runoff*. On a global scale, runoff has traditionally averaged approximately 37,000 cubic kilometers per year.[61] However, many human activities, including agriculture-related activities have altered this average figure, particularly in the last century.[62] A diagram showing the relationship between hydrological events is presented in *Figure 6-1*.

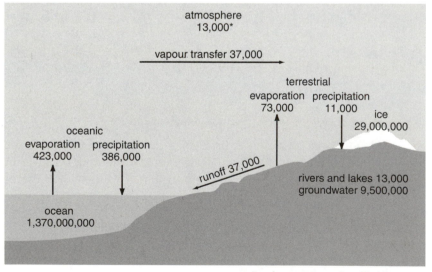

Figure 6-1
The hydrology cycle

Over the course of the last two centuries, farming practices in the U.S. have greatly increased topsoil erosion and water runoff. Over 30% of all farmland (approximately 100 million hectares, or 247 million acres) has been lost to erosion, waterlogging, or salination (excessive accumulation of salts) since the late 1700s.[63] Almost 90% of all cropland in the U.S. lost topsoil in early 1990s above the sustainable rate of 1 ton per hectare per year, and in certain areas like the rolling Palouse farmland in Washington state, approximately 40% of all topsoil has been lost since 1900.[64]

Researchers studying soil conservation have estimated that 1,064 pounds of nutrients are lost per acre of soil per year whenever erosion occurs at an annual rate of 17 tons per hectare.[65] For most farmers, this loss of nutrients signals the need for additional use of fertilizer, although the ability of the soil to retain the added nutrients is compromised by the very fact of erosion.

Deforestation

A variety of food-related practices affect basic groundwater quality, as well as above-ground runoff. One of these practices is the practice of deforestation (the destruction of forests). Deforestation has occurred for many reasons, but a primary reason during the last century has been large-scale food production. The creation of palm oil groves in Malaysia and cattle ranches in Central and South America are examples of food production areas that were created through the process of deforestation. (Both areas continue contribute to the content of U.S. food supply in the form of exported palm oil and beef).[66] Worldwide, approximately 40 million acres of forests are cut and cleared on an annual basis.[67]

Deforestation increases soil erosion and above-ground runoff. In addition, if newly-created agricultural areas are subsequently subjected to heavy pesticide and fertilizer use, the continuing erosion of soil and above-ground runoff can also lead to pesticide and fertilizer accumulations at sites very distant from the newly-created cropland. Agricultural activities along the Mississippi River, for example, have produced levels of uranium in the river that are 20 times higher than levels found in the Amazon River in South America.[68] These levels have been attributed to the heavy use of phosphate fertilizers on croplands adjacent to the Mississippi River, since mined rock used as a source of the phosphate in the fertilizer often contains significant concentrations of uranium.[69]

Waste Disposal

Industrial processes used to make fertilizers and pesticides can also contribute to groundwater contamination through the practice of waste disposal. Waste disposal occurs on a daily basis in the United States through a variety of mechanisms. Industrial surface impoundments are toxic waste disposal sites that involve ponds, pools, lagoons or pits. There are 181,000 industrial surface impoundments in the U.S., and over half of these sites are located above usable groundwater.[70] Other mechanisms of waste disposal include landfills, which number approximately 93,000 in the U.S.;[71] injection wells; and discharge into lakes and rivers. Use of sewage sludge as a crop fertilizer has also contributed to the contamination of groundwater. In the U.S., about 36% of all sewage sludge (or approximately 4 billion pounds) is used on farmland or forestland or mixed into plant-growing soils.[72] Most sewage sludge in the U.S. contains not only processed human waste, but also processed industrial waste discharged by local industries.[73]

Dams and Irrigation

Dams and irrigation constitute a third category of food-related activity that can significantly disrupt the hydrology cycle. On a global scale, humans have constructed approximately 800,000 dams. Included in this number are approximately 40,000 large dams, and 300 major dams. (A major dam is defined as a dam over 200 meters in height and holding over 43 million cubic meters of water). Since 1993, construction has begun on 1,240 new dams worldwide,[74] and irrigation is increasingly listed as the primary reason for this construction.[75] On a global scale, 40% of total crop production now originates in the 16% of cropland that is subjected to extensive irrigation.[76]

Approximately 85% of all fresh water consumed in the U.S. is used for crop production,[77] and net production of a single pound of corn can currently require over 635 liters of water.[78] Extensive use of irrigation can not only disrupt the natural distribution of water from surface deposits, but can also lead to salt build-up and waterlogging, particularly if extensive irrigation is carried out in arid regions.[79]

Gaseous Cycles

Nutrient cycles involving a major phase in which nutrients are present in the atmosphere as gases are typically referred to as gaseous cycles. In this section we will review two gaseous cycles and the impact of agricultural practices on their natural balance.

Carbon

Carbon is found in a variety of forms throughout the earth's ecosystems. In the atmosphere, carbon is found primarily in the form of CO_2 (carbon dioxide gas). In oceans and lakes, this carbon dioxide becomes dissolved and forms carbonic acid (H_2CO_3), carbonate (CO_3^-), and bicarbonate (HCO^-).

Carbon deposits in the ground often take the geologic form of $CaCO_3$ (calcium carbonate). After long periods of time, this form of carbon, when mixed with clay, can become compacted to form limestone. Also over long periods of time, carbon trapped in decaying organic matter can transform under high pressure and other necessary conditions into coal.(This process is reviewed in Chapter 3, page 93, under "Historical Perspectives: Petroleum and the Food Supply.") Finally, inside living organisms, carbon can be found in virtually all of forms the listed above (except coal and limestone), and can be further metabolized into a variety of other compounds, including proteins, carbohydrates, and fats.

Respiration and Photosynthesis. Uptake of atmospheric CO_2 by plants during the process of photosynthesis, and release of CO_2 back into the atmosphere by most living organisms during the process of respiration constitute the most critical balancing point in the carbon cycle. (see *Figure 6-2*). Worldwide, the release of carbon dioxide into the atmosphere by living organisms has been estimated at 100 billion tons per year,[80] and uptake of carbon dioxide through photosynthesis at 44–99 billion tons.[81]

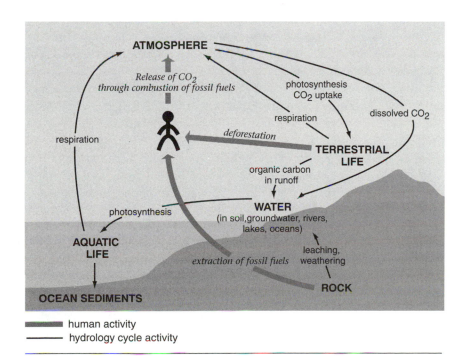

Figure 6-2
The carbon cycle

Natural daily and seasonal patterns in the carbon cycle have been well-documented. At night, when plant photosynthesis is large shut down, uptake of atmospheric carbon dioxide slows dramatically and atmospheric concentrations increase. Similarly, in winter, when plant activity is dramatically less than its summertime equivalent, atmospheric concentrations of CO_2 have also been found to increase. In parts of northern Italy, this increase in winter versus summer atmospheric concentrations has been estimated at approximately 20ppm (parts per million) CO_2.[82]

Not accounted for in the above equations is the impact of human activity on the carbon cycle. The burning of fossil fuels, production of cement, and clearing of forests all result in the net release of carbon dioxide gas into the atmosphere. When considered in combination, these human activities account for the release of approximately 5.1–7.5 billion additional tons of CO_2 per year.[83] Additional release of carbon dioxide into the atmosphere has raised worldwide concentrations from approximately 280ppm to 350ppm during the period 1750–1995, and levels as high as 700ppm have been projected for the year 2100.[84]

The "Greenhouse Effect." Increasing levels of carbon dioxide gas in the atmosphere have frequently been referred to as one component of the "greenhouse effect." Together with methane, ozone, nitrous oxide, and fluorocarbons, carbon dioxide is a gas that can absorb infrared radiation. Throughout the day, radiation from the sun (called solar radiation) warms the earth. This solar radiation is then re-radiated back into the atmosphere by the earth, primarily in the form of infrared radiation. Trapping of infrared radiation by carbon dioxide and other "greenhouse gases" raises atmospheric temperatures. Over the last 100 years, average global atmospheric temperature has been estimated to have risen approximately one quarter to one half degree centigrade.[85] Controversial projections of atmospheric warming up to an additional 3–4 degrees centigrade would have dramatic consequences on ecological events following melting of the earth's ice caps, rising of ocean levels, and alterations in climate.

Food production in the U.S. relies heavily on carbon dioxide-releasing activities. Fossil fuels are directly involved in the operation of most farm machinery, including tractors, harvesters, combines, and irrigation pumps. Production of fertilizers and pesticides also involves usage of fossil fuels. Further usage is required by transportation of food to processing, storage, and distribution sites. Considered as a whole, these food-related activities account for the use of approximately 850,000 billion kilocalories of fossil fuel energy each year.[86] This level of food-related energy consumption also represents approximately 17% of all energy consumption in the U.S.[87]

Nitrogen

Like carbon, nitrogen depends on the activity of organisms for its cycling, and is delicately balanced in the atmosphere as a result of organism uptake and release. In the atmosphere, nitrogen is found primarily in the form of dinitrogen gas (N_2). This molecular gas is uptaken by land-based and water-based organisms that convert the molecule into more complex organic and inorganic forms. These forms include ammonia (NH_3), ammonium ion (NH_4^+), nitrite (NO_2^-), nitrate (NO_3^{--}), nitrous oxide (N_2O), and nitric oxide (NO). Conversion of N_2 into other compounds is typically referred to as nitrogen fixation. (The fixing of nitrogen by microorganisms was described in detail in Chapter 1, page 9, under "Plant-Microbe Interactions"). Other nitrogen-based conversions also have common designations. The breaking down of carbon-containing nitrogen compounds into ammonia is typically referred to as *ammonification*, and the reduction of nitrate to any form of nitrogen gas, including N_2 or N_2O, as *denitrification*.

Like carbon cycling, nitrogen cycling shows patterned seasonal variation. The process of nitrification, for example, becomes most active in the winter. This increased activity allows for sufficient production of nitrate to be used in the spring by germinating plants. A diagram illustrating basic components of the nitrogen cycle appears in *Figure 6-3*, on the following page.

Manure and Fertilizer. A variety of food-related activities impact nitrogen cycling. These activities include deforestation and land clearance to provide for large-scale, machine-based crop production; production and use of nitrogen-containing fertilizers; agricultural practices that alter the presence of nitrogen-fixing microorganisms in the soil; and animal-rearing practices that create large concentrations of manure in a compact area or involve spreading of manure over cropland. The spreading of manure, for example, has been shown to increase atmospheric concentrations of ammonia, and this increase has been further connected with changes in plant diversity since plants differ in their ability to adapt to low-nitrogen and high-nitrogen conditions.[88]

In 1989, worldwide production of nitrogen-containing fertilizers from fossil fuels totaled approximately 132 billion pounds.[89] In the U.S., consumption of nitrogen-containing fertilizers rose from approximately 6 million tons in the late 1960s to 9.5 million tons in the late 1980s.[90]

Eutrophication. The presence of excess nutrients (like nitrogen) in an ecosystem can excessively accelerate biological activity in that ecosystem. This process of acceleration is typically referred to as *eutrophication*. (The term "eutrophication" is also typically restricted to the acceleration of activity in aqueous or water-based ecosystems).

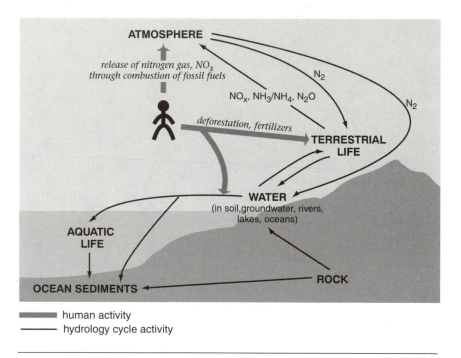

Figure 6-3
The nitrogen cycle

The Great Lakes region of the United States and Canada provides one of the best-researched examples of the eutrophication process. This region of North America contains the largest body of freshwater on the earth. It also houses approximately one third of the total Canadian population and one fifth of all U.S. citizens.

The Great Lakes region of North American has also been the site of extensive industrial activity. Nearly half of all Canadian industries, and one fifth of U.S. industries are located in this region.[91] Discharge of nitrogen- and phosphate-containing fertilizers into the Great Lakes ecosystem has contributed to an increase in phytoplankton (microscopic plants and animals that float and drift in bodies of water) counts from 81 per milliliter in 1929 to 4,423 per milliliter in 1962, and this increase has been largely responsible for severe depletion of dissolved oxygen in bottom water throughout the region.[92] Cumulatively, these changes have created dramatic shifts in the Great Lakes ecosystems, including loss of numerous water species that are unable to withstand low oxygen conditions.

Sedimentary Cycles

Nutrient cycles involving a major phase in which nutrients settle downward, become deposited, and begin to accumulate in soil or rock are typically referred to as *sedimentary cycles*. In this section we will review two sedimentary cycles and the impact of agricultural practices on their natural balance.

Sulfur

Sulfur passes through a variety of forms as it cycles through the ecosystem, and many of these forms involve combinations of sulfur with other metals (like potassium or calcium) or nonmetals (like oxygen or hydrogen). In the atmosphere, sulfur is found primarily in the form of sulfur dioxide (SO_2), elemental sulfur (S), or sulfides like hydrogen sulfide (H_2S). Sulfur dioxide becomes oxidized in the air to sulfur trioxide (SO_3). This sulfur trioxide subsequently combines with water (H_2O) to form sulfuric acid (H_2SO_4).

Sulfuric acid is routinely transferred by precipitation (in aerosol droplets) from the atmosphere to the soil, where bacteria routinely reduce it to sulfides (like hydrogen sulfide). Many plants specialize in the uptake of sulfur in the form of sulfate (SO_4^{--}) through their roots, and once incorporated into plant cells, sulfate can undergo a variety of transformations. Inside plant cells, sulfate can be converted into sulfite (SO_3^{--}), sulfhydryl groups (SH), bisulfate (HSO_4^-), bisulfite (HSO_3^-), potassium bisulfite ($KHSO_3$), and hydrogen sulfide. Plants, animals and microorganisms are often capable of reducing oxygen-containing forms of sulfur to hydrogen sulfide (H_2S), and this form of sulfur is commonly released back into the environment.

Geologic formations typically contain sulfur combined together with other elements in its sulfide or sulfate form. Rock sulfides include galena (PbS), acanthite (Ag_2S), chalcocite (Cu_2S), and pyrite (FeS_2). Barite ($BaSO_4$), celestite ($SrSO4$), anhydrite ($CaSO4$), epsomite ($MgSO4$), and gypsum ($CaSO_4 + 2H_2O$) are common rock formations contain sulfur in its sulfate form. Weathering of rock formations allows sulfur to leach into surrounding soils, and plants roots are frequently able to uptake leached sulfur when present in its sulfate form. A summary of the sulfur cycle is presented in *Figure 6-4* on the following page.

Acid Rain. The most common food-related disruption of the sulfur cycle involves release of excessive sulfur oxides into the atmosphere following the burning of fossil fuels. Although atmospheric emissions of sulfur dioxide are estimated to have decreased by approximately 17% between 1979 and 1988,[93] almost 23 million tons of sulfur dioxide were released into air space above the U.S. in 1988.[94]

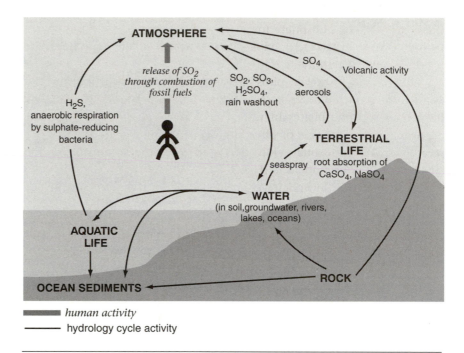

Figure 6-4
The sulfur cycle

Fossil fuel-derived sulfur dioxide emissions are directly linked to a variety of food-related activities. As described earlier in this chapter, in relationship to carbon dioxide emissions, the burning of fossil fuels takes place in the operation of most farm machinery, including tractors, harvesters, combines, and irrigation pumps; in the production of fertilizers and pesticides; and in the transportation of food to processing, storage, and distribution sites.

"Acid rain" is technically defined as precipitation that is characterized by an increase in hydrogen ion concentration. The relative acidity of rainfall typically varies between a pH of 4.5 and 5.5[95] Acid rains in the U.S. in the late 1970s and early 1980s were documented at pH levels of 1.4–2.2.[96] The presence of acid rain has widespread effects throughout the ecosystem. For example, nitrification by microorganisms that are pH-sensitive is typically inhibited by acid rain,[97] and bodies of water with little capacity to buffer changes in acidity may become unable to support marine life.[98]

Phosphorus

Like sulfur, phosphorus is found in a variety of organic and inorganic forms throughout the ecosystem. Rock deposits of phosphorus typically contain the element in its phosphate form (PO_4^{---}). These geological formations include apatite ($Ca_5[PO_4]_3$), vivianite ($Fe[PO_4] + 2H_2O$), pyromorphite ($Pb_5[PO_4]_3Cl$), and triphylite ($Li[Fe^{++}, Mn^{++}]PO_4$).

Unlike sulfur, however, phosphorus has no real atmospheric component to its cycle. Its incorporation into living organisms comes primarily from dissolved phosphates in water and leached phosphorus from soil deposits. Dissolved forms of phosphorus include phosphate ion (PO_4^{---}), monohydrogen phosphate ion (HPO_4^{--}), dihydrogen phosphate ion ($H_2PO_4^{-}$), and phosphoric acid (H_2PO_4).

Once dissolved phosphates are uptaken into microorganisms, plants and animals they can be converted into a variety of organic forms. A key repository of phosphorus in plants is the molecule phytic acid, which contains six phosphate groups attached to a cyclohexane ring (*Figure 6-5*). In humans, calcium phosphate ($Ca_3[PO_4]_2$) and hydroxyapatite ($Ca_{10}[PO_4]_6(OH)_2$) are also key repositories of phosphate. A diagram summarizing key events in the phosphorus cycle is presented in *Figure 6-5*, on the following page.

Fertilizer. As described previously in relationship to nitrogen, application of fertilizer is the primary food-related activity that contributes excessive amounts of phosphorus to the ecosystem. On a global basis, more than 13 million tons of phosphorus are added annually to croplands in the form of fertilizer.[99] Seepage into groundwater and runoff into neighboring streams carries excess phosphorus into nearby aquatic ecosystems, and creates the problem of eutrophication, discussed earlier in this chapter on page 271, under "Eutrofication."

Food Production as Biogeochemically Disruptive

The above-cited examples of disturbance in the hydrology, carbon, nitrogen, sulfur and phosphorus cycles point to U.S. food production as a fundamentally disruptive enterprise when analyzed from an ecological perspective. Reliance on irrigation and fertilizer application have contributed significantly to cycle disruption, as has deforestation in order to create large-scale, machine-accessible acreage.

In the maintenance of the U.S food supply, however, there may be no greater biogeochemical problem than the dependence on fossil fuel. It is difficult to find any phase of the food production process that does not rely heavily on supply of fossil fuel. This reliance begins in the very process of

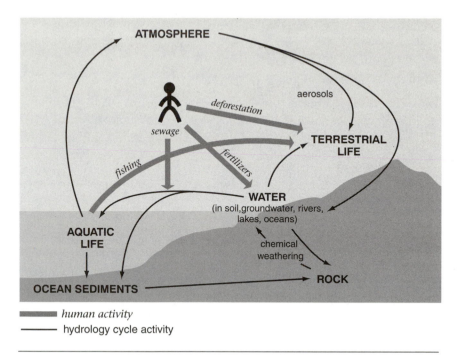

Figure 6-5
The phosphorus cycle

preparing cropland with bulldozers, backhoes, and graders. It continues with the operation of tractor-pulled plows, tractor-pulled furrow presses, and tractor-pulled seed drills. Fertilizers and pesticides depend on fossil fuel-derived components. Harvesters and loaders are put into operation once crops become ready for harvest, and grain cars are available to transport harvested crops via rail. The reliance on fossil fuel continues at food production and manufacturing facilities, where industrial equipment is essential for processing and packaging of food. The use of fossil fuels continues with distribution of factory products to retail outlets, and with storage and handling equipment used at those retail locations. In addition, all of the equipment listed above must be manufactured with the extensive use of fossil fuels.

As described earlier, numerous disruptions in biogeochemical cycles have been attributed to excessive combustion of fossil fuels. These disruptions include acid rain, the greenhouse effect, and eutrophication of lakes and rivers. (Added to these problems would be the health consequences of water and air pollution, which are described in more detail in Chapter 5). Collectively, these disruptions present serious drawbacks to ongoing maintenance of the U.S. food supply in its current form.

Sustainable Agriculture

The Concept of Sustainability

The word "sustainable" derives from the Latin *sub + tenere*, literally translated as "capable of being supported from underneath," "able to endure without failing," or "able to bear up." The word "agriculture" comes from the Greek *agros* meaning "field" or "pasture land" and the Latin *cutivatus*, past participle of the verb *colere*, meaning "to care for." When combined, the words "sustainable agriculture" literally mean "caring for the field in a way that is enduring and supported from underneath."

A more operational definition of sustainability has been proposed by environmental writer Peter Montague. Montague has defined "sustainable development" as "development without growth in throughput that exceeds the regenerative and absorptive capacity of the environment."[100] In this context, the word "throughput" is used to describe the totality of human economy. "Throughput" means everything people do or make, and it takes into account all materials and energy involved in the process. Throughput can be calculated by taking the total number of people and multiplying by their total consumption. Measuring the regenerative and absorptive capacity of the environment is a more complicated aspect of Montague's definition, but it is closely related to the biogeochemical cycles described earlier in this chapter.

According to either of the two definitions described above, maintenance of the U.S. food supply would be characterized as a non-sustainable enterprise. It is not difficult to understand how production processes leading to loss of topsoil or greenhouse warming represent non-sustainable approaches to food. Over time, loss of topsoil inevitably means loss of food and as a result, loss of potential for sustaining life. It is much more difficult, however, to understand how current approaches to the U.S. food supply could be transformed in such a way as to increase sustainability.

Organically-Grown Food

Organic Food Sales

Many individuals concerned about environmental aspects of nutrition have been strongly supportive of organic agriculture as a environmentally supportive enterprise. Alongside of these concerns has been a noteworthy rise in organic food sales in the U.S. during the last decade. According to the *Natural Foods Merchandiser*, a leading trade journal in the natural products industry published by New Hope Communications in Boulder, Colorado, total organic sales in the U.S. moved close to the $2 billion dollar level in 1996.[101] Included within the $1,950,000,000 total organic sales were $633,000,000 of sales in grocery and dairy; $395,000,000 in sales within a "miscellaneous" category including meat, poultry, seafood, personal care items, vitamins, and other supplements; $283,000,000 in sales of refrigerated and frozen products; $242,000,000 in sales of bulk foods; $191,000,000 in sales of herbs; $117,000,000 in sales of bakery products; and $89,000,000 in sales of produce.

The Organic Foods Production Act (OFPA)

Organic standards were first set forth in the Organic Foods Production Act (OFPA) of 1990, which was itself a section (Title 21) of the 1990 Farm Bill. Some of the highlights of OFPA included: use of approved seed and seedlings; non-use of fertilizers with synthetic or prohibited ingredients; use of raw animal manure on crops for animals only, or on human crops provided that the harvest occurs 60 or more days after application; use of organic feed for livestock that excludes plastic pellets or urea; non-use of antibiotics or internal parasiticides on a routine basis in the absence of illness; organic feeding of dairy cows at least 12 months prior to the sale of milk; non-use of nitrates, nitrites, or sulfites or any synthetic ingredients during processing or post-harvesting handling; and non-use of any non-organic ingredients during processing except ingredients included on the National List established by law. To date, all foods federally certified as organic must comply with all of the above regulations.

Limitations of Organic Production

It is not difficult to imagine ways in which biogeochemical balance could be restored through the widespread practice of organic agriculture. For example, discontinued use of artificial fertilizers and pesticides would logically result in decreased contamination of groundwater with pesticide residues and would lower risk of eutrophication through decreased nitrogen and phosphorus application. Discontinuation of these practices would also decrease agricultural reliance on fossil fuels and promote sustainabilty through this means.

At the same time, however, it is difficult to see how organic practices, in and of themselves, could assure sustainable food production. For example, large scale production of organic pretzels from 60% extraction, refined-wheat flour using current food supply production and distribution channels could easily produce nutrient cycle disruptions at a level virtually equivalent to disruptions currently being experienced in non-organic production. The wheat for such pretzels could still be grown in an area requiring intensive irrigation. Petroleum-powered machinery could still be used for land clearing and plowing, seed sowing and plant harvesting. The pretzels could still be produced in a way that required use of fossil fuel-driven equipment, packaged in a way that involved use of non-recyclable plastics, and then transported cross-country on fossil fuel-burning vehicles.

Community Supported Agriculture (CSA)

Community supported agriculture (CSA), also called subscription farming, is a relatively recent practice developed to promote sustainability and to increase a sense of community in local areas. CSA partnerships operate through the purchase of shares in a small local farm (typically organic) by individuals and families in the surrounding community. A CSA may sell shares to as few as 25 or as many as 500 subscribers. The cost of one share typically falls into a range of $250 to $500 dollars, and guarantees weekly access to food produced on the farm throughout a 6–8 month growing season. Shares are usually purchased well in advance of the growing season, often as early as January or February. There is no guarantee to subscribers of any fixed amount of any given food during the 6–8 month period. For example, if a broccoli harvest is particularly successful, larger-than-expected portions of broccoli will be distributed to subscribers. However, if a broccoli crop fails to mature, no distribution to subscribers will be made.

At an ecological level, CSAs work to eliminate the need for extensive transportation or storage of food, and thereby decrease the reliance on fossil fuel. When combined with organic production processes, CSAs also accomplish elimination of pesticides and fertilizers and thereby minimize contamination of soil, air, water and food. As of 1996, approximately 600 community supported agriculture (CSA) partnerships existed in the U.S. and Canada.[102]

Summary: The Challenge of Food Toxicity

Although response to food toxicity must be multi-dimensional and must involve the combined efforts of consumers, manufacturers, farmers, and healthcare professionals, the challenge of food toxicity is not only practical but also conceptual. The conceptual challenge of food toxicity lies equally within the two words. With respect to "food," the conceptual challenge involves re-integrating the features of wholeness, diversity, interaction, seasonality, and uniqueness into food as discussed in Chapter 1. These features have disappeared from view within the context of the U.S. food supply. With respect to "toxicity," the conceptual challenge is to move beyond a symptom-diagnosis-disease model in which symptoms can arbitrarily appear and disappear without providing a clue about their underlying origin.

The shift from an energy-based paradigm that focuses on food as fuel to an information-based paradigm that emphasizes food as messenger is a shift in thinking that will help restore the experience of food as a unifying moment in life. It will also help create an approach to health that treats toxicity as a root-level disruption of balance that underlyies many branches of disease. However, in and of itself, this shift in thinking will not be sufficient to pave the way for a restoration of environmental standards in nutrition. That accomplishment will rest equally on the adoption of ecologically-related values in the personal life of everyone who eats. From this perspective, the challenge of food toxicity is really two distinct challenges. The first challenge lies in understanding the link between environment, food quality, and disease. The second challenge lies in embracing that sense of connectedness in one's personal, everyday life.

1. Fortune Magazine. (1998). The Fortune 500. Fortune 137(8):F1-F70.

2. *Ibid.*

3. *Ibid.*

4. *Ibid.*

5. *Ibid.*

6. United States Department of Agriculture. (1998). Agriculture Fact Book 1998. Office of Communications, USDA Publication No. 7202791. Washington, D.C. (Website location: http://www.usda.gov/news./pubs/fbook98/content.htm).

7. *Ibid.*

8. *Ibid.*

9. *Ibid..*

10. *Ibid.*

11. *Ibid.*

12. *Ibid.*

13. *Ibid.*

14. Personal communication, Customer Service Department, General Foods Consumer Center, White Plains, New York.

15. American Dietetic Association. (1997). The American Dietetic Association (ADA) 1997 Nutrition Trends Survey. American Dietetic Association, Chicago, Illinois.

16. The Hartman Group. (1997). The Hartman report. Food and the environment: a consumer's perspective. Phase II. Winter 1997. The Hartman Group, Bellevue, Washington, Exhibit 7–5, p.53.

17. *Ibid*, Exhibit 7–4, p.52.

18. Washington Public Interest Research Group. (1989). Is beauty only peel deep? Consumers choose less pesticides. Organic Times, August, WASHPIRG, Seattle, Washington, p.1.

19. Dorland's Illustrated Medical Dictionary. (1965). 24th Edition. Philadelphia, WB Saunders, p.1482.

20. *Ibid*, p.411.

21. *Ibid*, p.428.

22. Ad Hoc Committee on Clinical Guidelines, American College of Rheumatology. (1996). Guidelines for the initial evaluation of the adult patient with acute musculoskeletal problems. Arthrit Rheum 39(1):1–8.

23. *Ibid*.

24. *Ibid*.

25. Lohr KN, Vanselow NA, and Detmer DE. (Eds). (1996). Summary from the nation's physician workforce: options for balancing supply and requirements. Committee on the U.S. Physician Supply, Institute of Medicine. Washington, D.C.,pp.1–13.

26. Nelson C and Woodwell D. (1998). National ambulatory medical care survey: 1993. Vit Health Stat 136(iii–vi):1–99.

27. National Center for Health Statistics. (1995). Fastats. National Center for Health Statistics, Centers for Disease Control, U.S. Department of Health and Human Services. Hyattsville, Maryland. (Website location: http://www.cdc.gov/nchswww/fastats/hospital.htm).

28. Bernard S. (1996). 1997 Standard ICD-9. International Classification of Diseases. Ninth Revision. Medicode, Inc. Salt Lake City.

29. Clarkson PM. (1995). Antioxidants and physical performance. Crit Rev Food Sci Nutr 35(1–2):131–141.

30. Mapp PI, Grootveld MC, and Blake DR. (1995). Hypoxia, oxidative stress and rheumatoid arthritis. Br Med Bull 51(2):419–436.

31. *Ibid*.

32. Joosten LA, Helsen MM, and van den Berg WB. (1994). Accelerated onset of collagen-induced arthritis by remote inflammation. Clin Exp Immunol 97(2):204–211.

33. Josefsson E and Tarkowski A.(1997). Suppression of type II collagen-induced arthritis by the endogenous estrogen metabolite 2-methoxyestradiol. Arthritis Rheum 40(1):154–163.

34. Kaur H and Halliwell B. (1994). Evidence for nitric oxide-mediated oxidative damage in chronic inflammation. Nitrotyrosine in serum and synovial fluid from rheumatoid arthritis patients. FEBS Lett 350:9–12.

35. Ledbetter WB. (1992). Cell matrix response in tendon injury. Clin Sports Med 11(3):533–578.

36. Mapp PI, Grootveld MC, and Blake DR, *op. cit. (see reference 30)*.

37. Ramasamy S, Lipke DW, Boissonneault GA et al. (1996). Oxidized lipid-mediated alterations in proteoglycan metabolism in cultured pulmonary endothelial cells. Atheroscler 120(1–2):199–208.

38. Zeeman F. (1991). Clinical nutrition and dietetics. 2nd edition. Macmillan, New York, p.737.

39. Mahan LK and Escott-Stump S. (1996). Krause's food, nutrition, and diet therapy. 9th Edition. WB Saunders, Philadelphia, p. 890.

40. Homandberg GA, Hui F, and Wen C. (1996). Fibronectin fragment mediated cartilage chondrolysis.II. Reparative effects of anti-oxidants. Biochim Biophys Acta 1317(2):143–148.

41. Maurice MM, Nakamura H, van der Voort EA et al. (1997). Evidence for the role of altered redox state in hyporesponsiveness of synovial T cells in rheumatoid arthritis. J Immunol 158(3):1458–1465.

42. Arnhold J, Sonntag K, Sauer H et al. (1994). Increased native chemiluminescence in granulocytes isolated from synovial fluid and peripheral blood of patients with rheumatoid arthritis. J Biolumin Chemilumin 9(2):79–86.

43. Sato M, Miyazaki T, Nagaya T et al. (1996). Antioxidants inhibit tumor necrosis factor-alpha mediated stimulation of interleukin-8, monocyte chemoattractant

protein-1, and collagenase expression in cultured human synovial cells. J Rheumatol 23(3):432–438.

44. Wasil M, Hutchison DC, Cheeseman P et al. (1992). Alpha-tocopherol status in patients with rheumatoid arthritis: relationship to antioxidant activity. Biochem Soc Trans 20(3):277S.

45. Kjeldsen-Kragh J, Mellbye OJ, Haugen M et al. (1995). Changes in laboratory variables in rheumatoid arthritis patients during a trial of fasting and one-year vegetarian diet. Scand J Rheumatol 24:85–93.

46. Rauma A-L, Torronen R, Hannainen O et al. (1995). Antioxidant status in long-term adherents to a strict uncooked vegan diet. Am J Clin Nutr 62:1221–1227.

47. *Ibid.*

48. Phillips RL. (1975). Role of lifestyle and dietary habits in risk of cancer among Seventh-Day Adventists. Canc Res Suppl 35:3513–3522.

49. Calkins BM, Whittaker DJ, Nair PP et al. (1984). Diet, nutrient intake, and metabolism in populations at high and low risk for colon cancer: nutrient intake. Am J Clin Nutr 40:896–905.

50. Colditz GZ, Stampfer MJ, and Willett WC. (1987). Diet and lung cancer: a review of the epidemiological evidence in humans. Arch Intern Med 147:157–160.

51. Eerhardt JG, Lim SS, Bode JC et al. (1997). A diet righ in fat and poor in dietary fiber increases the in vivo formation of reactive oxygen species in human feces. J Nutr 127(5):706–709.

52. Taber L, Chiu CH, and Whelan J. (1998). Assessment of the arachidonic acid content in foods commonly consumed in the American diet. Lipids 33(12):1151–1157.

53. Li D, Ng A, Mann NJ et al. (1998). Contribution of meat fat to dietary arachidonic acid. Lipids 33(4):437–440.

54. Bigazzi PE. (1997). Autoimmunity caused by xenobiotics. Toxicol 119(1):1–21.

55. Parke DV and Parke AL. (1996). Chemical-induced inflammation and inflammatory diseases. Internatl J Occup Med Environ Health 9(13):211–217.

56. Lundberg J, Alfredsson L, Plato N et al. (1994). Occupation, occupational exposure to chemicals and rheumatological disease. Scand J Rheumat 23(6):305–310.

57. Cuvelier C, Barbatis C, Mielants H et al. (1987). The histopathology of intestinal inflammation related to reactive arthritis. Gut 28:394–402.

58. Gordon W. (1984). A citizen's handbook on groundwater protection. National Resources Defense Council, New York, p.11.

59. U.S. Environmental Protection Agency. Office of Water. (1994). Class V injection wells and your drinking water. EPA 813-F-94-005, Washington, D.C.

60. Begon M, Harper JL, and Townsend CR. (1996). Ecology. Third edition. Blackwell Science, Oxford, pp. 763–764.

61. *Ibid*, p.764.

62. Vitousek PM, Mooney HA, Lubchenco J et al. (1997). Human domination of the earth's ecosystems. Science 277:494–499.

63. Pimentel D. (1994). Food, land, population, and the U.S. economy. Carrying Capacity Network, Washington, D.C., p.17.

64. *Ibid*.

65. Troeh FR, Hobbs JA, and Donahue RL. (1991). Soil and water conservation. Prentice Hall, Englewood Cliffs, New Jersey.

66. Gupta A. (1988). Ecology and development in the Third World. Routledge, London.

67. World Resources Institute. (1991). 1992 environmental almanac. Houghton Mifflin, Boston, p.13.

68. Spalding RF and Sackett WM. (1972). Uranium in runoff from the Gulf of Mexico distributive province: anomalous concentrations. Science 175:629–631.

69. *Ibid*.

70. Gordon W, *op. cit.(see reference 58)*, p.15.

71. *Ibid*.

72. Krauss GD and Page AL. (1997). Wastewater, sludge, and food crops. Biocycle (Feb):74–82.

73. Montague P. (1997). New U.S. waste policy, pt 2: sewage sludge. Rachel's Environment and Health Weekly, No.561. Environmental Research Foundation, Annapolis, Maryland. (Website location: http://www.monitor.net/rachel/).

74. McCully P. (1998). Silenced rivers. Zed Books, London.

75. Gardner G and Perry J. (1995). Vital sign. Big-dam construction is on the rise. World Watch (Sept–Oct):36–37.

76. Matson PA, Paarton WJ, Power AG et al. (1997). Agricultural intensification and ecosystem properties. Science 277:504–509.

77. Postel S. (1989). Water for agriculture: facing the limits. Worldwatch Paper 93. Worldwatch Institute, Washington, D.C.

78. Pimentel D, *op. cit. (see reference 63)*, p.18.

79. Matson PA, Paarton WJ, Power AG et al, *op. cit. (see reference 76)*, p.506.

80. Mooney HA, Vitousek PM, and Matson PA. (1987). Exchange of materials between terrestial ecosystems and the atmosphere. Science 238:926–932.

81. Kormondy EJ. (1996). Concepts of ecology. Fourth edition. Prentice Hall, Upper Saddle River, New Jersey, p.122.

82. *Ibid.*

83. Mooney HA, Vitousek PM, and Matson PA, *op. cit. (see reference 80)*.

84. Begon M, Harper JL, and Townsend CR, *op. cit (see reference 60)*, p.771–773.

85. *Ibid*, p.774.

86. Pimentel D, *op. cit. (see reference 63)*, p.20.

87. *Ibid*, p.21.

88. Berden M, Nilsson SI, Rosen K et al. (1987). Soil acidification—extent, causes, and consequences. National Swedish Environmental Protection Board, Report 3292, Stockholm.

89. Pimentel D, *op. cit. (see reference 63)*, p.20.

90. World Resources Institute, *op. cit. (see reference 67)*, p.34.

91. Kormondy EJ, *op. cit. (see reference 81)*, p.421.

92. *Ibid*, pp.421–426.

93. Harte J, Holdren C, Schneider R et al. (1991). Toxics A to Z. University of California Press, Berkeley, p.408.

94. *Ibid.*

95. Brandt CJ. (Ed). (1987). Acidic precipitation. Formation and impact on terrestial ecosystems. Kommission Reinhaltung der Luft. Verein Deutscher Ingenieure, Dusseldorf, Germany.

96. Kormondy EJ, *op. cit. (see reference 81)*, p.489.

97. Rudd JWM, Kelly CA, Schindler DW et al. (1988). Disruption of the nitrogen cycle on acidified lakes. Science 240:1515–1517.

98. Ember R. (1981). Acid pollutants: hitchhikers ride the wind. Chem Engineer News 59(37):20–31.

99. Begon M, Harper JL, and Townsend CR, *op. cit. (see reference 60)*, p.767.

100. Montague P. (1998). Rachel's Environmental & Health Weekly, Issue 624, November 12. (Website location: http://www.rachel.org)

101. Natural Foods Merchandiser. (1997). 16th Annual Market Overview, June 1997, New Hope Communications, Boulder, Colorado. (Website location: http://www.newhope.com).

102. UMass Extension. (1998). What is community supported agriculture and how does it work? UMass Extension, College of Food and Natural Resources, School of Public Health and Health Sciences, University of Massachusetts, Amherst, Massachusetts. (Website location: http://www/umass.edu/umext/csa/).

APPENDIX A: National Primary Drinking Water Standards*

Contaminants	MCLG (mg/L)	MCL (mg/L)	Potential health effects from ingestion of water	Sources of contaminant in drinking water
Fluoride	4.0	4.0	Skeletal and dental fluorosis	Natural deposits, fertilizer, aluminum industries, water additive
Volatile organics				
Benzene	0	0.005	Cancer	Some foods; gas, drugs, pesticide, paint, plastic industries
Carbon tetrachloride	0	0.005	Cancer	Solvents and their degradation products
p-Dichlorobenzene	0.075	0.075	Cancer	Room and water deodorants, and "mothballs"
1,2-Dichloroethane	0	0.005	Cancer	Leaded gasoline, fumgants, paints
1,1-Dichloroethylene	0.007	0.007	Cancer	Plastics, dyes, perfumes, paints
Trichloroethylene	0	0.005	Cancer	Textiles, adhesives, metal degreasers
1,1,1-Trichloroethane	0.2	0.2	Liver, nervous system effects	Adhesives, aerosols, textiles, paints, inks, metal degreasers
Vinyl Chloride	0	0.002	Cancer	May leach from PVC pipe, formed by sovent break-down
Coliform and surface water treatment				
Giardia Lamblia	0	*b*	Gastroenteric disease	Human and animal fecal waste
Legionella	N/A	*b*	Legionnaire's disease	Indigenous to natural waters, can grow in water heating systems
Standard Plate Count	N/A	*b*	Indicates water quality, effectiveness of treatment	
Total Coliform[a]	0	<5%[c]	Indicates gastroenteric pathogens	Human and animal fecal waste
Turbidity[a]	N/A	*b*	Interferes with disinfection, filtration	Soil runoff
Viruses	0	*b*	Gastroenteric disease	Human and animal fecal waste
Inorganics				
Antimony	0	0.006	Cancer	Fire retardants, ceramics, electronics, fireworks, solder
Asbestos (>10um)	7MFL	7MFL	Cancer	Natural deposits, asbestos cement in water systems
Barium[a]	2	2	Circulatory system effects	Natural deposits, pigment, epoxy sealants, spent coal
Beryllium	0.004	0.004	Bone, lung damage	Electrical, aetospace, defense industries
Cadmium[a]	0.005	0.005	Kidney effects	Galvanized pipe corrosion, natural deposits, batteries, paints
Chromium[a] (total)	0.1	0.1	Liver, kidney, circulatory disorders	Natural deposits, mining, electroplating, pigments
Cyanide	0.2	0.2	Thyroid, nervous system damage fertilizer	Electroplating, steel, plastics, mining,
Mercury[a] (inorganic)	0.002	0.002	Kidney, nervous system disorders	Crop runoff, natural deposits, batteries, electrical switches

[a] Contaminants with interim standards which have been revised
[b] Special treatment techniques required
[c] less than 5% positive samples
MFL=million fibers per liter

*U.S. Environmental Protection Agency. (1994). National primary drinking water standards. EPA 810-F-94-001. February 1994.

Contaminants	MCLG (mg/L)	MCL (mg/L)	Potential health effects from ingestion of water	Sources of contaminant in drinking water
Nitrite[a]	10	10	Methemoglobulinemia	Animal waste, fertilizer, natural deposits, septic tanks, sewage
Selenium[a]	0.05	0.05	Liver damage	Natural deposits, mining, smelting, coal/oil combustion
Thallium	0.0005	0.002	Kidney, liver, brain, intestinal	Electronics, drugs, alloys, glass
Organics				
Acrylamide	0	*b*	Cancer, nervous system effects	Polymers used in sewage/wastewater treatment
Adipate, (di (2-ethylhexyl)	0.4	0.4	Decreased body weight	Synthetic rubber, food packaging, cosmetics
Alachlor	0	0.002	Cancer	Runoff from herbicide on corn, soybeans, other crops
Atrazine	0.003	0.003	mammary gland tumors	Runoff from use as herbicide on corn and non-cropland
Carbonfuran	0.04	0.04	Nervous, reproductive system effects	Soil fumigant on corn and cotton, restricted in some areas
Chlordane[a]	0	0.002	Cancer	Leaching from soil treatment for termites
Chlorobenzene	0.1	0.1	nervous system and liver effects	Waste solvent from metal degreasing processes
Dalapon	0.2	0.2	Liver and kidney effects	Herbicide on orchards, beans, coffee, lawns, road/railways
Dibromochloropropane	0	0.0002	Cancer	Soil fumigant on soybeans, cotton, pineapple, orchards
o-Dichlorobenzene	0.6	0.6	Liver, kidney, blood cell damage	Paints, engine cleaning compounds, dyes chemical wastes
cis-1,2-Dichloroethylene	0.07	0.07	Liver, kidney, nervous, circulatory	Waste industrial extraction solvents
trans-1,2-Dichloroethylene	0.1	0.1	Liver, kidney, nervous, circulatory	Waste industrial extraction solvents
Dichloromethane	0	0.005	Cancer	paint stripper, metal degreaser, propellant, extraction
1,2-Dichloropropane	0	0.005	Liver, kidney effects; Cancer	Soil fumignt, waste industrial solvents
Dinoseb	0.007	0.007	Thyroid, reproductive organ damage	Runoff of herbicide from crop and non-crop applications
Dioxin	0	0.00000003	Cancer	Chemical production by-product, impurity in herbicides
Diquat	0.02	0.02	Liver, kidney, eye effects	Runoff of herbicide on land, aquatic weeds
2,4-D[a]	0.07	0.07	Liver and kidney damage	Runoff from herbicide on wheat, corn, rangelands, lawns
Endothall	0.1	0.1	Liver, kidney, gastrointestinal	Herbicide on crops, land/aquatic weeds; rapidly degraded
Endrin	0.002	0.002	Liver, kidney, heart damage	pesticide on insects, rodents, birds; restricted since 1980
Epichlorohydrin	0	*b*	Cancer	Water treatment chemicals; waste epoxy resins, coatings
Ethylbenzene	0.7	0.7	Liver, kidney, nervous system	Gasoline, insecticides, chemical manufacturing wastes
Ethylene dibromide	0	0.00005	Cancer	Leaded gasoline additives, leaching of soil fumigant

[a] Contaminants with interim standards which have been revised
[b] Special treatment techniques required

Contaminants	MCLG (mg/L)	MCL (mg/L)	Potential health effects from ingestion of water	Sources of contaminant in drinking water
Glyphosate	0.7	0.7	Liver, kidney damage	Herbicide on grasses, weeds, brush
Heptachlor	0	0.0004	Cancer	Leaching of insecticide for termites, very few crops
Heptachlor epoxide	0	0.0002	Cancer	Biodegradation of heptachlor
Hexachlorobenzene	0	0.001	Cancer	Pesticide production waste by-product
Hexachlorocyclopentadiene	0.05	0.05	Kidney, stomach damage	Pesticide production intermediate
Lindane	0.0002	0.0002	Liver, kidney, nerve, immune, circulatory system	Insecticde on cattle, lumber, gardens; restricted since 1983
Methoxychlor	0.04	0.04	Growth, liver, kidney, nerve effects	Insecticide for fruits, vegetables, alfalfa, livestock, pets
Oxamyl (Vydate)	0.2	0.2	Kidney damage	Insecticide on apples, potatoes, tomatoes
PAHs (benzo(a)pyrene)	0	0.0002	Cancer	PVC and other plastics
PCBs	0	0.0005	Cancer	Coolant oils from electrical transformers, plasticizers
Pentachlorophenol	0	0.001	Liver and kidney effects, cancer	Wood preservatives, herbicide, cooling tower wastes
Phthalate, (di(2-ethylhexyl))	0	0.006	Cancer	PVC and other plastics
Picloram	0.5	0.5	Kidney, liver damage	Herbicide on broadleaf and woody plants
Simazine	0.004	0.004	Cancer	Herbicide on grass sod, some crops, aquatic algae
Styrene	0.1	0.1	Liver, nervous system damage	Plastics, rubber, resin, drug industries, leachate from city landfills
Tetrachloroethylene	0	0.005	Cancer	Improper disposal of dry cleaning and other solvents
Toluene	1	1	Liver, kidney, nervous, circulatory	Gasoline additive, manufacturing and solvent operations
Toxaphene	0	0.003	Cancer	Insecticide on cattle, cotton, soybeans; cancelled 1982
2,4,5-TP	0.05	0.05	Liver and kidney damage	herbicide on crops, right-of-way, golf courses; cancelled 1983
1,2,4-Trichlorobenzene	0.07	0.07	liver, kidney damage	herbicide production, dye carrier
1,1,2-Trichloroethane	0.003	0.005	Kidney, liver, nervous system	Solvent in rubber other organic products, chemical production wastes
Xylenes (total)	10	10	Liver, kidney, nervous system	By-product of gasoline refining, paints, inks, detergents
Lead and copper				
Lead[a]	0	b,d	Kidneys, nervous system damage	Natural/Industrial deposits, plumbing, solder, brass alloy faucets
Copper	1.3	b	Gastrointestinal irritation	Natural/industrial deposits, wood preservatives, plumbing
Other interim standards				
Beta/photon emitters	0	4 mrem/yr	Cancer	Decay of radionuclides in natural and man-made deposits
Alpha emitters	0	15 pCi/L	Cancer	Decay of radionuclides in natural deposits
Total Trihalomethanes	0	0.1	Cancer	Drinking water chlorination by-products

[a] Contaminants with interim standards which have been revised
[b] Special treatment techniques required
[d] Action level 0.15mg/L
[e] Action level 1.3mg/L
pCi=picocuries

APPENDIX B: CERCLA Priority List of Hazardous Substances

The Comprehensive Environmental Response, Compensation, and Liability Act (CERCLA) section 104(i), as amended by the Superfund Amendments and Reauthorizetion Act (SARA), requires the Agency for Toxic Substances and Disease Registry (ATSDR) and Environmental Protection Agency (EPA) to prepare a list, in order of priority, of substances that are most commonly found at facilities on the National Priorities List (NPL) and which are determined to pose the most significant potential threat to human health. The CERCLA priority list is revised and published on a two-year basis, with a yearly informal review and revision. The following appendix provides the top 200 from the 1997 CERCLA priority list.

1997 Rank	Name	Total Points	1995 Rank	CAS Number
1	Arsenic	1627.32	2	007440-38-2
2	Lead	1522.67	1	007439-92-1
3	Mercury	1492.21	3	007439-97-6
4	Vinyl chloride	1397.67	4	000075-01-4
5	Benzene	1372.88	5	000071-43-2
6	Polychlorinated biphenyls	1340.07	6	001336-36-3
7	Cadmium	1315.14	7	007440-43-9
8	Benzo(a)pyrene	1285.71	8	000050-32-8
9	Benzo(b)fluoranthene	1257.85	10	000205-99-2
10	Polycyclic aromatic hydrocarbons	1251.50	New	130498-29-2
11	Chloroform	1249.95	9	000067-66-3
12	Aroclor 1254	1186.77	14	011097-69-1
13	p,p'-DDT	1183.50	11	000050-29-3
15	Trichloroethylene	1160.83	13	000079-01-6
16	Chromium, hexavalent	1152.07	15	018540-29-9
17	Dibenzo[a,h]anthracene	1141.98	17	000053-70-3
18	Dieldrin	1130.30	20	000060-57-1
19	Hexachlorobutadiene	1129.40	18	000087-68-3
20	Chlordane	1121.25	16	000057-74-9
21	Creosote	1121.05	23	008001-58-9
22	p,p'-DDE	1117.44	22	000072-55-9
23	Benzidine	1116-19	26	000092-87-5
24	Cyanide	1113.09	24	000057-12-5
25	Aldrin	1108.37	29	000309-00-2
26	p,p'-DDD	1104.19	19	000072-54-8
27	Aroclor 1248	1098.88	27	012672-29-6
28	Phosphorus	1094.63	30	007723-14-0
29	Aroclor 1242	1091.22	25	053469-21-9
30	Heptachlor	1087.81	39	000067-44-8
31	Toxaphene	1084.63	32	008001-35-2

1997 Rank	Name	Total Points	1995 Rank	CAS Number
32	γ-Hexachlorocyclohexane	1084.48	21	000058-89-9
33	Tetrachloroethylene	1082.21	28	000127-18-4
34	Aroclor 1221	1070.41	34	011104-28-2
35	β-Hexachlorocyclohexane	1054.20	31	000319-85-7
36	1,2-Dibromoethane	1052.88	35	000106-93-4
37	Disulfoton	1052.88	35	000298-04-4
38	Benzo[a]anthracene	1047.78	37	000056-55-3
39	Endrin	1040.58	38	000072-20-8
40	Aroclor 1016	1031.03	43	012674-11-2
41	Δ-Hexachlorocyclohexane	1029.75	44	000319-86-8
42	Di-n-butyl phthalate	1028-68	40	000084-74-2
43	1,2-Dibromo-3-Chloropropane	1027.45	33	000096-12-8
44	Beryllium	1023.27	46	007440-41-7
45	Pentachlorophenol	1022.95	45	000087-86-5
46	Carbon tetrachloride	1018.10	42	000056-23-5
47	Cobalt	1011.99	148	007440-48-4
48	α-Endosulfan	1010.08	52	000959-98-8
49	Nickel	1004.94	49	007440-02-0
50	Endosulfan sulfate	1004.02	50	001031-07-8
51	3,3'-Dichlorobenzidine	998.02	53	000091-94-1
52	Heptachlor epoxide	992.17	54	001024-57-3
53	Endosulfan	990.07	58	000115-29-7
54	Dibromochloropropane	987.92	59	067708.83-2
55	Aroclor	986.15	63	012767-79-2
56	β-Endosulfan	981.77	61	033213-65-9
57	Endrin ketone	978.82	56	053494-70-5
58	Aroclor 1232	974.72	60	011141-16-5
59	Benzo[k]fluoranthene	972.84	New	000207-08-9
60	2-Hexanone	970.35	65	000591-78-6
61	Toluene	969.44	55	000108-88-3
62	cis-Chlordane	959.77	66	005103-71-9
63	Methane	956.21	67	000074-82-8
64	trans-Chlordane	951.80	62	005103-74-2
65	Zinc	932.34	68	007440-66-6
66	2,4,7,8-Tetrachlorodibenzo-p-dioxin	928.58	69	001746-01-6
67	Di(2-ethylhexyl)phthalate	923.15	70	000117-81-7
68	Methoxychlor	916.15	51	000072-43-5
69	Chromium	908.93	72	007440-47-3
70	Methylene chloride	908.12	71	000075-09-2
71	Benzofluoranthene	907.82	48	056832-73-6
72	Naphthalene	902.82	73	000091-20-3
73	1,1-Dichloroethene	894.46	74	000075-35-4
74	1,2-Dichloroethane	871.62	77	000107-06-2

1997 Rank	Name	Total Points	1995 Rank	CAS Number
75	Cyclotrimethylenetrinitramine (RDX)	871.35	230	000121-82-4
76	Bis(2-chloroethyl)ether	869.02	78	000111-44-4
77	2,4-Dinitrophenol	867.30	79	000051-28-5
78	2,4,6-Trinitrotoluene	866.63	82	000118-96-7
79	1,1,1-Trichloroethane	858.26	76	000071-55-6
80	1,1,2,2-Tetrachloroethane	851.93	85	000079-34-5
81	Ethyl Benzene	847.51	80	000100-41-4
82	2,4,6-Trichlorophenol	845-69	86	000088-06-2
83	Total Xylenes	844.63	83	001330-20-7
84	Endrin Aldehyde	842.70	64	007421-93-4
85	Thiocyanate	842.29	New	000302-04-5
86	Asbestos	841.33	89	001332-21-4
87	4,6-Dinitro-*o*-cresol	837.64	90	000534-52-1
88	Uranium	831.94	92	007440-61-1
89	Chlorobenzene	829.90	91	000108-90-7
90	Radium	829.28	97	007440-14-4
91	Radium-226	829.10	93	013982-63-3
92	Ethion	827.76	98	000563-12-2
93	Hexachlorobenzene	827.25	94	000118-74-1
94	Dimethylarsinic Acid	826.85	87	000075-60-5
95	Thorium	824.99	96	007440-29-1
96	Fluoranthene	817.60	101	000206-44-0
97	Radon	817.53	100	010043-92-2
98	Barium	816.92	95	007440-39-3
99	2,4-Dinitrotoluene	816.26	105	000121-15-2
100	Diazinon	814.01	104	000333-41-5
101	Thorium-230	813.54	102	014269-63-7
102	Radium-228	813.21	103	015262-20-1
103	Uranium-235	812.64	109	015117-96-1
104	Uranium-234	811.75	111	013966-29-5
105	1,3,5-Trinitrobenzene	811.54	112	000099-35-4
106	Thorium-228	810.47	108	014274-82-9
107	*n*-Nitrosodi-*n*-propylamine	809.74	106	000621-64-7
108	Hexachlorocyclohexane, alpha-	809.46	118	000319-84-6
109	Tritium	809.15	188	010028-17-8
110	Cesium-137	808.35	119	010045-97-3
111	Radon-222	808.29	116	014859-67-7
112	Polonium-210	807.78	137	013981-52-7
113	Chrysotile asbestos	807.54	114	012001-29-5
114	Methylmercury	806.26	123	022967-92-6
115	Thorium-227	806.17	117	015623-47-9
116	Chrysene	806.09	113	000218-01-9
117	Thoron (radon-220)	805.93	121	022481-48-7

1997 Rank	Name	Total Points	1995 Rank	CAS Number
118	Plutonium-238	805.75	124	013981-16-3
119	Coal tars	805.52	New	008007-45-2
120	Chlorpyrifos	805.19	120	002921-88-2
121	Cobalt-60	804.86	205	010198-40-0
122	Lead-210	804.38	183	014255-04-0
123	Plutonium-239	804.29	129	015177-48-3
124	Potassium-40	804.29	129	013966-00-2
125	Strontium-90	804.05	223	010098-97-2
126	Americium-241	803.73	New	086954-36-1
127	Plutonium	803.73	209	007440-07-5
128	Iodine-131	802.92	New	010043-66-0
129	Amosite asbestos	802.59	128	012172-73-5
130	Guthion	802.59	191	000086-50-0
131	Bismuth-214	802.36	New	014733-03-0
132	Lead-214	802.36	New	015067-28-4
133	Kepone	802.03	187	000143-50-0
134	Plutonium-240	802.03	New	014119-33-6
135	Tributlytin	802.03	New	000688-73-3
136	Copper	797.77	110	007440-50-8
137	s,s,s-Tributyl phosphorotrithioate	790.05	New	000078-48-8
138	Manganese	787.11	41	007439-96-5
139	Polybrominated biphenyls	781.40	134	067774-32-7
140	Dicofol	779.80	136	000115-32-2
141	Heptachlorodibenzo-p-dioxin	778-15	99	037871-00-4
142	Selenium	777.71	135	007782-49-2
143	Parathion	772.49	142	000056-38-2
144	Hexachlorocyclohexane	770.93	140	000608-73-1
145	1,1-Dichloroethane	765.48	139	000075-34-3
146	Pentachlorobenzene	764.90	144	000608-93-5
147	Trichlorofluoroethane	762.34	218	027154-33-2
148	1,2,3,4,6,7,8,9-Octachlorodibenzofuran	760.87	88	039001-02-0
149	4,4'-Methylenebis(2-chloroaniline)	758.35	145	000101-14-4
150	Hexachlorodibenzo-p-dioxin	751.93	146	034465-46-8
151	1,1,2-Trichloroethane	750.84	155	000079-00-5
152	Chlorine	750.73	84	007782-50-5
153	Ammonia	748.21	147	007664-41-7
154	Heptachlorodibenzofuran	745-79	131	038998-75-3
155	Acenaphthene	743.04	150	000083-32-9
156	2-Methylnaphthalene	740.06	154	000091-57-6
157	trans-1,2-Dichloroethene	736.35	149	000156-60-5
158	Phenol	733.70	81	000108-95-2
159	Chromium (vi) trioxide	723.00	New	001333-82-0
160	Trichloroethane	714.58	133	025323-89-1

1997 Rank	Name	Total Points	1995 Rank	CAS Number
161	Bromine	709.92	New	007726-95-6
162	1,4-Dichlorobenzene	709.67	156	000106-46-7
163	1,2-Dichlorobenzene	707.59	157	000095-50-1
164	Lead-212	705.46	125	015092-94-1
165	Oxychlordane	705.35	115	027304-13-8
166	Radium-224	703.90	121	013233-32-4
167	Bismuth-212	702.51	125	014913-49-6
168	1,2-Dipheylhydrazine	700.49	158	000122-66-7
169	Tetrachlorophenol	695.54	132	025167-83-3
170	Carbon disulfide	695.24	152	000075-15-0
171	Hydrogen sulfide	694.52	159	007783-06-4
172	Chloroethane	693.13	160	000075-00-3
173	Acetone	692.84	151	000067-64-1
174	Hexachlorodibenzofuran	690.59	153	055684-94-1
175	Dibenzofuran	684.92	New	000132-64-9
176	2,4-Dimethylphenol	683.18	162	000105-67-9
177	Ideno(1,2,3-*cd*)pyrene	681.13	161	000193-39-5
178	Aluminum	678.54	164	007429-90-5
179	1,2,3-Trichlorobenzene	673.62	269	000087-61-6
180	Tetrachlorethane	668.57	251	025322-20-7
181	Pentachlorodibenzofuran	662.00	181	030402-15-4
182	Hexachloroethane (HCH)	655.93	171	000067-72-1
183	Butyl benzyl phthalate	651.38	170	000085-68-7
184	1,2,4-Trichlorobenzene	648.73	193	000120-82-1
185	Chloromethane	648.12	172	000074-87-3
186	Vanadium	633.08	176	007440-62-2
187	Tetrachlorodibenzo-*p*-dioxin	629.79	175	041903-57-5
188	Hexachlorocyclopentadiene	628.01	107	000077-47-4
189	*n*-Nitrosodiphenylamine	627.58	178	000086-30-6
190	2-Butanone	626.25	168	000078-93-3
191	Pentachlorodibenzo-*p*-dioxin	621.28	182	036088-22-9
192	2,3,5,6-Tetrachlorophenol	619.38	New	000935-95-5
193	2,3,7,8-Tetrachlorodibenzofuran	616.85	190	051207-31-9
194	Acrolein	616.25	165	000107-02-9
195	Chromic acid	612.79	195	007738-94-5
196	Silver	611.15	185	007440-22-4
197	Bromoform	609.55	216	000075-25-2
198	*trans*-Nonachlor	608.83	203	039765-80-5
199	1,3-Dichlorobenzene	608.33	202	000541-73-1
200	2-Chlorophenol	608.08	211	000095-57-8

Index